THE
E.I.
SYNDROME

REVISED

An Rx
For Environmental Illness

1995

by Sherry A. Rogers, M.D.

SK Publishing
Box 40101
Sarasota, FL 34242

The E. I. SYNDROME REVISED

Copyright © 1995

SK Publishing
P.O. Box 40101
Sarasota, FL 34242

For information address: SK Publishers, Box 40101, Sarasota, FL 34242

Library of Congress Card Catalog Number: 95-67456

ISBN: 0-9618821-7-4

Printed in the United States

1st Edition 1995

PREFACE

2ND EDITION 1995

In 1986, **The E.I. Syndrome**, was hatched after 3 grueling years. It was grueling because not only did I have a full- time private practice in environmental medicine, but I was teaching and lecturing around the country. But the thing that made this particularly trying was that I did it while I was still in the throws of "brain fog."

In fact, in 1986 even though I was infinitely better than I had been in the previous 1 1/2 decades with E.I., I was still so profoundly affected that when I lectured in Chicago that year, I had to rent 3 tanks of oxygen on wheels and wear it delivered through a ceramic mask just so I would know my name!

So a book in excess of 700 pages written by someone with absolutely no training in journalism is bad enough, but the brain fog makes this editing imperative. I was procrastinating for 8 years because I was hoping someone else would write something to cover the subject and I could refer people to that. But unfortunately there still exist many facts in here that do not exist elsewhere, so revise we must.

The second reason I held off was I was so frustrated by the fact that so much new information was coming out daily. I would feel compelled to sandwich it all into this piece so people could take advantage of it. But then this would have ended up in excess of 1000 pages, and I really wanted to slim it down!

So in the interim we have (and continue) to put all this newness in our Health Letter (subscription newsletter) and our on going books (I just started #8 and #9!) So **The E.I. Syndrome** can remain what it started out to be, a guide to people who have simple pollen, dust, mold, food and/or chemical sensitivities. And also for those who do not even

i

know they are reacting to the 21st century. We have in revising it, attempted to improve style, content and update resources and ideas.

As for the other books, you can for example, get yourself so well with diets, nutrient corrections and other techniques that you can truly heal the impossible. But regardless of what heights of wellness you chose to go to, everyone needs a fundamental knowledge of the principles in here. For to be unschooled in these would be like sending a surgeon to medical school but letting him skip taking anatomy.

I'm probably one of the luckiest doctors in the world, because I have the privilege of treating some of the smartest people. They know that somehow if they can learn enough, they can get themselves well, regardless of what anyone else has told them. And the vast majority dig in their heels and do just that.

I hope this work helps you attain your goals, and regardless of whether it does or does not, don't stop here. Keep reading. For you will amaze yourself at how much power a lot of knowledge can give you over your health.

FOREWARD

Dr. Doris J. Rapp is a dual board certified pediatric allergist who through numerous books like **Allergies and Your Family, Allergies and the Hyperactive Child**, and **The Impossible Child**, has saved many childred from the fate of being labeled learning disabled. Dr. William J. Rea is a thoracic, cardiovascular, abdominal, and general surgeon who partially from needs and interests arising from his own environmental illness established the work's largest and most comprehensive environmental unit, the Environmental Health Center in Dallas. He also authored the world's first 4 volume medical textbook, **Chemical Sensitivity.**

Both these pioneeers in environmental medicine have carried on the groundwork laid by Dr. Theron Randolph, the founder. Dr. Rea and Dr. Rapp have lectured throughout the world for years, have published many scientific papers that are landmarks in the field, and their dedication has added immensely to the quality of life for thousands of victims of E.I. On the following pages are their comments about this patient manual:

FOREWARD

A potpourri of practical advice presented in a humorous forthright manner to help the many who suffer needlessly from unrecognized environmental illness. This book is full to overflowing with valuable essential facts to relieve medical problems which range from mild to devastating. Dr. Rogers is not reluctant to say what needs to be said. She explains why you may not need "to learn to live with it", and in simple language, what you can do to help make yourself feel better. If you have gone from doctor to doctor and have not been believed or helped, this book may provide the answers you need.

Doris J. Rapp, M.D.
F.A.A.A., F.A.A.P.
Buffalo, New York
October 9, 1987

FOREWARD

Dr. Sherry Rogers clearly demonstrates her dramatic recovery from devastating environmental sensitivities. In doing this , she conveys hope to many people who are wounded by toxic elements in their environment. Many of the people will be enlightened as to a clue for their diagnosis and for others — details of how to obtain and maintain good health will be achieved. Understanding the principles of evaluating cause and effect of environmental incidents appears to be essential in understanding how to prevent disease and promote optimum health. Dr. Rogers details her understanding of total pollutant load, the adaptation and bipolarity phenomenon and the biochemical individuality (our uniqueness of response) — all of which are paramount to understanding environmentally triggered disease. The knowledge of where, how, and when we are exposed to toxic elements in our environment helps the reader relate to his / her own exposure and environmentally related problems. It is most important that each individual understands his surroundings and his reaction to them. The book should help the reader to better obtain optimal health.

William J. Rea, M.D.,
F.A.C.S., F.A.A.E.M.
Dallas, TX
October 6, 1987

THE E.I. SYNDROME
Table of Contents
Preface to 2nd Edition

I

DEDICATION

To Rob: May this work give others as much life as you have given me.

ACKNOWLEDGEMENT

Whenever an author is called upon to give thanks, it becomes a very difficult task. However, my number one thanks must go to the most wonderfully loving person that I've ever known in my entire life, my husband Rob. Simply, he created me (the good parts that is, the bad ones I came equipped with). He is responsible for all of my accomplishments, for without his nurturing and guidance I would have floundered by the wayside. He is God's only mistake, for He wasn't supposed to make any of us mortals perfect. But He goofed; He made just this one perfect.

Also, I owe a great deal, not only for contributions to this book but also contributions to my life-long health, to Dr. William J. Rea of the Environmental Health Center in Dallas, Texas. He's the second greatest teacher I ever knew as he makes you feel like you just discovered whatever it is he's been trying to drill into your head for the last few moments. He has opened himself to share his philosophy and is particularly tolerant of our blindness.

I also extend thanks to Dr. Doris Rapp of Buffalo, New York, whose unselfishness, dedication and enthusiasm left me spent. She and Dr. Rea showed me what dedication meant. Before that, it was just an empty word. I really wanted her to adopt me, but she's too young.

Dr. Joseph Miller holds a special place in my heart since he took a virgin conventional allergist and showed her that provocation-neutralization works. He also cleared up her face. There are many other physicians who unknowingly influenced and educated me. I ran into them at courses or in their books or through personal communication. They are that rare breed with unprejudiced and inquiring minds who have the courage to use methods that are contrary to orthodoxy.

Thanks to Dr. Bedros P. Mangikian for giving me the time away so that I could write this work. Thanks to Dr.

Fred Terracina, Ph.D., taxonomic mycologist, who did the impossible — taught a medical doctor a little about the real world of science. And to Rika VanderWalt who unknowingly helped nurture my writing tendencies by promoting lectures and editing my material for publication in her Western New York Ecology Newsletter, and to Cindy Thompson for her tireless typing of the manuscript. And thanks go to Richard Short, Professor of English at Erie Community College for the frustrating job of correcting language technicalities while being denied license to alter the doctor's personality.

Last but not least, thanks to Rosalie Muehlberger, R.N., who kept me healthy with produce from her organic garden, and who lent me the very first clinical ecology book I ever saw. She, herself, was the first clinical ecology patient I ever treated. Actually, there were probably hundreds before her, but I didn't know it. You see, the only reason I knew she was one is she told me so. It is to all these people, many of my patients, and our dedicated office staff that I owe a great deal of thanks, for they all show constant courage and faith. Many of them are victims who have persisted and hung on and found a way to adapt to the 21st century.

ABOUT THE AUTHOR

Sherry A. Rogers, M.D., F.A.C.A. is a Diplomat of the American Board of Family Practice, a Fellow of the American College of Allergy and Immunology, a Diplomat of the Board of Environmental Medicine, as well as a former board director. She is a Fellow of the American Academy of Environmental Medicine.

She has published 15 scientific articles and numerous lay articles in health magazines (**Let's Live, Spectrum**, etc.), newspapers and newsletters. She has appeared on many TV and radio shows. She has lectured for over a decade in seminars such as the Advanced Instructional Courses for Physicians in Environmental Medicine, the international symposium Man and His Environment in Health and Disease Featuring Chemical Sensitivities in Dallas, and presented scores of lectures for organizations such as the American College of Allergists in New Orleans, the American Academy of Environmental Medicine; the American Academy of Otolaryngic Allergy, the Pan American Allergy Society; the American College for Advancement in Medicine, and more. She has presented at the Upstate Medical School in Syracuse New York; the Halifax Medical School Family Practice Refresher Course; the St. Joseph's Hospital Family Practice Refresher Course; and at Morristown Hospital, a teaching arm of Columbia College of Physicians and Surgeons, as other examples.

In 1985, she accompanied Dr. William Rea of the Dallas Environmental Unit and Dr. Theron Randolph of the Chicago Environmental Unit on a scientific exchange program where they lectured in six medical centers in the People's Republic of China.

She has lectured in 4 major international indoor air symposia, in over 6 countries and over 50 U.S. cities, in medical schools, churches, universities, colleges, and convention centers, taught the advanced courses for physicians for over a decade, published 15 scientific papers, 8 books, been the sole editor for the environmental medicine column in 1992-1993 for **Internal Medicine World Report**, and much much more.

She has a solo private practice in allergy and environmental medicine, nutritional biochemistry in Syracuse, New York and is attending physician at Community General Hospital.

DISCLAIMER

In this office we are going to be focusing on nutritional and environmental causes for your symptoms. Therefore, we will assume you have already had a thorough physical by your family physician to rule out any common conditions (diabetes, hypoglycemia, hypothyroidism, brain tumors, etc.). The potential environmental causes are far too many and too complicated and highly individual in many cases. To have to go back and do basic medicine is not my interest, nor do I have the luxury of time for it. I leave that to people more qualified and who do it daily. I look for the things that they rarely know exist. If at any time you feel you would like further conventional medicine evaluations, do not hesitate to ask, and we will get you the appropriate referrals.

Also, the staff are all at various levels of sophistication in terms of their knowledge of allergies. Some of them have accompanied me around the United States when I have lectured and even to scientific meetings in Australia and Europe, and we have available consultations with them for you to save time and money. If you at any time prefer to see the doctor or feel you are not getting better or your questions are not satisfactorily answered, it is your obligation to schedule to see the doctor.

We will assume you have begun to take responsibility for your health and have read and retained the facts in this book. We prefer to help you where this book leaves off, not reiterate what you can just as easily and more inexpensively read. We get several hundred calls a week from our patients from all over the world. In order to help each person to the best of our abilities, we prefer to limit questions to those not already answered in this material.

Each patient must also have a family doctor, since Dr. Rogers, is often out of the state lecturing and currently the next closest certified specialists in environmental medi-

XV

cine are in Buffalo, New York City, and Pennsylvania. Emergencies and prescriptions will need to be dealt with by your family physician.

Note: At this point, read all references under these 3 categories: Caution, Disclaimer, and Warning. You are responsible for your body and what risks you decide to take with it. Furthermore, since I am frequently out of the country (one year alone I lectured in 4 different countries and over half a dozen U.S. cities), you might want to give your family doctor, or whomever you will be seeing for check- ups and emergencies, a copy of this manual and **TIRED OR TOXIC?** so that he/she may better understand what you are doing. In this way, he will be more prepared to assist you. And who knows? He may start coming to the courses and become the leading environmental medicine specialist in your area. In over a dozen years of teaching the advanced course for physicians, there has never been one doctor from Syracuse. But we keep hoping. Hence, of necessity, we leave your coverage up to the person who knows you medically the best.

DOES YOUR ENVIRONMENT MAKE YOU SICK?
EASY SOLUTIONS
TO DIFFICULT MEDICAL PROBLEMS

1. Did you know that many patients with arthritis don't hurt if they don't eat any beef, tomato, pepper, or potatos?

2. Did you know that many patients with inability to concentrate and muscle weakness are reacting to chemicals such as natural gas and formaldehyde?

3. Did you know that children with hyperactivity or unharnessed aggressiveness may be reacting to foods most frequently eaten, such as milk, wheat, corn, cane sugar, food dyes, and preservatives?

4. Did you know that many people with asthma, chronic colds and eczema are clear when they stop eating mold-containing foods, such as breads, cheese, alcohols and vinegars?

5. Did you know that many patients with psoriasis can clear with the correct fatty acid supplementation?

6. Did you know that many people with headaches are totally clear after they have gotten off coffee for a week?

7. Did you know that people with chronic tiredness are sometimes universal reactors and sensitive to many types of dusts, molds, foods, and chemicals?

8. Did you know that many people who feel depressed or have symptoms at the office may be reacting to formaldehyde from the furnishings, supplies, and

cleaning solutions?

9.   Did you know that people with colitis often times
     have hidden food allergies and low blood levels of
     many vitamins?

10. Did you know that depression can be caused by
     chemicals from a sofa or carpet or by a yeast growing
     in your body, or because you've have too many birth
     control pills or antibiotics?

11. Did you know that many people with diagnoses like
     chronic EBV (mono) and SLE (systemic lupus
     erythematosis) actually are universal reactors to
     many foods, chemicals, and Candida?

12. Did you know that many people with a host of
     symptoms who just never feel great have multiple
     vitamin and mineral deficiencies?

13. Did you know that no two people with arthritis have
     the exact same causes? A revolution in medicine has
     begun where we realize "cookbook" medicine is
     archaic for we have staggering individual biochemi
     cal, genetic, and environmental variability.

14. Did you know that E.I. classically attacks several
     organ systems at a time, leaving specialists who limit
     themselves to one organ baffled?

15. Did you know that many can be exposed to the same
     chemical, but they may all exhibit different symp
     toms or target organs? Some reactions will also be
     delayed or not manifest until combined with other
     exposures later o

16. Did you know that when the precise balance for an individual body is restored, it has the potential to heal anything including cancer?

PHYSICIAN:
HEAL THYSELF, IF YOU CAN!

During the summer of 1976, I developed a sudden and severe skin condition known as eczematous or atopic dermatitis. It was so disfiguring that often my patients, upon entering my office for treatment, would cry out involuntarily, "Oh my God, what happened to your face!"

My affliction began with large, red, painful cysts, which eventually drained and merged, leaving my face looking scaley, red as a beet and lumpy. I tried everything I know to look more presentable, at least during office hours. Convinced that something I was eating cased the reaction, I just about starved myself, limiting my diet to foods that I knew were harmless. I ate lots of carrots, and every night I lathered my face with gobs of a potent steroid cream. These steroids cause blood vessels to dilate , a condition known to doctors as telangiectasias and described by lay people as "broken blood vessels".

Even though I kept dropping foods from my diet, it seemed that more and more of the things I ate caused me to break out; finally 50 different foods were on my "hit" list. The trouble was it took 18 to 24 hours after eating before I realized I'd ingested the wrong food. Back came the red bumps and ugly cysts, which itched, burned, and ached for several days.

Until the first outbreak in 1976, I'd never had a skin problem in my life. True, as a child I'd snuffled and snorted a lot, but my complexion was normal. Then, after I left medical school and began my practice, I started having such terrible headaches I was sure I had a brain tumor. My husband, Rob, who had been working as an allergy consultant to physicians, diagnosed it as an allergic condition, tested me and gave me injections. The headaches stopped almost immediately. But, like most physicians who tend to disparage injections for allergies, I stopped this treatment as soon as the headaches disappeared. Sure enough, they came back stronger than ever. I continued this off-and-on approach to my allergy program until other serious problems began to surface, including severe asthma attacks, and finally, the disfiguring skin problem.

My fellow allergists kept insisting there was no such thing as food allergy injections for this condition. "If you know that certain foods are causing you to break out," they'd admonish, "then don't eat them. Live on carrots!" The dermatologists, meanwhile, kept prescribing more steroids and facial creams, which did more damage than good. I developed glaucoma from them. Gradually, in a desperate effort to solve my own problems, I became an expert on food allergies. I took special courses in immunology and clinical allergy, read volumes of medical journals, and worked closely with prominent physicians in the field. Through it all, I simply ignored the medical establishment, which continued its dogmatic assertions that food allergies were unproven and improbable at best.

By far the most intelligent and open minded advice I was given during this period came once again from Rob, who urged me to visit Dr. Joseph B. Miller in Mobile, Alabama. Dr. Miller had been practically excommunicated by his peers in the medical profession. He became a master in food allergy because no other doctors could solve his incapacitating migraines. His published works and numerous lectures on the subject were all dismissed as unfounded doctrine.

So he just kept healing himself and his patients. In June of 1981, I went to see Dr. Miller both as a patient and student, with faith and confidence. And miracle of miracles, within two weeks my face was clearer than it had been in six years. I could now eat foods to which I had been wildly allergic, such as pears, which heretofore had caused violent skin eruptions. Now I could eat three or four whole pears at a sitting with no problem.

The Treatment

The first thing Dr. Miller did upon my arrival in Mobile was to record my entire history (I had already filled out dozens of questionnaires in advance of my arrival there). "The first thing we're going to do", he announced early in the second day, "is test you to the foods you consider safe." Whatever skepticism remained in my mind came bubbling to the surface. "Yikes!" I moaned, "What a waste! I came all the way down here to be tested to foods I already know were safe!" But there was a method to Dr. Miller's apparent madness. He quietly explained that for people who, like me, are extremely sensitive, a neutralizing dose is required for every food we ingest. He later turned to those foods I could not tolerate;the ones that turned my face into such an awful mess. Later on, I will explain Dr. Miller's testing methods, which I have adapted in large part for my own practice. It is enough to state that Dr. Miller performed a small miracle. In just a few days, he isolated the foods to which I was sensitive and prescribed a neutralizing dose for each, thus enabling me to function without fear of recurrence. It was like being reborn.

Upon my return to practice in Syracuse, New York, my friends and patients were openly astonished by the change. "What happened?" they exclaimed. "Your face is beautiful!" As pleased as I was by their reaction, I was dismayed by my medical colleagues who insisted that it was not possible to cure my ailments with food injections, and I had believed them. They had, in fact, made me feel like a common quack for having the nerve to question their traditional approach to the treatment of allergies. I was like some unwritten law that says nothing of any value can possibly originate outside the ivory towers of academic research. I couldn't believe the stubbornness of their closed minds. Strengthened in resolve and fortified with new knowledge about the causes and effects of allergies, I contacted several former patients whose symptoms I'd been unable to treat and urged them to come in for food allergy tests. One was a 27 year old victim with what had been diagnosed as Crohn's disease (similar to an ulcerative colitis) For years this man had experienced as many as fourteen bloody bowel movements each day, until finally he was sent to surgery where part of his bowel was removed. They wanted him to have a colostomy next(surgical removal of the diseased part of the colon), and wear a collostomy bag for the rest of his life.

I told him what had happened with me and that I was certain I could improve his colitis. We tested him to the foods, taught him how to give his own injections at home, and within two weeks he was markedly improved. What's more, he continued to improve over the years. Since then I have continued testing patients in this manner. These are people suffering from insomnia, depression, chronic fatigue, and countless other symptoms. Most have improved, and they have been able to discard the potent chemical medications they'd been taking for years. As a bonus, they also experienced renewed energy, better sleep habits, fewer headaches, less fluid retention, and the like.

I do not know if everyone with colitis or arthritis is allergic. But I do know, that if you have any common allergic symptoms such as migraines, hayfever, asthma, eczema, chronic sinusitis, and so on, that you should definitely explore the possibility of food hypersensitivity. If you are at the end of your diagnostic rope and have nothing but undesirable options to look forward to, it behooves you to check out food sensitivity as the root cause of your symptoms. It could mean the difference between wearing a colostomy bag for the rest of your life or following a four-day rotation diet and an injection of food extract twice a week.

I have since discovered a multitude of people who had defied diagnoses by conventional medical techniques and who were forced to ferret out the causes for themselves, then locate a rare physician who is trained in these techniques who could help them (we are indeed a scarce commodity). I have read a whole library of books and articles on the subject of allergies and learned all I could about people with conditions previously considered medical in origin, but which proved otherwise. I am now convinced that the constant invasion of our environment by noxious gases, such as phenol from plastics, heating fuel, and formaldehyde, to name a few, has produced a vast array of symptoms from asthma and sinusitis to crippling arthritis and phlebitis;the latter so severe at times that amputations of limbs have actually resulted.

Finding out from Dr. Miller how to control my eczema with food injections and a rotation diet was just the beginning. Through my interest in his work, I was exposed to a group of people, I had never heard of, called clinical ecologists (nowadays they are called specialists in Environmental Medicine). At first I was even more skeptical of them that I had been of Dr. Miller because they thought that people reacted to (get this!) their city drinking water and the "chemicals" in the air; in general they were very anti-pollution. Little did I know they would save my life, and the lives of thousands of my patients.

Since the beginning of my quest for the truth about allergies and their proper treatment, I have met and talked with a prominent thoracic surgeon, a psychiatrist, a Harvard internist, a Yale pediatrician, and numerous other members of good standing in the medical profession who, like me, have "seen the light" and adopted the methods of clinical

24

ecology or environmental medicine outlined in this book. The psychiatrist, for example, placed several of his mentally ill patients on the four-day rotation diet for two weeks and found to his amazement (and consternation) that most of them returned to "normal" within that period and were able to discard their usual medications.

It is my strong conviction, based on personal experience and careful observation of others, that the revelations and techniques embodied in this book (and those written by my colleagues in recent years (see supplementary reading list in Section X, Resources) will eventually bring about a revolution in health care. Slowly but surely the tide is turning. The doubting Thomases are becoming believers, and sooner or later all the world will be turned on to the tested methods and procedures I am about to present in this manual. I wish you all good health and a life in control of your allergies. (Note: Physicians who are board certified in environmental medicine can be located by contacting the American Academy of Environmental Medicine, Box 16106, Denver, Colorado 80216. Physicians board certified by the American College of Occupational and Environmental Medicine, or by the American Academy of Allergy & Immunology do not teach and use these techniques.)

INTRODUCTION TO ALLERGY & ENVIRONMEN-
TAL MEDICINE
Audio Cassette Transcript:

Allergy comes in many disguises. I'm going to start with the undisguised form and progress toward the most difficult, and you can see where you think you fit in. Remember, anyone can become allergic to anything at any time. It's no trick to diagnose hayfever. You can recognize the misery a block away with constant itchy eyes, runny nose, cough, facial pain and congestion; but the sneaky symptoms are in people who maybe had hayfever as a child

25

and now gradually develop low grade chronic sinus problem as an adult. It's frequently not bad enough that they would seek medical help, but gradually other symptoms develop such as chronic tiredness for no reason, or sinusitis that gradually gets worse and more unbearable. By this time, the victim is so accustomed to ignoring or tuning out his sinus problems, that he has forgotten that he has allergies. He has many physicals each year only to be told he has to learn to live with his tiredness; or the headaches are chalked up to stress and a tranquilizer is prescribed. And if he does complain of sinus problems, he is told everybody in Syracuse has them.

Those aren't the only symptoms of allergy that are missed every day. Besides chronic sinusitis, headaches and tiredness for no reason, there are repeated ear infections, dizziness, and recurrent hearing loss requiring PE tubes. Whenever ear, nose, and throat operations such as PE tubes, deviated nasal septal repair, sinus operations or nasal polyp removals are required, it's good to question why the condition is occurring in the first place. If it's because of constant mucous formation, as it frequently is, there can be underlying allergy that no amount of surgery will permanently correct.

Ignoring a low-grade chronic sinus allergy with mild symptoms is possible for many unless they get to the next stage of chronic fatigue, headaches, or even asthma. One out of every three people with sinus allergies, whose allergies are untreated with injections, will progress to get asthma. This has many forms. Sometimes there's just a tight chest as though an elephant were sitting on it and shortness of breath; but frequently the person has a normal chest x-ray and blood tests, then the doctor listens and says that everything sounds fine and that probably it's chronic cough and "nerves". When there is overt whistling and musical wheezing that even your grandmother could diagnose, it's finally called asthma; and multiple drugs are prescribed.

26

The most dangerous drug is prednisone. It can cause cataracts, ulcers, diabetes, weight gain, abnormal menstrual periods, death of the adrenal gland, high blood pressure, depression and aseptic necrosis of the artery in the hip necessitating a metal hip joint replacement. The other drugs prescribed have side effects of nausea, shakiness, or palpitations, and they don't do a thing to correct the tiredness that accompanies this form of allergy or to stop its progression. It's only logical that you can't have all that phlegm and congestion in the lungs day after day without a small amount of cumulative and irreversible lung destruction called emphysema. After years of allergic asthma treated only with drugs, such as is done by pulmonary specialists, it's not at all uncommon to see someone enter with over $200 of medicine a month; and what do they have to show for it? Better Health? No! Only permanent destruction of part of the lung from chronic asthma that has been untreated in terms of its basic cause: allergy. Only allergy injections, diet and environmental controls can simmer asthma down to where drugs are no longer required. And only these can treat the exhaustion that accompanies asthma.

Mold Allergy

Allergy can disguise itself in the form of chronic diseases that seem undiagnosable; I'll give you some examples. I was a sniffly, snorting kid, and no one ever took me to a doctor for it or even dreamed I had allergies. Then in my 20's I had such headaches I thought I had a brain tumor. I didn't even dare tell my husband because I thought surely anyone with headaches like this was not long for this world. But I was clear within a couple of months with injections and environmental controls, so I prematurely dropped my injections. Of course, within two years all the symptoms recurred, and I now had asthma as well. I didn't mind the asthma as much as the chronic tiredness that accompanied it. It was interesting for me to see how a patient felt with asthma and how he felt on the various drugs; but awakening exhausted after 10 hours of sleep was incompatible with a practice, and I recovered after restarting injections.

Bob was a 41 year old chairman of the theology department who for two years had headache, body aches, tiredness, and felt like he had a constant flu with tremendous weakness. He had a work up at the medical school including lumbar puncture and CT scan of the brain. He was told no reason could be found. When we retested him, we found that he was sensitive to housedust and several types of mold. Within two weeks of his injections and doing the environmental controls we suggested, all of his symptoms were gone for the first time in two years. When he was late for his injection, his symptoms recurred, but they would clear within 20 minutes of receiving his injection.

Edith was 49 and had been disabled with attacks of dizziness the last 10 years. She couldn't even work and never went out of the house without a cane. Within two months of dust and mold injections, she served Thanksgiving dinner to 32 people and has never since used her cane in the last few years. (I'm not sure you could give me enough injections to ever have me able to serve Thanksgiving dinner to 32 people!) Anyway, these molds that most people respond to were the result of our research published in the world's leading clinical allergy journal, the **Annals of Allergy** (July, 1982; January, 1983; and May, 1984).

In short, I was curious why still many people didn't get better when they had allergy injections. Obviously, they were sensitive to antigens which they tested positive to and which were in their injections; but something else was missing. Sure many were better, and it cleared my chronic sinus, severe headaches, and asthma; but I was worried about those who were no better. In many cases, as you've just heard, the reason was mold sensitivity. You know that if we layed a piece of bread on the table and returned in a few days, it would be moldy. Mold is everywhere. You can't escape it. Just as some people breathe microscopic ragweed and grass pollen and get stuffy and congested, the same thing happens when others breathe mold. Our research showed that doctors and hospitals all over the country use an inferior growing media in petri dishes. If they would use another media or a different type of agar, they could grow and identify 32% more molds in the air than they ever knew existed. We also learned the highest mold counts for the year occur in the spring and the fall; this is the time of year when the pollens are blamed for everyone's symptoms. Testing for these molds and giving the necessary shots produced some of the dramatic results that you have just heard about.

Serial Dilution End-Point Titration for Skin Testing

Another reason our results occurred so quickly is the method of testing. As you are probably aware, all of us were trained to test one dose of tree and one dose of grass and so forth as they are injected on your forearm. Whatever you react to is put in your injection. They start with one unit of all the antigens they reacted to and the dose schedule mathematically increases with every injection until they reach a predetermined dose or when you have a reaction. It includes the erroneous assumption that you are just as allergic as I am because we all are on the same dose schedule. It's a "convenient" or simplistic approach and very mass applicable and many people get better, but I was concerned about those who do not.

In the 1970's this concern got to me, and I was very concerned about the people who could not tolerate these "convenient" or simplistic dose schedules, and I was concerned about the people we actually made worse with them. So I went around the country to many courses and meetings and learned there was a much more logical method that had been done for over 30 years; and you don't have to be an allergist to see that it makes more sense.

To test, we put on one strength, for example, of house dust. This is done the same as the other allergy tests with a small amount being injected just under the very first layer of skin, and it generally disappears in 20 minutes. We observe whether there is any immunologic reaction for that dose. In other words, is there any redness or swelling around it. If not, we test with the next dose five times stronger.

Then every 10 minutes we test with another five times stronger. If there is no reaction, the person is not sensitive to that antigen, and we know he produces no antibodies. When a strength is found that causes redness and growth around it or symptoms in the patient, the test is stopped. The last one not to react is the dose we put in the injection for treatment. Hence, we end up with a highly individualized dose schedule for each person and for each antigen that he is sensitive to. This results in quicker relief of symptoms, and there are far fewer reactions than in the old days. In fact, we have never had a serious reaction in over 24 years now, as opposed to the non-individualized method.

How do allergy injections work? The body is an amazing piece of machinery. If it receives the same ragweed in a small amount injected under the skin, it makes a protective or IgG antibody, as opposed to the allergic or IgE antibody made when ragweed is breathed. It is as though someone up there knew we were going to need a way to combat allergies.

Provocation-Neutralization Testing for Foods

Another beauty of this method also is that it allows us to take one giant step forward and test foods and chemicals as well. You can imagine how thrilled I was after six years of horrible eczema on my face to be cleared in two weeks and gradually become able to eat many of the foods to which I was allergic. You see, most doctors in the field of allergy still claim to this day that there are no injections for food allergies. In fact, if I had believed this myth, I would still have severe facial eczema and be unable to eat over 50 different foods and unable to eat any fruits. But the specialty of environmental medicine tests and treats food and chemical allergies. Being fully indoctrinated by my medical education, even though it was no secret my eczema was much worse whenever I ate, I never dreamed it was possible to be clear with injections to foods. Many doctors told me if I just calmed down I could get rid of it! I'd like to see them "cause" eczema by being "nervous!"

After years of going to bed in tears because my face was so bad, I finally took my husband's advice, "Why don't you go work with this doctor who claims to treat food allergy with injections?" In spite of my skepticism, I went as a patient and as a physician to learn. In two weeks I was clearer than I had been in 5 years and able to eat many of the foods which previously caused reactions. Before I went I had spent months on water and sugar diets, and many other diets equally unappealing and unhealthy.

I was an eager student and brought back all I had learned. I quickly phoned the six worst patients I could think of and announced, "I just learned to test food allergy and my eczema is totally clear for the first time in 5 years." From what I learned, I think we can now clear your condition as well. Sure enough, in two weeks another gal who looked as bad as I did was clear. That's the way we all were: several migraine cases, asthmatics who never totally got off medicine, and cases of severe depression for no reason. It turned out that food allergy requiring injections was the answer for many of us.

The Brain is a Common Allergy Target Organ

We should never forget that the brain is the commonest allergic target organ and the one most frequently overlooked. Alexander was eight years old and had been on three amphetamines a day from the medical school pediatric neurology department. This controlled his hyperactivity fairly well, they thought, but they didn't have to live with him. He threw the iron at his father, poured scalding water on his baby sister, failed in his school work, and made life a nightmare for his family. Within the first month of his food and mold injections, he was a totally different person, off all medicines and getting A's. But if he missed any injections or got into the wrong foods, he was back to his old self in minutes or hours. A year later I was curious if he really needed the mold injections any more, so I substituted water for a couple of weeks with the intent of calling his mother and asking if anything had been different during those two weeks. I didn't have to call her, however, because she came in wearing a black eye he had given her in an unprovoked attack.

On an older note, Daniel was depressed for 20 years and now at 39 had spent the last eight years and thousands of dollars with many psychologists and psychiatrists and a chronic prescription of Elavil. Two weeks of food injections and he was able to throw away the Elavil and discover he had a keen mind as well as no depression. Months later he tried to stop them and all his symptoms recurred so he got right back on.

Food Allergy Has Many Disguises

The examples go on and on. Many people are lucky and don't even need to test foods, but just go on a special diet which is described later.

Sandra was amazed to discover chocolate caused her asthma. Monica found that wheat and mold foods caused her asthma and Mick found coffee was the cause of his intolerable headaches that made him feel suicidal.

It turns out that when a certain percentage of a person's symptoms are better with inhalant injections to pollens, dusts and molds (the commonest form of allergy), but that some symptoms persist, it pays to evaluate the diet to see if hidden or unsuspected food allergies are the cause. It's a rare bird who doesn't have a hidden food allergy, but has migraine, eczema, emphysema, hyperactivity, depression or chronic tiredness. Nearly all of these diseases have hidden food allergies as part of their trigger.

Also, for every food allergy a person knows he has, there are usually half a dozen other food allergies that he is not aware of.

Chemical Sensitivity Also Masquerades As Many Mysterious Symptoms

Now remember all of the hoopla that urea foam formaldehyde insulation caused? As with my years of anguish over having my severe facial eczema, there's always some good that comes from the bad. The cases of formaldehyde hypersensitivity taught us a tremendous amount about chemical sensitivity. You see, most of the victims had an insidious or gradual onset of headache, dizziness, nausea, inability to concentrate, muscle aches, muscle spasms, and depression; and virtually all medical exams, blood tests and x-rays were negative. Some had a host of other symptoms, but these were the commonest.

Some started symptoms immediately and got progressively worse. Others took years to develop their chemical symptoms. Many patients exhibited a snowball effect; they developed other allergies to ragweed, hayfever, foods, or worst of all other chemicals such as natural gas.

So when we started seeing people with the same symptoms of headache, dizziness, muscle aches and spasms, depression and extreme tiredness, and all the tests were negative, we began to question formaldehyde. The problem was that these people didn't have any foam insulation. So we had to find the culprit now that we had the classic symptoms of chemical hypersensitivity. Our diligence paid off, for we found that many 20th century materials that we all take for granted outgas more formaldehyde than a recently foam-insulated house. This is especially true when the building itself has been tightened to conserve energy. Normally a building exchanges inside air with the outside every 2-4 hours. Now with tightening to conserve energy with vinyl siding and vapor barriers, insulation, paneling, caulking, and tighter construction, a house might take 1 or 2 days to exchange air. The mechanisms and scientific references for all this are in **TIRED OR TOXIC?**

We Are the First Generation of Man
Exposed to so Many Chemicals

Not only do we get a buildup of incomplete combustion products from gas heating systems and appliances, kerosene heaters and wood stoves (all of which put out formaldehyde), but we've added many new materials that constantly outgas formaldehyde. These include particle board in kitchen cabinets, particle board or plywood flooring, shelving and dressers, new carpeting, draperies, furniture, stuffings, laminates, glues, upholstery, plastic containers, books and mattresses.

In short, we've created a monster. We've created a

disease that only a few hundred physicians are specialists in. It is a disease that is so new and difficult to learn that it is not taught in medical schools yet. And there are no x-rays or blood tests to diagnose it. Also, it is a disease that breaks many of the rules of conventional medicine, thus blocking the thought patterns of conventionally trained physicians and actually leaving them frustrated, angry and hostile toward learning more about it. We've tightened up houses and cut down on air exchange with the outside, and at the same time we have introduced hundreds of new chemicals a year into the home which outgas chemicals to create baffling symptoms. As the person's exposure continues, he becomes increasingly sensitive to the chemicals. Even if the level of chemical exposure is lessened by getting rid of some of these materials, he still reacts because it takes much weaker levels now to create even worse symptoms than he ever had before. In other words, he has become much more sensitized.

There are people now who, because of their increased sensitivity, can't even come in our office. One gal becomes comatose in 2 hours. One nurse gets glassy eyed and appears drunk in half an hour. Another lady used to get severe asthma in 20 minutes from the chemicals when we still had carpeting, plastics and carbonless copy paper. This is partly why we must have such strict rules for admission to the office. The slightest odor of left-over perfume or smoke on your clothes can throw some of these patients into a backslide for days.

We were going to hire one chemically sensitive nurse to make house calls and point out to patients where the chemical problems in their houses were, but it took her two days to recover from symptoms she developed from entering other patients' homes.

35

Testing for Chemical Sensitivity

Fortunately, we are well-versed in the only method to diagnose chemical sensitivity since it is the same as for food testing. When proof is needed, we test chemicals single-blind. In other words, the patient doesn't know what is being tested until the session is over. Some of the tests are placebos or water; others are chemicals. By randomly mixing the order of the chemicals being tested with interspersed placebos, we can prove chemical sensitivity. And with random single-blind tests, no unknowledgeable "authority" can accuse the victim of faking or malingering. Just as the body recognizes one dose of thyroid as causing hyperthyroidism, nervousness and diarrhea, and another dose as too low, causing hypothyroidism with weight gain constipation, tiredness, and still another dose as just right, so too, the body reacts in a similar fashion to chemicals. I have now published this for doctors in the United States government's National Institutes Medical Journal (Environmental Health Perspective, 76, 195-198, 1987).

One dose can produce overdose symptoms, and another dose can produce under dose symptoms, and another dose can turn the symptom off. For example, we filmed Irene many times. She lost her voice for two years after her house had been insulated with urea foam formaldehyde. One dose of formaldehyde restores her voice in seven minutes. We can mix these up in any order, but can turn her on and off like a switch whenever we use the doses specific to her system. Likewise, we can turn on and off asthma and measure it with a peak flow meter during testing, or we can turn on a host of symptoms that people complain of and never dreamed were the result of allergies. Not all chemically sensitive people respond as easily as Irene does because she has no other allergies. She is only sensitive to formaldehyde. Charles was an engineer who just ached. A work-up by rheumatologists and their many prescribed trails of different anti-inflammatory drugs did not relieve him. But, being out of town on a consulting job did. We could turn on and off his arthralgia in the office when we tested him to formaldehyde. A weekend at home gave him twice as high a blood level of formaldehyde as a day at work. The source? The particle board sub-flooring and carpeting in his 2 year old house.

I use to get many symptoms from prolonged form-aldehyde exposure, but testing did nothing immediately because I had too many other sensitivities as well. I was too overloaded for one more chemical to make much differ-ence. And we learned that no test is 100% perfect.

Note: All of the techniques in this book have finally been researched and proven valid. There is a 130 page book of scientific explanations complete with hundreds of refer-ences available from this publisher. People have used this information to help small claims court attorneys under-stand that they are being unfairly discriminated against if they are denied reimbursement for this type of medical treatment. The book is **THE SCIENTIFIC BASIS FOR SELECTED ENVIRONMENTAL MEDICINE TECH-NIQUES.**

Total Load is Crucial to Understanding
Multiple Sensitivities

This brings us to the concept of total load. If a man comes in the office complaining of a painful foot and I examine him and remove four out of five nails for his shoe, he's going to leave saying, "She's a lousy doctor, my foot still hurts!" So it is with the highly allergic person. A person may have migraines or asthma or chronic sinus from dust and mold allergies. If injections and environmental changes in the home only bring 80% of the relief, he won't find total relief until he discovers the hidden foods or chemicals that he has a minor sensitivity to. For some the missing ingredient could be a vitamin or mineral deficiency.

Now the conventional allergist who does the convenient one-dose for all form of testing does not test for the new molds we discovered, and he does not utilize the individualized doses. He does not test chemicals and foods by the provocation method; he does not treat the Candida syndrome; he does not look for vitamin, mineral and essential fatty acid deficiencies. He has had no training in the complex or comprehensive form of environmental medicine. So no wonder allergy has a bad reputation among doctors of being inconsequential and they consider it of no consequence that they are unknowledgeable about diagnosing the new disguises that allergy has. They are unaccustomed to seeing serious undiagnosable conditions get better because when one does simplistic allergy, only the simplest allergies get better. The severe ones remain a mystery and one is often told they are not even allergic. So the symptoms are never suspected of having an allergic origin. There are well over 4,000 conventional allergists in the United States and many more dabblers who practice it without training. There are by contrast about 400 comprehensive allergists and they are at various levels of training. I know, because I teach yearly at the Advanced Courses for physicians learning these techniques.

Common Versus Comprehensive Allergy Investigations

Mary had eczema for 14 years. We found she was sensitive to many pollens, dusts, and molds; and her blood levels of vitamin A and B6 were abnormally now. She was clear for the first time in 14 years within one month, but she had been to three other very good allergists with no results. The secret? They didn't use the more sensitive testing method. They didn't test to the newer molds we discovered. They didn't use our media as described in our research papers and see what molds are growing in her environment. They didn't use our accelerated technique for giving injections, and they do not do blood levels for vitamins. Had she not been better, I would have looked for a missing food or chemical sensitivity, and they do not even have the tools to do that, namely, the provocative- neutralization technique just described. In fact, the official position of the American Academy of Allergy and Immunology today is that the technique should not be used. John had 57 years of psoriasis and was clear for the first time with four dollars worth of the right missing essential fatty acid that does not even require a prescription. He can buy it in any health food store. When the store runs out, his psoriasis returns until he gets more. So there are many hidden vitamin, mineral, fatty acid, and amino acid deficiencies that contribute to symptoms, as well.

Phenol Sensitivity Can Make Common Allergy Injections Intolerable

Another nail in the shoe is phenol. You may have never heard of this chemical. Another name is carbolic acid. Phenol out-gases from many plastics that also outgas formaldehyde. Phenol also is an excellent preservative, and it's in many medicines and all allergy injections around the world. There are, at this time, about a dozen of us in the United States who have a special set of extracts that are phenol-free because patients like myself are too sensitive to it.

Lenny had asthma for 27 years. He had injections from three different allergists, but thought he was allergic to the shots because they made him worse. I was pretty sure I wouldn't make him worse because we would use the individualized dosage or titrated method. You can imagine my surprise when I made him worse just like the others! Then I suspected the real problem. So we tested him to phenol and precipitated a grand slam asthma attack. Giving him phenol-free injections has him without asthma and on no medication for the first time in 27 years. Most people who already know they are very sensitive to other chemicals like formaldehyde, auto exhaust, smoke or perfumes eventually exhibit what is called the spreading phenomenon. They start developing symptoms to other chemicals or foods. Therefore, we usually have to give them phenol-free extracts as well, thereby reducing their body's chemical overload.

The ultimate in pure extracts for the most exquisitely sensitive people are phenol-free, glycerine-free extracts that are costly to make. Less than half a dozen offices in the world make them. But there are scores of people we could never have helped get better without them.

Controversy in Allergy

I practiced conventional allergy for nine years the way all allergists are taught. There's nothing wrong with it, for many people with simple allergies are helped. But it can't help the person whose sensitivities require precise fine-tuning, or who have food, chemical, or Candida problems and require comprehensive allergic and environmen-

40

tal management. I'd still probably be doing it if I had not been forced by my own food, chemical, and Candida allergies to know everything possible about the disease and explore new horizons. In fact, I'm ashamed to admit that before I learned these techniques (when I knew absolutely nothing about them), I also told others with all the authority that a physician carries that the techniques to test food and chemical sensitivities were unfounded. How illness humbles us and makes us infinitely more inquisitive and honest. In fact, at this time there appears to be a silly feud going on between simplistic allergists who don't do these tests to foods and chemicals by the provocation-neutralization technique and ecologists or specialists in environmental medicine who depend upon these techniques to diagnose complex allergies.

Part of the argument lies in the fact that the conventional or simplistic allergists attempted to do a study to show that the PN technique does not work, but they never came to any of our offices to learn it. So, of course, the technique did not work for them, and they published a paper showing the technique did not work. They claimed that our patients were hypochondriacs and good actors. I got a little tired of this petty squabble so I proceeded to settle it. You know, of course, we humans do not have a monopoly on allergic diseases.

So we did a double-blind study on horses with heaves which is just like human asthma. We didn't tell the horses, the testers, the veterinarian who examined them, or myself who was filming them, what they were being tested to. We had a university professor immunologist run the study. We turned on and turned off the horses's asthma complete with wheezing and coughing with their appropriate doses of mold and timothy grass which is in their hay. In fact, the worst horse with heaves was able to be ridden for the first time in six years after his injections had been started. This study was published (and is still the only study on animals using P.N.) and should lay the controversy to rest and allow us to practice medicine to the best of our abilities using the tools we are trained in, free from denigrating remarks from those untrained in these techniques.

The Candida Controversy

Another nail in the shoe is the problem of Candida. If you carefully question some people as to when they last felt well, you can find their downfall was preceded by a pregnancy, surgery, even dental work, or maybe an antibiotic, the birth control pill, steroids, or some factor which fosters the overgrowth of a particular yeast called Candida albicans. Once it is growing in the body, it produces toxins to which some hosts react or become allergic. The most bizarre symptoms can arise; they can be either totally inexplicable such as mental fogginess, inability to concentrate, or unprovoked mood swings; or they can mimic known diseases like colitis, sterility, endometrosis, depression, urethritis, asthma, Sjogren's syndrome, or arthritis so that no other cause is sought. It is only after this yeast is treated that the symptoms can be annihilated. A white tongue can be one that's loaded with Candida; a normal healthy tongue is pink.

Hormone Sensitivity

Some people are sensitive to their own hormone levels. Premenstrual syndrome is a good example. We have filmed several gals who complained of severe premenstrual depression and violent mood swings. With one dose of hormone we can duplicate the crying that turns on for no reason and the inability to make a decision, and with another dose we can bring about smiles and happiness. There are a host of other substances, many naturally produced by the body, which we are constantly finding that

42

people react to. Histamine and serotonin and even the flu virus are sometimes the antigens that allow people freedom from their unusually aggravating symptoms.

One lady was bedridden for three months with rheumatoid arthritis. We've filmed her several times because within four minutes of the phenol injection (like formaldehyde, phenol is everywhere in your home and abounds in plastics) she goes from barely able to get out of the chair to dancing down the hall. For days prior she was unable to even comb her hair, but for some unknown reason a particular dose of phenol (which we tested and filmed double-blind on three occasions) relieves her pain and stiffness as she waves her arms about, squats, gets in and out of the chair effortlessly, and touches her toes. This effect lasts for two days. If she feels extremely edgy or panicky, we found that a dose of histamine relieves this. No two patients with the exact same diseases have the same causes.

But I'm even the one who is often pleasantly surprised. One lady with 28 years of rheumatoid arthritis said she could not stand the last two years of Sjogren's syndrome. Her eyes were so dry she had to use artificial tears every 15 minutes. Her lips were dry, cracked, and peeling; her tongue looked like that of corpse. In two months of Candida treatment she was so clear she got a job for the first time in 18 years and resumed a social life. She started it off with flying colors in time to attend her daughter's graduation. Before, she could never be in public. Now you can understand some of the motivation for my long hours. Every day brings such unheard of happiness for someone, that I am driven.

The people I have had the privilege of treating have helped us unlock the secrets of the body. There is suddenly hope where there was none, partly because one of those secrets is known. We are all biochemically unique. Simplistic medicine is still in search of one cure for rheumatoid arthritis, for example. But in the scores of people that we have helped improve, no two have the exact same set of responsible hypersensitivities. They are all uniquely different individuals, each with different causes. One exciting aspect of this specialty of environmental medicine where complex allergies are diagnosed and a comprehensive treatment is prescribed is that it is growing at a rapid pace, and there's constant hope and newness. Patients from around the country make it a point to check back yearly to see what is new that may pertain to their condition. Also, I keep in touch personally with the other leaders in this field as I lecture around the country in the courses and meeting for physicians learning this specialty. I have worked with Dr. William Rea in the Environmental Unit in Dallas, and Dr. Joseph Miller in Mobile, and I have also learned from the office visits with Dr. Theron Randolph in Chicago, Dr. Doris Rapp in Buffalo, Dr. Sidney Baker at Yale, and Dr. Marshall Mandell in Norwalk. With scores of lectures each year to give as well, the pace may be a bit demanding, but the constant discoveries provide the fuel!

Universal Reactors

Many people do not have sensitivities limited to just molds or pollens or foods or chemicals. They have a mixture. Those who react to everything, such as I did, are called universal reactors. This makes the field complicated and difficult. But it's exciting that we no longer need to consider many conditions as something one has to learn to live with such as eczema, adult acne, migraine, phlebitis, colds, cardiac arrhythmia, lupus, Tourette's syndrome, arthritis, colitis, ulcers, learning disabilities, inability to concentrate, lupus sarcoidosis, Sjogren's syndrome, thyroiditis, and more. The list of chronic illnesses responding to comprehensive allergic and environmental management grows yearly. Sometimes we use laboratory tests to help us with our diagnosis. An IgE or allergic antibody level helps us know whether to suspect hidden chemical allergies when it is very low. A CBC helps uncover hidden infection when it is elevated. A Chemical profile can show liver or kidney dysfunction. A formic acid measures formaldehyde. And, of course, many vitamin deficiencies can be found in analysis of the mineral and vitamin levels that we do. Mineral toxicities can be suspected by hair analysis. Some people have had many thyroid tests but never a test to see if they make antibodies against their own thyroid. And many people have hidden asthma but never had a comprehensive pulmonary function to measure how much of the lung is asthmatic, how much is destroyed, or what percent represents emphysema from years of asthma untreated with allergy injections, or how much of the lung is normal. After the first reading, an injection for asthma is given, and the lung function test is repeated. This measurement shows us now how much of the lung can be restored to normal once the allergies are treated.

Some need x-rays of the sinuses to enable us to see scar tissue that plugs the drainage openings. This scar tissue also results from years of chronic sinusitis untreated with injections. Some need chest x-rays, TB skin tests, or patch tests to chemicals to determine which chemicals they are touching that are causing their skin to break out. Many asthmatics, we were startled to find who had had years of prednisone and antibiotics for repeated infections, had never had a sputum test for possible overgrowth of fungi such as Candida (who's growth is fostered by both medications). There were several dramatic cases of asthmatics treated with hundreds of dollars of drugs a month who were found, by culturing the chest phlegm on our special mold plates as described in the **Annals of Allergy**, to have actual yeasts or molds growing in their chest sputum. By treating them for just one month, they were off all medicines and had no asthma for the first time in years. Other people have dangerous levels of accumulated chemicals and pes-

45

ticides in their systems. They can now be measured by blood tests. So there are increasingly more exciting diagnostic techniques.

But much more crucial than any lab tests, is the story each person has to tell of his symptoms. Many clues may not seem worth mentioning to the uninitiated, as I wrote in **Bestways** magazine, February, 1984. For example, many people purchased new furniture, a new bed, new carpeting or renovated the house within five years of the onset of their symptoms. It's the overload from these chemicals that damaged their immune systems enough to turn on their allergies. Why do you think 20 years ago one in 20 people had allergies, and now it's one out of every four?

Also, a contributory factor is the destruction of vitamins such as B6 in our food through processing as I wrote in the March, 1983, issue of **Let's Live** magazine. Also, the repeated commercial growing of foods on the same soils has lowered our essential body minerals as well. Zinc and selenium and magnesium are just a few that are essential to a healthy immune system. And vitamin E, as I wrote in the January, 1986, **Let's Live**, is crucial to help the body detoxify chemical pollutants. This knowledge is not so new, but is still ignored.

How Long Will It Take to Get Better?

How long will it take to get better? How long will you be on injections? That's highly individual. One lady with a 20 year cough who had had bronchoscopy and several pulmonary and ENT specialists was clear in two weeks. She just removed all we told her to after testing, and she didn't even need injections. People who crash into their environmental controls get better quicker and are able to go off injections sooner. Some can go off in two years. Others have so many sensitivities they will probably never go off, unless they plough through the additional techniques in

46

our subsequent books. Those who procrastinate in following suggestions for a more hypoallergenic home take longer to get relief and have difficulty staying symptom-free once off injections.

You can think of me as just a mechanic for your car. I can find the trouble spot and many times I can patch it up. But I'm not responsible for how you drive the car. As you can see, we don't have all of the answers, but it certainly is exciting seeing what every day brings. Sometimes a person's improvement comes quickly and dramatically so that we can film him and use it to teach doctors about this phenomenon; in other cases it takes months or even a couple of years to bring symptoms under control. Unfortunately, very few attain full control over their symptoms without measures at home to reduce the total antigenic or stimulatory load. We will address this problem and teach you how to control the environment at home.

Many of the patients are more than happy to talk with new patients to help them reduce the loneliness, confusion, and frustration that having this new 20th century disease brings. The best exposure is to join the HEAL group (see resources). As we begin to unravel your sensitivities we may find that they are limited only to ragweed, hayfever or pollens, or you may have all year round symptoms and have dust and mold sensitivities as well. For others, their allergies extend further; they have chronic symptoms, such as tiredness and depression for seemingly no reason, which seem undiagnosable, and it turns out they have hidden food or chemical sensitivities or sensitivities to chemical mediators within the body. Others have hidden vitamin, essential fatty acid, or digestive enzyme deficiencies. Other like myself have all of these problems and are termed universal reactors. Until each culprit is identified, your system cannot be fully relieved of this 20th century overload.

Others have much more serious conditions like end

47

stage forms of cardiovascular diseases and cancers. Whatever you have, from hang-nails to cancer, every malfunction of the body can be improved upon by application of the techniques that promote relief from E.I., or environmental illness. For the basic principles of clean air, food and water and the correction of biochemical effects is now the forefront of the new era in medicine. No longer is a headache a Darvon or aspirin deficiency. We no longer use merely drugs to chronically cover up or mask symptoms. Instead, we shoot for the underlying causes and real health.

Whatever your sensitivity is, we look forward to teaching you as much about allergies and your body as possible and to help you discover how you can feel your very best.

My goal is to first help you get rid of symptoms. Then to get rid of medications, and finally to get rid of me. For as you will see, there is seemingly no limit as to how healthy a person can be. His biggest limiting factor is motivation. Some are lucky and have to do very little. Others, like myself had to do everything I have written about to get free of symptoms, medications, and injections.

THE ALLERGY STORY

We take up where conventional medicine leaves off. The ideas that will be presented here will be very new to many people. The fact that there is now evidence that people with diagnoses of early multiple sclerosis, depression, diabetes, phlebitis, angina, arthritis and a host of other degenerative and auto-immune diseases are actually triggered by a type of allergic reaction may seem preposterous. In fact, it probably seems like some fly-by-night bit of quackery that one disease could be responsible for so many problems. You will find yourself in a strange situation. As you learn and grow you will discover that you know more about this new field of medicine than probably most other doctors you'll ever meet again. Even though some may react with anger, hostility, and disbelief, avoid reciprocating in kind. Instead show them that you're willing to lovingly teach them, no matter how long it takes for them to accept and learn. This is the medicine of today.

The actual conceptual problem lies in the nomenclature of medicine. We have taken, for example, groups of symptoms such as pain, swelling, and tenderness; and we have erroneously termed them a disease diagnosed as arthritis. The problem is that this is not the name of a disease, but merely a collection of symptoms. One of the disease states that can cause this complex of symptoms is an adverse reaction in some people to inhaled antigens such as dust, mold and pollen plus adverse reactions to foods that are ingested as well as chemicals that are in the environment. As I'll show later on, there is an immunologic explanation for all of this.

In short, we differ from the rest of medicine in that we look for the causes, and attempt to avoid prescribing drugs to mask symptoms. Instead, ecologists back up to a more fundamental level and try to determine what it takes to unload your body so that it can now heal itself. This point in very perplexing to physicians accustomed to practicing medicine where one specific chemical stops one particular symptom. It seems like quackery or voo doo to them, when by putting a group of people on the Candida program and mold injections we are able to turn off about a dozen different symptoms in each of them. This is simply because we have just relieved part of the total body burden, and in doing so the body has become healthy enough to heal itself. As Dr. Rea says, surgeons do this all the time. They would never think of suturing a wound without washing it first. They try to lower the total load, by scrubbing, giving tetanus injections and immobilization to promote the best opportunity for healing.

We don't know at this point if all arthritis or all multiple sclerosis cases have environmental triggers, but we know that if you are at the end of the diagnostic road and have a dead-end diagnosis such as rheumatoid arthritis where there's no place else for you to go, you owe it to yourself to investigate the possibility of an allergy. You may find an environmental trigger and learn to manipulate this either through avoidance, or environmental controls, or injections so that you can turn your disease and symptoms off before irreversible damage occurs.

This is not a new concept, and I'm not the first one to write about it. It has been proven time and time again in places called environmental units. The best to my knowledge in the world is the Environmental Health Center in Dallas directed by Dr. William J. Rea, a cardio-vascular surgeon. Dr. Theron Randolph, the first physician to discover that people really do have a host of symptoms in response to chemicals, created the first environmentally controlled hospital unit. Even though he retired his unit this year, from living with good ecologic principles, he still practiced in his eighties just outside of Chicago.

The Environmental Control Unit

The knowledge that environmental triggers have caused the symptoms listed came about through careful avoidance and provocation coupled by observation. The unit consists of a specially constructed hospital wing in which the air is meticulously controlled. Many types of odors and chemical gases that you take for granted as being totally innocuous have been diligently removed from the air. When a person enters, he is showered and given cotton gown washed in spring water. He is not allowed to bring any materials in the room that could cause allergic problems, such as toiletries or even newspapers. Visitors are likewise scrupulously screened for odors and allergens on their person.

The patients fast for a week, and what has happened typically in this controlled environmental setting with fasting was that not only did the patients clear traditionally allergic symptoms such as asthma, headaches, and sinusitis, but also symptoms that we never dreamed of as being allergy related. This included symptoms of MS, arthritis, colitis, multiple dermatoses, dizziness, muscle cramps, lupus, vasculitis, depression, exhaustion, seizure disorders, schizophrenia, recurrent phlebitis, recurrent angina, idiopathic fluid retention and many more.

And, when common everyday foods were added back one day at a time and patients were exposed to common, everyday chemicals one at a time, some miraculous things happened. Not only were they able to turn on their classically allergic symptoms, but they were also able to turn on these other symptoms. Later, by removing these incitants from their environments, they were symptom free again. These symptoms, again, included such things as convulsions, diabetes, arthritis, colitis, schizophrenia, depression, angina, etc. These are the maladies for which conventional medicine provides medications with dangerous side effects and implies that if you don't take them for control of these symptoms that medicine has nothing more to offer. So in this way, we were able to diagnose symptom complexes or disease states that were caused by foods and chemicals that we all take for granted as impossible to cure. And we were able to turn the symptoms on and off by controlling the exposure.

You Do Not Have to Learn to Live With It.

One problem is that not everyone has symptoms severe enough to warrant going into a unit, and yet they are troublesome enough that they interfere with their lifestyle. Many people go through life at half-mast, feeling chronically tired or depressed for no reason at all. They wouldn't dream of taking these symptoms to a physician because they have already had thorough physicals and been told that they are in great shape and that these symptoms are due to nerves or working too hard. Or they have been told, "You have to learn to live with it."

But one thing E.I. or environmentally- induced illnesses have in common is that as diverse as their symptoms are from person to person, nearly all patients have a common denominator of tremendous tiredness and depression for no reason that is secondary to their allergies. There are two types of patients that I'm trying to address here with this message. One type knows who they are. They have silently struggled with their environmental illness for years, trying to maintain a low profile and adapt to a world that seems to be their enemy. They try to hurry through stores and avoid elevators where they might come into contact with people wearing perfumes and aftershave. They try not to linger in public places where many types of chemicals and fumes abound. They limit the foods that they ingest and they try to have organic or chemically less contaminated foods because they know that all of these different exposures produce symptoms in them. They dare not tell anyone because it would sound too unconventional, and they don't want to be thought of as any stranger than they already seem. In fact, they struggle to put on a normal front because they can't bear the isolation they feel when they divulge their allergies.

The second type I'm addressing is just the opposite. They don't have the faintest idea that there is anything wrong with them, least of all an allergy or hypersensitivity to the environment. They think that they are perfectly healthy and only when pressed or upon taking a very thorough medical history would one find that they indeed go through life at half-mast, never feeling truly vivacious and energetic, always craving cigarettes, coffee, coca-colas or pastries.

When we have a sick plant, we ask ourselves if it needs more water or better light; but when man is sick, we irradiate him with x-rays and drug him with chemical prescriptions. Many a modern doctor, whether due to insecurity or training, relies first on evidence from lab tests and x-rays, second on his own knowledge, and third on what the patient has to tell him. Unfortunately, this is just the exact opposite order of what we need to use in order to understand ecologic illness. We first must rely extremely heavily on every piece of information that the patient is able to offer. Second, we rely on our own knowledge of environmental medicine to synthesize a working hypothesis from what we have just gained from the patient. Third, laboratory aids are just an adjunct; and with appropriate testing, we can obtain treatment doses of antigens to be used in our patients.

This is why so often a patient will say, "I have these horrible headaches but my doctor did x-rays and blood tests and says there's nothing wrong with me." If we reverse our priorities and acknowledge that here is a patient who has headache, we can commit ourselves to a different approach. Here is a patient with headaches, and even if his blood tests and x-rays are negative, I'm going to persist and find the cause. It's an ego-centric, lazy, irresponsible and dishonest cop-out to say that just because I can't find the cause by lab tests, the patient must be a hypochondriac.

Another problem with conventional or laboratory-based medicine is that it has an arbitrary breakdown into anatomical and physiologic areas of specialization. One man takes care of your bones; one man takes care of you head; one takes care of the right kidney; and seemingly, one, the left. Unfortunately, ecologic illness is a multi-system disease, so that when a person consults a physician, he only hears that part of the complaint which refers to his area of specialization. Very often, people with ecologic illness go from doctor to doctor. They start with the family doctor; then go to an internist, an ear, nose and throat doctor, a neurologist, a neurosurgeon, and possibly a pulmonary specialist. They all tell him that, "Whatever you have, it's not in my field." Some may suggest that there is nothing wrong and perhaps they should see a psychiatrist. After a while, even the most stoic and persistent individuals can begin to doubt his own sanity. After all, how can four out of four doctors be wrong? Very easily.

You see, it's the basic way in which medicine is set up that is erroneous. We doctors are programed just like a computer. We are programed to think of the body in compartments or physiologic organ systems; and if a disease has multi-system involvement, this does not fit into the computer. As with any computer system, GIGO holds true. In computer language this stands for "Garbage In, Garbage Out," and what it means is you only get out of the computer what you put into it. I shudder to think of all the people I was unable to help before I developed environmental illness.

Likewise, you only get out of physicians what has been programed into them during medical education.

Consider a typical person who has exposure to formaldehyde and natural gas (for example, formaldehyde in clothing, building and paper products, and natural gas in trace amounts in the home or business from the heating system), and who is hypersensitive to a few foods; he may experience a variety of symptoms, the commonest constellation being severe headache, dizziness, nausea, achiness of joints, chronic tiredness, depression and chronic sinusitis.

When he goes to the physician complaining of all of these, the physician is overwhelmed and the patient is immediately intimidated and made to feel like a hypochondriac so he only concentrates on the worst symptoms one at a time. He attempts to minimize his list of complaints and hone in on the worst one. So perhaps if during the last few weeks his sinusitis has been bothering him the most, he will go to an ear, nose and throat specialist. He will be checked over and told, "Well, there doesn't appear to be any infection. Perhaps an antihistamine-decongestant would help you" and he prescribes another chemical to overload the system of someone who is already multiply chemically sensitive.

And so we have worked ourselves into a corner with the way in which we have designed medical education. Now, however, we have changed our thinking and see the body as a whole. We can step back and get a different perspective on the individual and realize that environment plays a large part in disease in many people.

Even before all of this was known, allergic patients have classically gotten the short end of the stick through history. People who wheezed and had severe asthma were thought to have induced it by their own volition and it has been taught that it is a manifestation of their anxiety state.

Even to this day, many people with asthma are referred to pulmonary specialists as their sole treatment. They are excellent in prescribing capsules and aerosol inhalers to mask the symptoms, but many disregard allergy as the major cause of asthma and so they rarely refer an asthmatic patient to an allergist. Or worse, they dabble in allergy often relying on the result of a few insensitive blood and skin tests to come to the erroneous conclusion that the patient is not allergic.

As a rule, they load them with medication and when they get progressively worse, which they eventually will, they then put them on more potent and harmful medications of steroids like prednisone (a relative of cortisone).

And everyone knows this class of dangerous drugs can eventfully cause glaucoma, cataracts, diabetes, ulcers, hypertension, osteoporosis and more! You see, asthma is a genetically-linked allergic disease, and it has only one way to go. If it is left with the underlying allergic cause untreated, it can only get worse. Obviously, something has to trigger the formation of all this mucous and spasm and tightening of the breathing tubes. And you can only have so much accumulation of phlegm and bronchospasm in the lung before you start developing permanent irreversible destruction. This destroyed tissue is called emphysema, and it is a one-way street. It does not get better with a treatment that just covers up the symptoms.

Also, all these medications do nothing for the chronic state of tiredness that accompanies most allergic problems such as asthma. Avoidance of the antigens that cause it and injections to make the person synthesize or manufacture blocking antibodies to turn the allergy off are the only ways to improve these people.

By synthesizing blocking antibodies in their bloodstream in response to administration of allergy injections and by avoiding many of the things that were found to trigger their asthma, eventually many asthmatics can be off all medication and free of wheezing. Nothing relieves the chronic tiredness that accompanies this disease except avoidance of known allergens, diets and/or injections. Likewise, the hyper- irritability of the asthmatic system is markedly improved. People who wheeze will know what I mean. If they jog, get exposed to the cold or just laugh, they can precipitate asthma, a tightening of the chest, cough or copious throat phlegm. But after I had injections, I no longer had any asthma; I require no medication, and I can no longer trigger the wheezing with uncontrolled laughter.

There is a Difference in the Way Allergies are Diagnosed and Treated

People constantly ask us after they are off their medications and their asthma is markedly improved, "Why didn't my doctor send me here years ago? Why did he tell me in fact not to go to an allergist—that it would be a waste of time and money?" Partly he told them that because indeed it may have been the truth. You see, the way in which allergy is practiced differs tremendously from individual to individual. It is one of the least standardized areas of medicine at this point in time. (See the explanation of various methods of testing in "How to Choose an Allergist.")

Most physicians doing allergy do what we call conventional allergy. I did it too, for nine years, because it's the way we're all trained. They test everybody to one or two strengths of the different antigens such as dust and mold; then whatever gives a positive reaction on the skin test is included in the extracts. The dose schedule for administering this starts out with a tiny dose which is slowly increased to an arbitrarily predetermined large dose. It's a "one dose for everybody" type of situation, a very canned approach. It reminds me of a panty-hose commercial, where one size fits all.

The problem is that in no way are we as individual as we are in our allergies. We all are very different and biochemically unique; we all have different allergic triggers or causes. We also have very precise requirements for the dose of each antigen that we need to turn off our symptoms.

Whoever said that just because you are allergic to trees and grasses and dust and mold, that you are just as allergic to trees as you are to grasses or dust or molds? Therefore, why should we all have the same dose in our injections? And who says your dose to these should be the same as mine? And yet, this is why many pulmonary specialists do not think that immunotherapy (allergy injections) has a very good track record in terms of asthma. They are right. It doesn't have a great past because it is not individualized enough to serve the needs of many highly allergic individuals. Conventional allergy does treat well many types of allergies, but not the complex ones that require comprehensive treatment. Also, conventional allergy does not address food allergies, chemical hypersensitivities, or newly researched molds; and they are not trained in the techniques to test hormones, Candida, nutrition, and much more.

Instead, there is another system which we will explain later on whereby, for example, one strength of house dust is applied to the arm by injection under the skin; then another does five times stronger is put on. Then another dose five times stronger is put on. When the point of reaction is found by redness and a growing bump, this tells us where the treatment dose is for this particular antigen in this particular patient at this point in time. It is much more fine-tuned and therefore gives quicker and better results.

You have only to ask yourself—do you want someone to use the same test and treatment dose on you that they use for everyone? Or do you want it individually calibrated or titrated according to your body's own unique response?

Many people with classic allergic symptoms complain, "I have chronic sinus problem, headaches, and tiredness. I'm always carrying a Kleenex and people are always asking me if I have a cold. But when I went to the allergist, he tested me and said I wasn't allergic." Having done conventional allergy myself for nine years, it wasn't until I learned the individualized or titrated method, that I was able to find the dose for these people to relieve their symptoms.

I already knew they had to be allergic, because if I gave them a nasal provocation, in other words a bit of dust or mold or pollen to sniff on the end of a toothpick, they'd stuff up or say "That's the headache I've been telling the neurologists about!" Some opponents of this method argue if you test with strong enough doses, everyone will react. But we use a control to which the patient responds negatively to be sure they don't just indiscriminately react.

Mold Allergy Has Been Improved

Aside from not using serially diluted end-point titration, another reason that many people do not improve with conventional injection therapy as much as they would like, is that they have hidden mold allergies.

Molds are invisible, microscopic particles that float around in all air constantly. They are not seen, but you know if you left a piece of bread on your desk for a couple of days, it would be moldy. These molds cause a host of symptoms in people. They can cause any allergic symptom that you can think of from eczematous dermatitis to hyperactivity to sinus to headaches to asthma, vasculitis, and arthritis as well as symptoms that are attributed to multiple sclerosis. One of the problems is that only a very minute percent of the molds in the air are tested for by many allergist.

We have completed some research which enable us to find many more molds that are commonly in the air at all times; and by applying this individualized testing method to these newer molds, we have been able to expand the treatment repertoire. This research is published for all physicians in the **Annals of Allergy,** July, 1982; and January, 1983; and May 1984.

Differences in the Practice of Allergy

Doctors in general have been hesitant to refer to allergists for years. And in view of the fact that it was sort of an art in search of a science for many years I can understand why. But it is time that they now realize that there are many differences in the way that allergy is practiced. They need to find who in their area is practicing the most up-to-date form of allergy with emphasis on environmental hygiene so that they can appropriately refer patients for treatment via the simple allergy or comprehensive allergy route.

Ear, nose, and throat specialists see people with chronic sinusitis, post nasal drip, and rhinitis day in and day out. If one in five, or 20%, of normal population is allergic at some point in their lives, probably 80 or 90% of those that the ENT specialists see are allergic. Instead, they x-ray, load up with drugs, then sometimes operate to correct hyperplastic sinusitis or deviated nasal septums. Many patients tell us they are not better after all this or report they went to an ENT doctor for 2-5 years but never once did he suggest that they see an allergist. In fact, some patients actually asked if maybe they should see an allergist and where told it wouldn't help.

And yet, many of these people are able to be markedly relieved of symptoms within several months of starting their injections. These people are furious because many of them had been operated on and were not any better. They ask us, "Don't they teach about allergy in medical school? Why don't people who specialize in diseases of the sinuses know about allergy, the number one commonest disease of the sinuses?" Knowledgeable ones will not be afraid to consider the possibility of allergy with you.

On the other side of the coin, some ENT's realize how prevalent allergy is. Some go to a one-week crash course and call themselves allergists. To dabble in allergy is as serious as dabbling in neurosurgery. Not only do the failures give allergy a bad name, rob people of their money and discourage them for seeking further consultations, but allergy can be fatal. When a patient does poorly with one "allergist," he is loathe to try another and may become severely ill in the interim. Pick a dedicated ENT-allergist who insists on you reading and learning.

Often times by applying an intradermal test to a mold or a dust, we can turn on a patient's profuse sinusitis and make him very stuffy and constantly clearing his throat. Then by putting in the next or treatment or neutralizing dose, turn his symptoms off just as dramatically so that in this way we can prove to him what antigens trigger his symptoms. At other times we can give him nasal provocation tests. In other words, we can have him sniff certain species of pollens or molds and give him the very symptoms which he has been complaining of, so he has the proof that he would benefit from an injection program.

The purpose of this manual is only one. That is to help people who cannot afford to wait ten or twenty years while many doctors catch up with this new area of knowledge, environmental medicine. It takes over where medicine and allergy leave off.

Very possibly in ten or twenty years there will no longer be specialists such as a neurologist or endocrinologist or a diabetologist. Doctors will not be able to concern themselves with one narrow niche of medicine, but will have to encompass a broader range of immunologic reactions that can occur in any target organ of the body or any endocrine receptor site on a cell. In other words, these will all be one melting pot, and the physicians who treats any symptom within these specialties will need to be well-versed in immunology, toxicology, nutrition, allergy: environmental medicine is all of these related sub-specialties. It will take several decades to train a new generation of doctors who see the patient as a whole, unique being, not as a diseased liver or as an inflamed knee joint. In the meantime, not only are there people suffering with a multitude of symptoms, but some people are actually dying. And they can't afford to wait. They need to know what to do to help themselves now.

Look at how many years it took to ban DDT after its harmful effects were known for a long time, and yet it is still floating around in my bloodstream in very measurable amounts even though I have not had exposure for a long time. And most people are still ingesting it unknowingly because we have given many third world countries the benefit of our technologic knowledge by shipping barrels of carcinogenic and highly toxic chemicals to countries where some illiterate peasant farmer cannot read his own language much less the English directions on the barrel. Often the farmers come with bowls and jugs to a central supply area to pick up their aliquot of poison to use on the crops. And many of these countries buy our illegal cast-off pesticides. Then our ignorance comes full circle because we buy the produce back from these countries and feed it to our families. Also, a recent analysis if some California crops show that it is still being used illegally. So with an appreciation of how long it takes to make change, and how often things can go astray when efforts have been made to change something, you can easily understand why I feel an urgency to take matters in my own hands to try to set the record straight.

It may seem futuristic or resemble a flight to paranoia to find that chemicals can cause allergic reactions, but there is solid, firm, immunologic data in the world literature showing that chemicals cause disease. For example, toluene diisocyanate (TDI) is a chemical commonly encountered in the plastic industry, and it is able to cause a minute change in the proteins in the bodies of some susceptible individuals. They then make an antibody to this new protein; and the combination of this new protein, their antibody and the TDI causes a variety of symptoms. The first symptom they discovered was asthma. And so, we have evidence of a chemical causing asthma and other symptoms; so it should not be too hard to realize that in a world where a new chemical is synthesized every minute, there are many other chemicals out there causing a vast array of changes in those of us who are genetically susceptible.

Cookbook Medicine Treats Diseases as Though They Were Drug Deficiencies

Currently, the medical school journals are full of examples of hundreds of everyday chemicals found in homes, offices, schools, stores, and churches that cause any disease one can think of. But the most confusing part for doctors is the individuality of symptoms and target organs. In medicine we're trained like Julia Child—to follow a recipe. It's easy to do cookbook medicine; everybody with a sore throat gets a throat culture. If the culture grows Strep, give penicillin for 10 days. If the patient is allergic to Penicillin, use Erythrocin or Tetracycline. Easy! Or for more complicated diseases such as diabetes, lose weight, go on a diabetic diet, use glucose-lowering pills if necessary. If not successful and the sugar is still high, go to insulin. Medicine does not yet look for the cause even though we know, for example, that juvenile diabetes can come from milk antibodies that attack the pancreas (NEJM 327: 302, 1992).

The problems are much more complicated than that. For a person with recurrent sore throats, it may be due to a hypersensitivity to molds, dust, pollen, foods or chemicals. Or they could have a Candida sensitivity or nutritional deficiency that wears their immune system down making them even more susceptible to new triggers. And the triggers are all different for each person.

As you can read in Philpot's **Victory Over Diabetes**, the causes of diabetes are just as individually varied. But once you have them all nailed down, you have a person who is healthier, off drugs, and in total control of his health.

So you might ask what my motivation is in preparing this unique manual. Could it be notoriety? I hardly think so. I'm not the first person to write about environmental illness and I won't be the last. Could it be money? Obviously not, since the audience to whom this is directed is most likely too select. Could it be fame? I certainly doubt this since I can't conceive of anyone wanting to admit they've slept rolled in aluminum foil and have pistachios for breakfast, avocados for lunch and oysters for dinner. Certainly, it is leaving myself vulnerable to ridicule by the myopic members of the medical community to admit these facts.

No, the purpose is actually to save lives. It may sound a bit dramatic, but indeed there are those already whose lives have been saved with the very principles that will be outline in this manual.

Medicine fails to recognize that as well as looking different, we all are immunologically and biochemically very different. Medicine prefers the cookbook or simplistic method: treat everyone with anti-inflammatory drugs for an inflamed ankle. It does not want to look further at the causes. Instead, it is much easier to prescribe an aerosol inhaler for everyone with asthma rather than to try to find the individual cause for each person's wheezing.

Most people for whom this has been written have been everywhere, have had every test and still either have no diagnosis or have a diagnosis which is a dead-end diagnosis. They have been told they have to learn to live with it. They have been to a host of physicians, all of whom had one thing in common. In the differential diagnosis in their computer minds, environmental illness was not one of the possibilities. They were unaware of it, and therefore, no matter how much you complained of various symptoms or even if you suggested that your problem might be due to chemicals or foods, he most likely discounted your information because it was not one of the diagnostic possibilities in his programing.

Fortunately, there are very few physicians who have come out of medical school without having annihilated that mystical part of the brain which questions and has curiosity. Somehow, along the road in our course of medical education, our teachers made sure that we were highly programed. This ensures uniformity, predictability, and control. Then they destroy a certain part that must have been innate in all of us to make us want to go into medicine in the first place. A part that is left in scientists but is taken out of medical doctors. A part that makes people want to question and find out why, rather than just apply cookbook techniques to the practice of medicine. Fortunately, there are many physicians in the world who escaped the dogma and they have been instrumental in expanding our knowledge in clinical ecology or environmental medicine.

The Changing Tide in Medical Knowledge

Very few people realize how ill a person with environmental illness can be. And, indeed, it can be fatal as you will learn. You are now, by the very fact that you are reading this book, part of a revolution in medicine. A revolution that is bigger than Semmelweiss or Pasteur ever imagined. When Semmelweiss suggested hand washing after autopsies before delivering babies, women would endure anything to be sure they would be delivered on the days he practiced, because they saw his mortality rate was vastly lower than the other doctors! Being a greedy, jealous lot, they, rather than investigate or adopt his techniques, got rid of their competition by kicking him out of the medical society! That'll teach you, Semmelweiss! He died ostracized of suicide. And, as usual, the patient suffered.

Pasteur suffered equal grief as doctors derided the idea of vaccination being able to confer immunity.

One of Semmelweiss' and Pasteur's problems was that doctors couldn't expand their imaginations well. This is understandable, because we're mostly machines with a great memory but little creativity. So they said it seemed preposterous that unseen germs were causing the diseases they treat. And even if they were, how could one ever come up with a different antibiotic or a different immunization for them all? Well, a hundred years later we have, and we take it for granted as part of everyday life.

Now, we have evidence that many chronic diseases are caused by idiosyncratic reactions to foods, hormones, chemicals, inhaled dust, molds and pollens.

Again, doctors are at first loathe to believe it and react by showing their economic jealousy. The American Academy of Allergy and Immunology is currently trying to have all food testing labeled as experimental so that insurance companies will not cover it. If they succeed, people will not be able to afford to have it done, and so it will die. And those who enjoyed its benefits will suffer.

Those who are a little more receptive say, "Even if you're right and chemicals can cause disease, how can we possibly get away from them all?" As you will read further, many people have solved that problem long ago—out of the sheer necessity to stay alive.

You can be instrumental in the revolution and in improving the quality of your own health care by giving a copy of this manual to your doctor to read. Start his wheels going and cross your fingers that he is one of the few who

66

is genuinely interested enough in your welfare to open his mind and evaluate the evidence. Remember, it's very easy to coast along on old knowledge and not change your practice around. So be patient with him; for it may take a while, and he'll need to prove much of it to his own satisfaction. If he is not open, pass him up, for you'll eventually find those who are.

How do you choose a specialist in environmental medicine? You need to check out how he approaches a patient, how much he wants to know about you, how much of a well-verse staff does he have, and if he has phenol-free extracts. Most of all, he will encourage you to read and educate yourself.

How I Approach a New Patient

Here's a logical approach to patients with 20th century disease. First and foremost, is the story they come with. My first encounter tells me many things. It tells me if they are intelligent, motivated, and organized enough to work hard in getting clear. If they skimp on filling out the questionnaire, I suspect they'll be lazy in doing environmental controls and reading. This tells me they won't do very well and will always be grumbling because they are not better. They'll always have an excuse why they haven't done environmental controls. The amount I can do for a patient is directly proportional to the amount they are willing to do for themselves in return. I have little patience with the person who wants to "buy" health with a "Take me, I'm yours" attitude. They erroneously think all they have to do is show up for injections and they'll be better. Fortunately, there are a number of people with that attitude who are correct. But people with chemical and food sensitivity never fall into that category. They have to sink or swim in terms of educating themselves.

Fortunately for them, I was full of denial for several

years, but because my husband and Bill Rea had tireless patience, I got over that hump. But it does point up the fact that without a good support system, it makes it extremely difficult for anyone to succeed and improve.

So having assessed the intelligence, motivation, and support system I now hone in on the medical history, per se. This is where I decide whether it's merely a seasonal pollen and mold problem, or more complicated. With many patients it's a matter of whittling away at the total load until they are finally better. As careful as we try to be, there are always tons of surprises. No one ever knows how multiply sensitive a person will turn out to be. On three occasions I even saw people get their immune systems turned on more potently after chemical or mold testing; they were suddenly more sensitive. Why should this happen when the doses we test are nothing compared with daily home-office-traffic exposures? This is a complication all should be aware of in deciding whether to have any testing. It is extremely rare and just points to the need to do environmental controls meticulously. No one knows why it happens, except that it was probably the final straw after a lifetime of exposures that left them progressively more compromised.

So in general, we first assess whether we should use phenolated or non-phenolated extracts. Then we begin to attack the first part of the total load by testing and giving inhalants. If environmental controls are done during the first month of injections, the majority of the symptoms that are due to inhalants dramatically simmer down. So the fourth step is to do the diet and see what other symptoms simmer down. These are presumed due to the foods; and you prove it by adding them back, one new food every day or two and see if you can reproduce the symptoms you just got rid of. If you find you have far too many food allergies and only feel best fasting, then we can test you to foods and have you give yourself injections to foods to increase your tolerance.

Fifth, chemicals can be tested because people often need evidence before they are motivated enough to do the tough environmental controls necessary for the chemically sensitive.

At this point before steps four or five, sometimes people are so highly inhalant sensitive we need to test them to the individual molds, trees and grasses that are in the mixes. A simple treatment dose to a mix is not enough to hold them symptom-free. They need a dose to every individual component of the mix. Fortunately, these people are rare.

So after the six stages are covered, if a person still has symptoms, what can we do? We can look for a Candida sensitivity by doing the diet, taking Nystatin, or optionally, Nizoral as a trial. We can test for hormone or mediator sensitivity, or we can look for a hidden heavy metal toxicity or pesticide level stored in the body.

Last, but not least, if all your machinery isn't in good working order, you'll never heal your immune system. So we need to assess whether there is a vitamin, mineral, essential fatty acid, amino acid, hormone, or enzyme deficiency. And we need to reduce the amount of stress.

So this is a stepwise approach that could be used in an office work-up. Just watch out for the physician who is stuck at one stage. You know, the fellow who thinks every patient has Candida or every patient needs $500 worth of amino acids. It's very easy to get hung up on one stage just because you've had a few miraculous successes with it. These people have lost sight of the tremendous individual variability among people. They can't see the forest for the trees.

For the very worst patients, the stepwise whittling away won't work. They need to lower their total load fast. The easiest way is to go to the unit. But many have been highly successful in following our advice. They merely go home and create a mini-unit there, for a lot less money.

69

The serious ecologist will also have a local support group, H.E.A.L. These are invaluable for a multitude of reasons. An example is the person who arrives at the office with one year of intolerable headaches, nausea, dizziness, muscle aches, depression and brain fog. He has been to many specialists and doesn't even have a diagnosis. He comes to our office not even knowing what we are all about and just thinks it will be more wasted money, but he's desperate. We tell him what he has, we prove it to him, and then he is absolutely stunned. He can't believe it. He worked all his life to get a new home, new carpeting, new furniture. His dream finally materialized; a year later he is a sick as a dog, and now we tell him that these are the causes. He doesn't know whether to rejoice that the cause has been found or to kill himself; what's he supposed to do? Does he sell the house? Where does he go? How does he make his current home a healing home? Will his friends now be thoroughly convinced that he's nuttier than a fruitcake?

This poor guy needs to be invited to the home of H.E.A.L. members and see how they live, symptom-free. How they, too, were in the same boat and recovered. He needs to see that people do manage to re-prioritize their lives in order to heal their immune systems.

You'll notice the victims of E.I. need to shift gears. They have spent years trying to ignore or tune out symptoms. Now they need to listen to their bodies and become aware of what exposures are inducing symptoms.

SECTION I
INHALANTS
THE ALLERGY PLAN

You know you have hayfever if you emerge from a field with red, swollen, draining eyes, snorting, sniffling, coughing and wheezing; you know you're allergic to strawberries if every time you eat strawberries you break out in hives. No one has to tell you that you have an allergy.

But did you know that chronic hidden allergies could cause headache, migraine, dizziness, burning eyes, constant colds, sore throats, sinusitis, itching, depression, pain, exhaustion, arthritis, asthma, bronchitis, colitis, phlebitis, spastic colon, eczema, cystic acne, schizophrenia, cystitis, premenstrual syndrome, severe muscle weakness, Tourette's syndrome, learning disability, extreme lethargy and tiredness for seemingly no reason, backache, hyperactivity and much more?

Since allergies can masquerade as just about any symptom it's very difficult to prepare one manual for everyone. That's why this one has been partitioned into categories that most commonly affect people, and in the order in which most people develop their sensitivities.

Because many allergic people have had exhaustive medical exams and tests and sometimes surgeries only to be told that there's no known cause or they will have to learn to live with their symptoms, this manual has been prepared to help you learn as much as possible about allergies. With a solid understanding of allergies you will have the tools that will enable you to control your health.

Regardless of whether you think you just have pollen allergies or food allergies or chemical allergies, the fact is that when a person's immune system starts breaking down and producing allergic symptoms, it rapidly undergoes the spreading phenomenon. In other words, the impaired or allergic immune system rarely directs itself toward one substance or antigen. Instead it goes wild and develops abnormal reactivity to a number of unrelated substances or antigens.

Because dust and mold allergies are universally common to nearly all allergic people, we must first test you to this and cover this aspect of your total load first. For without doing so, there is slim hope of ever getting all the other allergies controlled. And frequently we find that in testing the dust and molds we have already reduced the initial symptoms significantly. You see we have no way of knowing what part of your total load it contributes to until we have treated it.

At your first consultation with the doctor, a general plan will be mapped out to begin to uncover the most likely environmental causes for your symptoms. Since dust and mold sensitivities are almost universally present, we begin with those. Fortunately, environmental controls on your part (there is an audio tape on this plus the manual covers it) and injections from your doctor or the office usually controls this part.

You'll be given some mold plates or petri dishes to see how heavy the mold actually is in your environment and whether any unusual types are present. Since food sensitivity is often a source of hidden, unsuspected allergy, we'll ask you to give yourself a two week trial of the rare food diagnostic diet (also on cassette and in this manual). Basically, you'll be eating foods you rarely eat to see if any symptoms lessen. If they do, you have a hidden food allergy. For some, adding the food back will uncover the culprit, and then mere avoidance of it for a few months may restore tolerance for it. In others, like myself, the diet only brings partial improvement, and we need to give ourselves injections to the foods and rotate our diets to get total relief. For many, they may need to rule out hidden Candida sensitivities, chemical problems or nutritional deficiencies. As soon as you get your inhalants (dust and molds) tested, have the nurse order them to be prepared and sent to your family doctor. Start them twice a week. A month or two later you will have scheduled a consultation (termed a "history" by the staff) with the doctor. Don't forget a spouse, or tape recorder if you like, and a pad and pencil for sure. At this time we will sit down and determine what else may be needed.

Basically, we will see what symptoms are improving and what the most likely cause of their improvement is. Then we will see what, if any, symptoms remain and determine what the most likely cause would be and map out an appropriate plan of attack. In other words, for most people we go in stages to whittle away at the most likely causes and the more easily treated causes first. In this way many people are clear and do not need to look for more elusive and difficult to treat causes. The universal reactors, like myself, however, need everything and may as well jump in and start.

How to Start

Summary of Unloading Steps:

1. Assess vitamin/mineral levels by blood and urine tests.
   Schedule to go over the results and get your nutrient prescription in 6 weeks.

2. Schedule pollen/dust/mold testing.

3. Culture bedroom, etc, for mold overgrowth.

4. Read this manual and do environmental controls.

5. Start Vital dophilus, Vital Plex, or ProBionate-C, do rare-food, diagnostic diet for one to three weeks,

then add back foods to find culprits.

6.   Stay sugar-free, yeast-free if starting yeast program. Read Candida section for all directions.

7.   Test pollens/dust/molds, start injections twice weekly until symptoms are clear and medicines are no longer needed, then go weekly.

8.   See doctor to assess what may be needed further (foods, chemicals, xenobiotics, hormones, nutrients, etc.) A lengthy appointment called "A History" is scheduled in 3 months to see what has improved and what has not, so a plan of attack can be mapped out. Everyone is different. For example, hayfever patients only need steps 2, 3, 4, 7, and 8.

CRITERIA FOR ADMISSION TO THE OFFICE

In order to be admitted to the office, patients first have to be checked by one of the nurses to be sure they are hypoallergenic; that is, they are not wearing or carrying something that might cause others to have allergic reactions. If they do not pass, they cannot be allowed to enter this area regardless of how urgent their sensitivities are, how far they have traveled, or regardless of the fact that they were scheduled for that day.

The reason is that the more chemically sensitive a person is, the more acute is his sense of smell and the more rapid is his reaction. If someone is in the test room with aftershave, scented makeup or cigarette smoke on his jacket, others will be affected in various ways. Some will have symptoms and erroneously attribute them to what they're being tested to. Some testers will have severe headaches and an inability to concentrate. Other patients may have a fulminating asthma attack; others may become comatose within half an hour. It is unfair to allow someone with chemical odors into the testing room when other patients have traveled thousands of miles to be tested and have scrupulously followed the admission criteria.

Therefore, the following guidelines must be followed for admission:

Shower: Use Ivory soap, oilatum, or Nivea Basis soap.

Hair shampoo: Use Henna Care, Jhirmack, Gelave, Suave, or Johnson's Baby Shampoo, Almay or Ar-ex.

Conditioner: Use Rainsilk (Shaklee), Unicure (Fay's), Johnson's baby, lemon, or none.

Hair spray, setting gel or mousse: Use sugar and water, or none.

Toothpaste: Use Arm & Hammer baking soda. Do not use mouth fresheners, gum, lozenges or life savers while in the office.

Deodorant: You can splash baking soda in the axilla (under arms area).

Preshave: Use ice cubes

Cosmetics: Use Almay, Ar-ex, Marcelle, or Indian Earth. Under no circumstances will perfume, cologne, or aftershave be allowed on the person or as a residual odor left on clothes previously worn. Do not bring a purse that has had perfumes or fragrant cosmetics in it into the office. There are lockers for these. It is easier to just forego the makeup.

Clothes: Cotton is preferable. The testing shirt must easily expose the top of the shoulder. An oversized cotton T-shirt is fine. Clothes should be washed in Borax and/or baking soda, and a vinegar rinse may be used for static. Arm & Hammer liquid detergent is acceptable and also Yes and Neolife. No fabric softeners, no anti-cling dryer sheets, no dry cleaned clothes, and no fresh shoe polish should be used.

Smoking: Smoking must be stopped 12 hours prior to entering the office and testing area and the mouth should be brushed with baking soda. You must wash hair after the last cigarette. Do not wear clothes that have been in a car or office with other smokers present. If you must travel in a car with a smoker to come to the office, or if you must stop at your office or a restaurant where there are smokers, cover your head and wear an outer coat; outer garments can be left in the mud room of the office. Hair and fibers are porous, and they hold odors for hours. You won't notice them, but we will.

No patients under 18 will be tested without an adult present. All of the above criteria apply to anyone entering the area, whether he is being tested or not. For appointments with the doctor you are invited to bring your spouse or a tape recorder. However, the spouse must follow the hypo-allergenic guidelines if he wants to accompany you to testing. Also, always bring a pad and pencil so you can take notes. You are going to learn a great deal and cannot possibly remember all that is recommended.

In summary, a pair of cotton jeans, a T-shirt and a flannel shirt for warmth washed in baking soda and/or borax would be fine. Bathe in Ivory soap or Nivea Basis, and you're all set.

No food is allowed in the test area. Glass bottled water is allowed. Try to avoid loud talking and do not distract others who are concentrating on recording their symptoms on the testing sheet. Try to remain in the testing area throughout the testing period; use the bathroom before.

coming into the testing area.

Coats and other articles should be left downstairs. We have lockers available so that nothing will be brought into the test area.

If you want a permanent record of your results, be sure that your testing results are recorded in your work-book at the end of each session. This is your responsbility, not the nurse's, and it will not be done at other times if you forget.

Also, for any copies of laboratory results that you want, they will not be honored without a written request specifying which labs (by name or date of test) and the inclusion of a self-addressed, stamped envelope. That goes for any prescription and other items you want mailed to you. We are busy trying to meet the needs of some of the most highly sensitive people in the world, so we expect your cooperation in the "pitsy" stuff. Also, be aware that mail takes about 2 weeks to reach my desk (orders are taken out, etc), and I detest FAX paper. So learn to plan ahead.

Also if there is anything in the testing room that bothers you, it is up to you to tell the nurse. If someone got through with smoke odor, for example, and it interferes with your testing, we are not embarrassed to ask them to leave. We know you are not trying to be difficult.

By creating as clean an environment for you as possible, we hope to obtain the most reliable results for both you and others who are being tested. Than is our goal.

ALLERGY INJECTION INFORMATION

The allergy injections advised for you are the only specific means of trying to control your condition. Pills, sprays, filters only treat your symptoms, not the cause of them. Another reason for advising such a long and in-volved treatment is that this is the only means of attempting to prevent further severe complications. Medicines do not prevent the progression of the disease nor the chronic accompanying tiredness. Only by training your body to make IgG blocking antibodies to fight off your IgE allergic ones can you simmer down your symptoms. You've already prevented yourself from getting lockjaw by getting tetanus shots. These shots trained your body to make the antibody against Clostridia tetani, the causative agent.

This specific treatment involves **twice-weekly injections** for approximately three to six weeks, or **until your symptoms and medicines are none**. Then your treatments are reduced. If you are worse, go back to twice weekly as long as needed: whether on once or twice weekly continue without interruption until your first clear season. When you have obtained a good degree of benefit at that time and require no medication, the treatments are then reduced to every 10 days, then every two weeks, then every three weeks. All of this depends on the control of your symptoms.

At no time should you be on an injection less than once or twice a week if you still require daily medication. Depending on the person, many can go off injections after four to ten years and remain clear. For others, with more severe allergies, the injections seem to help only as long as they are taken. You should not interrupt the injections. If three months of injections are missed, it is usually necessary to test again because your dose changes with environmental overload. Never go beyond a weekly interval until you are totally off medication. As long as you require medication, you need weekly or twice a week injections.

These treatments may produce reactions, especially when you have become overloaded by your environment; sneezing, runny nose, tickling of the throat, asthma, or hives. These reactions usually occur within twenty minutes after your injection. They are relieved by the administration of adrenalin and occasionally other medications. For this reason, it is very important for you to remain in the doctor's office twenty minutes after every treatment. If you do have a reaction, I am available to guide your doctor in determining what to do with the next injection. Having a reaction is not a reason for stopping treatment, but you should notify us so that we can evaluate your next injection. We must emphasize again that you must remain in the doctor's office for twenty minutes after each injection.

You will be billed from the clinic for the extracts. We have to insist upon receiving payments for the extracts before we mail them out. The extracts will be mailed to you directly.

When you have had your fifth injection, make sure you send your order blank to us for refills so that we have time (3 weeks) to make them; indicate how many more injections you wish. (Made in multiples of 10 doses)

Also, equally important, let us know what your symptoms and reactions are from the injections. We need all the questions answered on the extract order sheet. It is permissible to take, under your doctor's supervision, antihistamines, inhalers, and other allergic medication. It is better, however, on the date of your injection not to take any antihistamines until after you have received your injection. The reason is that the antihistamines may mask a reaction that might prove larger later on.

Many people experience striking and early improvements in their symptoms. But it might take as long as six to nine months before you see any change. There are many individual factors that bear on this, most important of which is how fast you do your environmental controls. By no means should you stop treatments during the first year because you feel it has been ineffective. Give yourself at least one year of continuous treatment before making any decision to stop, and then only after going over your particular situation with the doctor.

When you require absolutely no medications, you may extend your interval between injections to 7 days.

After a symptom-free and medication-free year, you may extend your injections to two weeks. After another year of no symptoms and no medications you can extend them to three weeks, etc. Only change the intervals during the winter when the environment is more stable and after you have had your evaluation with the clinic. Remember that spring and fall are double-headers. Not only are they the peak pollen seasons, but also the peak mold seasons. Many people need to return to twice a week during a bad season. Remind your doctor the dose is never altered when you go back to twice a week for a heavy season.

Many people don't get a return of their initial symptoms as the clue that they need to shorten their interval between injections. They just feel exhausted or begin to encounter recurrent sickness or infections. Any time the total load or life stress increases, do not hesitate to put injections back on twice a week to help the body cope. There is no dose change, and you can resume your prior interval whenever the stress is over.

You were given a copy of the order sheet or plan for your workup. It is up to you to be sure all the items are done and checked off. For example, the environmental controls can be reviewed by VTR, audio cassette, or read in this manual before an overall history/evaluation is done. And if the history/evaluation is not done within three months of initiation of injections, the injections will be automatically discontinued. This is one of the measures we need to assure quality control.

The overall history/evaluation is a time for you and the doctor to go over all the questions you have written down , to review all your test reactions and to decide if further tests are needed, and plan for your treatment. Most people at that time rate themselves as 50-100% better.

The field is changing so rapidly that there are new developments every 3-4 months, many of which may be pertinent to your allergies. For this reason, you are reminded to make an appointment after three to six months of injections in order to check your individual program and make sure all allergens have been added and environmental controls have been taken care of. Many patients do feel better after a short time and they choose not to see the doctor. It should be pointed out that you may be "out of season" or that you are having good results earlier than norman. However, if allergens are left out of your program, you will not achieve the best control. New antigens become available, allowing control of a problem that possibly a year earlier had no treatment.

If at any time you do have any questions reqarding your treatment or anything you have read about, write them down and feel free to drop us a line (written double-spaced, easily legible with a space following each question in which an answer can be written. Make the questions "yes" "no" types. Anything requiring a lengthy expanation requires seeing the doctor. Also enclose a self-addressed stamped enveloped; or if you are coming into the office make sure to bring them to the attention of the staff. The most efficacious treatment of allergic disease is through a comprehensive knowledge of allergy, good observation of the patient's symptoms, and meticulous control of the patient's environment.

EXAMPLES OF
SYMPTOMATIC MEDICATIONS

Medications are for symptomatic relief to tide you over while you are getting all of your environmental causes figured out. As you uncover many of your triggers and learn how to control them, you should require progressively fewer medications until you are entirely off. (The letter "q" stands for every; "h" is hours; "sig" means directions for taking; "gtts" is drops; "b.i.d." is twice a day;

81

"t.i.d. is 3 times a day; and "q.i.d. is 4 times a day.)

Eye problems:

Naphcon-A, 10cc, sig 2-3 gtts in each eye q4-6h.
This is for burning, swollen eyes.

Opticrom 4% solution, 10ml, sig 2-4 gtts q4-6h in each eye as an allergy prophylaxis. It needs to be taken regularly to be effective, but is exceedingly safe.

General antihistamine-decongestant combinations: Trinalin, Tavist D, Seldane D, Drixoral, Naldecon; sig 1/2-1 q12h Caution: can cause urinary retention, cardiac arrhythmia, drowsiness and other side effects.

Antihistamines without decongestants;
For those who get too dry.
Optimine, 100, sig 1/2-1-2 tabs q12h
PBZ 25mg, 1-3 q6h
Seldane 60mg 1 q12h (produces less sleepiness than others)

All of these 4 antihistamines are unrelated to the Actifed, Dimetapp, Ornade group of antihistamines, so that if those are known to cause sleepiness, perhaps these may not, since they are in different pharmacologic classes.

Remember to use an antihistamine or an antihistamine-decongestant whenever you need ophthalmic or nasal medication since you usually need coverage systemically.

Decongestants alone:
Sudafed, phenylephrine, Entex

Nasal medications:
Afrin nasal spray and Neosynefrin are obtainable over the

counter, however, they can be addicting and you'll develop rebound phenomenon, as well as tachyphylaxis (this is where more and more is required because it does less and less).

Prophylactic medications are better; for instance, the prophylactic nasal medication of Nasalcrom. (The prophylactic ophthalmic analogue is Opticrom, or the prophylactic inhaled analogue in the lung is Intal.) They take at least a week or two to build an effective level.

Nasalcrom, 1 inhaler, sig 2 puffs each nostril q4-6h

The beauty of Nasalcrom, Intal, and Opticrom is that they are not systemically absorbed and rarely have side effects. They are probably the safest medications ever made since they just inhibit the allergic cells in the nose, lungs, and the eyes from releasing as much histamine as they normally would when the patient contacts an allergen.

Beconase or Vancenase (Beclomethasone)
Use 2 puffs each nostril 3 times a day. Try to aim down the middle of canal or toward sides, not toward middle septum. These are nasal steroids and are far safer than oral steroids.

Note: These are prophylactic medications. This means to become effective they require regular daily doses. They take at least 3-10 days to become effective, so don't pitch them because they don't work right away.

Nasal saline lavage for painful sinuses and to avoid antibotics:
Nasal saline lavage to remove infected material from plugged sinuses. Put 1/2 tsp salt in 1 cup of warm water. Fill nose with this by either of 2 methods:
a) Lie with head hanging upside down over edge of bed and use dropper to fill nasal canal. Stay in that position 2-

4 minutes, or

b) Standing, put nose in cup and sniff water until it drips down throat and nose is full. Spit out the salt water, do not swallow it. Or for best results, cover the nostril on the good side and snort water into the open one 3-4 times. Then alternate. Once the nose is filled with the salt solution, quickly hold your nose so water doesn't run out the front; Standing, keep your knees straight and bend down so the top of your head is pointing down at the level of your knees and your nostrils are pointing up. Stay there 2-4 minutes.

After a or b is done for 2-4 minutes, stand and gently blow. Thick and sometimes bloody and infected mucus is pulled from the sinus that cannot be removed by normal blowing. This is because the salt solution first pulls moisture out of the swollen sinus canals so they are now open and able to drain. This is much like the wrinkled finger tips you get when swimming in the ocean. Excess moisture has been pulled out. Next the salt creates an osmotic pressure, as swimming in ocean water does, and pulls the trapped mucus out. This helps to relieve the pain and also make the sinusitis heal faster. Getting the infected trapped mucus out promotes healing just as draining an abscess does. Check the color of mucus, because if it is green or yellow or foul smelling, antibiotics will be needed if the condition persists. See your family doctor for all antibiotics.

Note: At all times a PDR (Physicians Desk Reference) is available to be read in the office. Page copies can be made $1.00/page, not chargeable). This book has the side effects of all prescribed medications.

Management of Asthma Medications:
Theophylline, Theodur, or Somophyllin CRT, 100 mg, sig 1-6q8-12h. Build the dose slowly, adding one more capsule each time to find your top tolerated dose. Stop and back off

by one when you get nausea, palpitations or shakiness. Some people are fast drug metabolizers and need their 12-hour theophyllines really every 8 hours. If you feel it wears off in 8 hours, take it every 8 instead of every 12 hours.

Inhaled bronchodilators:
Albuterol, Proventil Ventolin, Tornalate, or Alupent inhalers: 2 puffs q4h; but q6-8h for Tornalate.

Inhaler use: Tip head back in a sword-swallower position. Hold inhaler 2 inches from lips. As you squirt, take a long, slow, deep inhalation and hold it as long as you can. Wait 5 minutes, then take the second inhalation. In essence, you let the first puff open you up and make way for the second puff to get deeper. If inhalers bother you, try squirting it down a rolled up piece of tablet paper placed between inhaler and your mouth. It slows the force and velocity of the medicine. The staff can explain this technique of using a spacer.

Beclovent Inhaler, Vanceril, or Azmacort: 4 puffs after inhaled bronchodilator inhalation. Inhaled steroids are used 2-4 puffs twice a day for severe asthmatics.

Intal: Inhale 2 puffs q.i.d. (Nurse can give instructions if you prefer to use the spinhaler).

Prednisone is a last resort, and it is always temporary; use as few as needed and as short a course as possible. If worse comes to worse a temporary trial of oral steroids can be given: Prednisone 5mg. You may start with up to 40-60mg (8- 12 tablets all at once first thing in the morning) a day depending upon the severity. Usually that dose is held for three days. Then wean down by 10mg every other day. Remember, steriods have many dangerous side effects if used for months on end, so we always save them for

85

emergencies and then get off as quickly as possible. They can cause glaucoma, cataracts, ulcers, diabetes, aseptic necrosis of the femoral artery (so it dies and a total artificial cap and ball hip joint is required), weight gain, permanent stretch marks, decrease your body's resistance to infection, and deplete many vitamins and mineral like B6 and magnesium. Fortunately, these side effects usually take years of high doses to appear and even then you may still escape problems. However, there are on record people, for example, who developed aseptic necrosis of the femoral artery after only a month of steroids. (Although not technically correct, most of the time the words "prednisone", "cortisone", "medrol", and "steroids" are synonymous).

All medications have side effects. Somewhere there is someone who will have a symptom from a medicine that no one ever thought possible. The commonest symptoms from antihistamine-decongestants are drowsiness and dryness. More dangerous symptoms are inability to empty a full bladder (called urinary retention), worsening of problems with blood pressure, prostate, thyroid, cataracts, etc. If in doubt about a medication, stop it and see if the symptom goes away. Remember, all medication is just a temporary crutch. Our goal is to teach you enough environmental controls so that combined with your injections you will be medication- free and symptom-free.

There is always a copy or two of the PDR in the waiting room. If you need one and can't locate one, ask an allergy nurse. In it you can look up any prescription drug and read all the side effects. If you take any medication, part of your responsibility is to be aware of the adverse effects it could have on your body. Also, all drugs constitute another aspect of chemical overload. However, they are indeed necessary at various stages before total wellness is achieved.

You may think we're pretty dogmatic with all these rules, but remember: you are learning how to take respon-

86

sibility for your body so you can get well. Medicine made an error when it intimated you could eat, drink, smoke, and breathe anything you want because we had a magic pill for everything. That's not the way to wellness. **A headache is not a sign of Darvon deficiency**. In general we've seen from past experience, the smarter you are, the faster you get well. So **we're here to educate, not medicate**. We don't have all the answers, but we can show you how a lot of us got better.

GENERAL ALLERGY INSTRUCTIONS

Proper use of medications for asthmatic:

1. Start appropriate medications at the first sign of even mild symptoms. Do not wait until symptoms are so severe that even good medications become less effective.

2. Do not skip any doses. Do not stop taking your medications when you get a little better. Be totally clear for 3 days

3. If any medication is affecting you badly in any way, or if you cannot afford the medications prescribed, please let us know.

4. For wheezing, coughing, or chest congestion; take EVERY dose as directed on EVERY day that you have any of these symptoms. Continue the medications for three additional days after the symptoms are gone. In other words, you may stop your wheezing or asthma medication, but only after you have been completely clear of wheezing, coughing or chest congestion for 3 days. These medicines should be started immediately at the first sign of chest congestion, wheezing or coughing. Do not wait a day! It is

much easier to stop an attack early; it is much more difficult to stop wheezing after it has been present for some time. One bad exposure can produce enough reaction in the lung to keep you wheezing for weeks. Several missed doses can produce enough chest phlegm that you need hospitalization.

5. For nasal congestion, sinus symptoms, posterior nasal discharge, nose running, eyes running, itching and burning, the feeling of congestion in your ears or mucus in the back of your throat, take your antihistamines—every dose as directed. Don't skip doses and don't stop your medicine until symptoms are gone for a least 24 hours.

Hydration:

1. Drink 8 glasses of extra water a day to keep chest secretions liquid and from becoming sticky.

2. You may count fresh-squeezed juices, herb teas, and other mildly flavored water as water.

3. Milk, sodas, canned and prepared juices, and alcohols, especially beer, commonly cause more congestion and allergy in many people.

4. Increasing your fluid intake is particularly important when you are wheezing, or have nasal congestion or related symptoms.

5. If your fluid intake is adequate, your urine should be clear and not color the toilet bowl water yellow (but vitamins can color it yellow, so see what color it is while off vitamins a few days.) If your urine is naturally yellow, you need to drink more water.

6. The purpose of hydration is to keep your nasal mucus

and/or your bronchial secretions thin and loose. If you drink enough liquids, it will be easier to get relief by coughing up the mucus and/or clearing your nose by blowing it. If you don't drink enough fluids your secretions will get thick and sticky, and they tend to stay in your nose, throat, sinuses or bronchial tubes. If you have difficulty clearing the secretions by coughing or nose blowing, then your congestion tends to remain longer; germs are more likely to grow in the stagnant mucus and this may result in infection—colds, sinusitis, bronchitis, and pneumonia.

Environmental Controls:

1. Avoid or dispose of the things that cause or aggravate your symptoms. If complete avoidance is not possible, then reduce exposure to them as much as possible. Definitely do not have them in your bedroom.

2. Please read and follow the instructions concerning the environmental controls.

3. Now that you have been told some of the allergens that are likely to be contributing to your symptoms, taking appropriate measures immediately may help reduce your symptoms considerably.

Additional Suggestions:

1. If you are wheezing, coughing or have chest congestion, remember that any hand spray inhaler (mouth inhaler) that you have may give immediate relief; but, if taken too frequently, it may indeed make the symptoms worse after initial improvement. If needed more than every 4 hours, see the doctor immediately to avoid hospitalization.

2. Over the counter nose drops or nose sprays should be avoided if possible (except prescribed Intal, Nasalcrom, Beconase or Vancenase). All that they give is immediate relief. After continued use, they may irritate and cause swelling of the nasal membrane resulting in worse nasal blockage. Using sprays on alternate days may help this situation.

3. **STOP SMOKING**. Smoking is an irritant. It causes inflammation and swelling of the mucous lining of your nose and bronchial tubes. The swelling causes increased blockage of the airways.

4. Remove from your house, if sensitive, any furry or feathered pets. Definitely do not bring them into your bedroom. If there is a strong emotional need, we can hyposensitize you to them if it's absolutely needed.

5. Vaporizers and humidifiers should be washed out thoroughly once a week. If not, they can accumulate mold which is often dispersed into the air. Zephiran, vinegar or baking soda and borax will generally clean them.

6. If you have a hot air heating system, change the filter on your furnace at least once a month. If necessary, change it even more frequently. Space-Guard is a good one.

Note: Pets are often like a member of the family and we realize that special concessions may need to be made. If you do not intend to keep all animals from the house, be sure to discuss this with the doctor so the best alternatives can be found to keep your symptoms to a minimum.

In essence, as you clean up your environment and reduce the overload of dust, molds, and animal danders that you are exposed to, you'll be able to wean further down the scale from your medications. But asthmatics must do this cautiously. When in doubt, see the doctor.

Inhalant Allergies

In subsequent chapters, you will learn of allergies that cause disease that defy the current conventional medical diagnostic armamentarium. In order that you will be able to more fully comprehend these allergies, it would be best if you first learned about inhalant allergies, even if you don't think you have any.

Anyone can diagnose hay fever. We've all seen the typically swollen, teary eyes, and congested, drippy nose of the mouth breather.

Anyone can diagnose the person with obvious cat sensitivity. His eyes swell and itch and he wheezes. Anyone can recognize hives from ingesting strawberries or shellfish. Many physicians tell people, "Don't worry about your hayfever symptoms. Just take antihistamines." Some lax physicians even prescribe steroids throughout the season of pollination. But steroids impair your body's ability to fight off infection, leaving you vulnerable to any infection that comes along.

What they fail to realize is that by masking the symptoms, they don't stop the progression of the disease. If not treated with the proper injections, one out of three people with hay fever will progress on to get asthma. Also, antihistamines have a side effect of making people sleepy, and the allergy itself causes such tremendous tiredness in most people, that they do not need their symptoms compounded. Only injections will impede the progression of the disease as well as turn off the tiredness.

Many people are not aware of the symptoms of inhalant allergies. Many people with chronic sinus problems go year in and year out to ENT specialists and are subjected to surgeries, only to finally show up in our offices saying that these operations never helped. Some have a history of having recurrent surgeries for nasal polyps, but they were not told that if allergic causes are taken care of , they rarely re-grow.

Many people are puzzled when within weeks or months of injections, their symptoms are markedly improved and they realize that they could have done this years earlier, if only it was recommended. They ask over and over again, "Why doesn't he know about allergies?" Finally, today our 20th century immunology is catching up and revealing the mysteries of the body chemistry to us. Now we are beginning to understand. There is often a 20-50 year lag between science and the changing of the medical school curriculum, rewriting textbooks and educating a new generation of physicians. For those of us who are afflicted now, we can't wait 20-50 years.

Headache is a common symptom of allergy. I, for one, had such severe headaches that I thought I had a brain tumor and didn't dare tell my husband for many months. I remember sitting in a car and suddenly having the feeling as though someone had driven a knife through the right posterior section of my skull and then encircled the head with a tight metal band.

Some people with inhalant allergies only have tiredness as their chief complaint. Other people have recurrent earaches, sore throats, colds and infections.

In the twenty four years that I've been practicing medicine, I have seen so many mothers who have said that they knew there was something wrong with their children, that it wasn't right that they got so many infections. And yet when they would plead with the pediatrician to even consider the possibility of an allergy, they were intimidated and made to feel as though they were overly worried and undereducated.

Likewise, many children have recurrent otitis, or infection of the ears, and secretory otitis, or fluid buildup behind the tympanic membrane with resultant decrease in hearing. It causes permanent deafness if not treated in time. The pediatrician sends them to the ear, nose and throat specialist who recommends insertion of little plastic tubes to put a hole in the membrane so that it can now drain out. Often, the pediatrician neglects to send them to an allergist to try to find the real cause of the extra secretion of fluid. As a result, the child has to undergo unnecessary anesthesia and the risk of infection that could spread into the mastoids and even into the brain itself. Again, this mechanical treatment does nothing to prevent progression. Nor does it help correct the chronic tiredness and resultant poor learning which follows the child through life, if the cause is allergy.

Another disease which is all too infrequently referred to the allergist is eczema. It can be on the hands, the feet, in the crease of the arms, behind the knees, on the face, or scattered over the whole body. Most people, thinking it's a skin disease, go to a dermatologist. He prescribes brand after brand of steroid cream. When these are used on the face, they cause not only atrophy or premature tissue-paper-like thinning of the skin so that the skin looks like it's 90 years old; but also telangiectasias, a condition where tiny broken blood vessels break and disfigure the skin.

When these patients proceed to get worse, they are given steroids orally or by injection that last a month. The side effects from these are many. Because of years of steroid injections from a dermatologist, my own mother had two cataract operations before she was even 55, and there had never been a family history of cataracts in 4 generations. The other effect from steroid injections that we commonly see is that it can upset a woman's periods, causing her to have abnormally heavy bleeding or irregular periods or cessation of menstruation entirely. Because the dermatologist usually fails to warn the woman of this, she ends up with needless worry and spends much time and money at the gynecologist's office, sometimes even having a D&C. Also, steroids have a host of bad side effects leading to high blood pressure, diabetes, ulcers, necrosis or death of the arteries supplying the neck of the femur (which is the long bone of the thigh), not to mention atrophy or degeneration and death of the adrenal glands which are necessary for life.

Asthma is yet another very serious form of allergy which is often incompletely treated. Many times when a person feels short of breath, tight or heavy in the chest, he seeks out a pulmonary specialist. If the specialist is knowledgeable about the mechanisms of allergy injections, he will suggest that the patient look for environmental causes.

Sometimes people come to our offices using at least $200 worth of medication a month; there is nothing being done to find the cause of their problems, nor is there anything done to prevent the progression of their asthma. Some are spending $2000/year in breathing treatments at home, depending upon the severity and duration of the asthma. Oftentimes, we can have a person off all medication within six months of starting injections.

I recently saw a 69 year old lady who had had severe asthma for 10 years. She was completely off all medication after six months of treatment. This was the first time she had been off any medication (including steroids) in 10 years. She was furious with the pulmonary specialists who she had seen in Florida and New York State because none of them had recommended allergy treatments and none had ever suggested that it was possible she could be free of her asthma and without medication, and enjoy the return of her normal state of energy. But they are not at fault. They are only practicing to the best of their current knowledge. And we can't help all the cases, either.

Currently, there is more and more evidence now that many of the inhalers that are used for asthma have adverse effects on the lungs. It only makes sense that the inhaling of high-pressured hydrocarbon aerosols and chemical preservatives adversely affects the lung tissue of some people. Sometimes, this may be caused by the medication; sometimes, the preservative; sometimes, the vehicle used.

Many children and young adults have large dark

circles under their eyes. These are called allergic shiners. They are the manifestation of swollen, congested veins that are not able to drain properly through the sinus area because of untreated allergy. I looked older at 29 than 39 because of dark circles under my eyes due to untreated allergies.

The brain is probably the commonest allergic target organ, yet environment and nutrition are commonly discounted. Hyperactive children oftentimes have inhalant allergies that vastly alter their behavior. Many are dangerously aggressive or pathetically retarded at intervals. Smart mothers who tell the pediatrician that there are periods of normalcy are thought by pediatricians to be dreaming! These doctors can't conceive of these conditions being turned on and off by the ingestion of foods or exposure to chemicals, and they assume these problems are chronic. Rarely will they ever exhaust allergic possibilities first before prescribing harmful amphetamines like Ritalin. Depression as well as migraines can be the only manifestation of an inhalant allergy in others.

Even people with seemingly clear-cut emphysema have been mis-diagnosed. There have been several medical studies done in the last few years to demonstrate that one in five people with emphysema has been incorrectly diagnosed, and that they really have chronic allergic bronchitis or asthma, which has now gone on to form irreversible permanent lung destruction, or emphysema. I have personally seen the progressive destruction in emphysema patients come to a halt because their allergies were brought under control. Indeed, when asthma is not turned off and corrected through injections, emphysema will be the result. You cannot have tremendous secretions of mucus and phlegm in the delicate tissues of the lung year in and year out without having some permanent irreversible scar tissue and damage. This is slowly cumulative and in time causes emphysema. Many people just have a chronic cough, and they chalk it up to smoking or a nervous tic. Usually, however, a chronic cough is the precursor of asthma. Asthmatic bronchitis is simply constriction in the higher tubes or bronchi.

The basic pathophysiology in allergy is that the person develops an antibody towards something that he inhales, such as dust, pollen, or mold. This antibody attaches to cells in the lung or the nose or wherever the allergy is. When it attaches to basophil cells or to mast cells, this triggers the release of chemicals which create the symptoms.

One of the chemicals is histamine. That's why we take antihistamines to try to simmer down the allergic reaction. Histamine opens up holes in between cells in membranes so that now fluid and other chemicals can leak into areas that were not normally exposed. This leaking can occur in any tissue. When it occurs in the skin, it's a dermatitis, like eczema or acne. When it occurs in the cerebellum of the brain, it can be mood swings, depression, hyperactivity, or the allergic-tension-fatigue syndrome. When it occurs in the lung and fluid leaks in and there is constriction of the bronchials due to the chemicals released, it's called chronic bronchitis. When it occurs in the nose, it's rhinitis. Sometimes polyps are formed was well. When it occurs in the sinuses, it sinusitis.

But it can occur in just about any part of the body. For some unknown reason, we are genetically predisposed to have particular target organs or places. Many people like myself have different organs for different antigens.

For example, my face would break out when I ingested certain foods. I would cough if near a dog. I would wheeze when exposed to carbon monoxide fumes, barns, or horses. I would get stuffy and have a congested nose and sneeze when exposed to molds. These abound in the air at all times. The whites of my eyes would swell violently if I touched my eyes after having touched a cat or horse. It looked like jelly oozing out between swollen lids. Or I had severe depression from overdosing on wheat, or tremendous tiredness by overdosing on sugar. If I sat in a plastic chair with foam formaldehyde stuffing or slept on a conventional foam mattress with permanent press sheets, I had severe inflammation of an old back injury. I cried for no reason or became severely depressed when breathing natural gas, diesel fumes or glue. I had many other triggers as well. The symptoms go on, but this shows you that there are a variety of target organs that can be present in just one person.

Other people have sneakier symptoms. Their leakage is in organs that have not been identified as having anything to do with allergy by the majority of physicians. Some women have irregular menstrual periods only during the fall ragweed season, or they have toxemia of pregnancy, or uterine hemorrhaging. Just as the ragweed antigen can cause leakage in vessels in the nose or in the lung, it can also do it in vessels in the uterus. And just as this same ragweed antigen can cause a muscle spasm in the bronchus causing asthma, it can affect the smooth muscle of the intestine causing colitis, diarrhea and cramps, or it can affect the smooth muscle of the uterus causing cramps and bleeding.

How Do Allergy Injections Work?

It was discovered years ago that if in the genetically susceptible person an antigen, such as dust, mold, or ragweed, is presented, he will make an allergic antibody called IgE. When this antibody attaches to the mast cell, chemical mediators such as histamine, S-RSA, or kinins are released. The reactions that occur create multiple symptoms that can occur in any target organ in the body. If this same material is injected intravenously, it can cause anaphylaxis.

If it is injected subcutaneously, that is under the skin,

98

in just the right amount, an IgG or blocking forms. These antibodies are very helpful because they block allergic reactions. Depending upon the amount that a person's body is able to synthesize, he can obtain as much as total relief from his symptoms through injections only. Other people make large amounts of IgE (allergic antibodies) to so many other allergens that they need other measures as well, such as stricter environmental controls and sometimes medications.

Controlling the Environment

About 35 million people in the United States have pollen allergies. One in five people has an allergy that he is aware of at sometime in his life. But many others have hidden hypersensitivities that go forever undiagnosed. Some people just go through life at half mast, never feeling great, but afraid to complain about how they do feel for fear of being thought of as a hypochondriac. They never would dream that an allergy to dust or mold could give perennial headache or tiredness.

Pollens, however, are a little more difficult to miss because they have such a definite season. Showers of pollens occur in our area in April when the trees (actually March through June) start budding, in May and June when the grasses start coming out, and again when the various weeds pollinate throughout the summer. Then ragweed hits in early August to October. House dust is a ubiquitous antigen because we cannot get away from it. It is everywhere and is probably the commonest allergen. The house dust mite is an antigen that was discovered in the 70's. It is a little microscopic animal that lives in mattresses, bedding, sofas and other areas and goes usually hand in hand with a person's dust allergies. There was a definite improvement in many people when this antigen was added to their injections.

Molds are the sneaky part of inhalant allergy because they are often grossly underestimated. They are the "pollens" that last all year long because not only do they flare during times of high pollination, but they are present in all seasons, indoors and outdoors. And there are thousands of types. Some molds send showers of millions of spores into the air every night at a precise time; others at noon, others do so when the climatic conditions are just right for that particular species. So what we end up with are countless massive showers of mold spores occurring throughout a day; each individual type is dependent on some crucial change in temperature or humidity or light to trigger its occurrence. These showers can cause symptoms far more severe than pollens, but their causes are not as obvious nor as facile to prove.

Normally, allergists test primarily to Aspergillus, Hormodendrum, Penicillium and Alternaria. Some add a handful of other molds, either individually or in a mix. In the **Annals of Allergy**, (July, 1982 and January, 1983 and May, 1984) we showed that there were indeed many more molds that no one was aware of since our plates picked up 32% more molds (special growing media). Also, we found that their plates were being prematurely discarded before the appearance of many molds that grow only after several weeks of incubation.

We also did a study of the molds growing in people's 24 hour environment for over a year. We divided their lifestyle up into three 8-hour segments, culturing the bedroom where they spent a third of their lives, their work environment where they spend another third, and then wherever they spent most of the rest of their time, such as the kitchen, family room, basement, barn, etc. We found that there were many more molds than are commonly tested to.

We cultured their environments, grew out these newer molds, tested to them and included those in the allergy injections of people that reacted to them. The proof of the pudding was, of course, that the patients' symptoms were indeed better. We had an excellent opportunity to test this out when people who had been on injections for quite a while came for evaluation and said they were improved but had room for further improvement.

We would culture the molds that were in their environment by giving them petri dishes to set out for an hour, and then tested them to the molds to find their exact treatment dose and administered it.

Many people would continue to do very poorly in October and could not determine why, since the ragweed had ceased pollinating. Mold was the cause. September was the next commonest month of mold prevalence. Then May and June were the next heaviest months of mold growth; and, of course, these are times of heavy tree and grass pollination, and many people's spring symptoms are probably erroneously blamed on this. They would benefit by testing to these newer molds

One lady with sudden severe asthma owned a bakery. She was found to be highly wheat allergic. On the basis of this, many allergists would recommend she stay out of the bakery. But we exposed petri dishes in her home and found excessive levels of Sporobolomyces. This mold usually will not grow on the agar put in petri dishes by hospitals and allergists. But it does grow on ours (a malt extract agar). We gave her injections to this, and she has no asthma, is on no medication, and is still a happy baker!

Candida is a particularly interesting mold. In fact, when we studied over 400 plates, the most prevalent mold at all times was any member of the yeast family, and Candida is one of these members. Yeasts are not well-studied, nor well- tested for by conventional methods. We eat yeast every day in the form of bread, pastries, crackers, alcohols, fermented foods, beverages, vinegars, cheeses, salad dressings, etc. Also, we inhale it constantly because it's in our environment all the times, both indoors an outdoors.

With the increased use of antibiotics in this century, Candida has grown in unprecedented numbers in the intestines of many people. Many people start becoming allergic to the very yeast or mold, Candida, that they are wearing in their intestines. The target organ for this allergy can be anything. We have seen Candida sensitivity cause years of chronic diarrhea and/or constipation, depression, exhaustion, headaches and other symptoms. It is in most women's vaginas and worsens periodically causing itching and a fishy odored discharge. More on that in the Candida section.

There are a few other antigens which have been tested and found to provide great relief in certain people. For example, one gal had extreme somnolence and tiredness, and one of the antigens which caused this in her was algae. Algae is a plant that is in lakes and waterways, but it also is dispersed in the air.

Goldenrod is another pollen which was not formerly tested to because in traditional allergy we were always taught that anything that is brightly colored is probably insect pollinated. Mother Nature gave goldenrod bright color to attract the birds and bees. The ugly things like ragweed which are dull brown are not very attractive, and so depend on the wind for pollination. It's the wind-borne pollens that create our symptoms when they land on our respiratory cells. However, when we started testing people to goldenrod, lo and behold, they were usually more sensitive to it than ragweed; and we have, needless to say, now included this in our armamentarium.

If a person's symptoms persist even with coverage of the inhalant antigenic load, then it's time to investigate foods, chemical sensitivities, and the more bizarre.

Before a person begins injections, he should first want to be sure he has done all that is possible in terms of environmental controls. If he cannot even awaken totally clear and without symptoms, or if he is definitely worse after he goes to bed or in the evening, then it's more than likely that there are neglected changes that can be made in the bedroom.

Often times the presence of an animal is the main reason for lack of improvement. He will rationalize, "Well, it's okay because the dog is only in the house a few minutes a day to eat," or "He's only inside when I'm not there." What they don't realize is that the dander from the skin and the hair float around in the air and become imbedded in the carpet and the furnishings; then people walking through track this into other rooms. Children are often guilty of rough-housing with animals and then wearing the same clothes to lie down on their beds or on the floor, thereby spreading the animal's dander.

Or they will say, "I'm not worse when I'm around the dog." They don't understand that it provides the last drop that makes their allergic barrel of symptoms overflow, causing their sickness. It's the last straw analogy. Allergic people down deep hope they only have 1-2 allergics. But we have many. And if they are not all controlled, we don't do well.

If you're definitely worse in the evening and when you awake, then your bedroom is the culprit. You want to create an allergy-free oasis in your bedroom. This can be done to a variety of extents depending upon your sensitivities. The quickest and most ideal thing would be to choose a room in the house where you could have only your bed. Seal off the forced air duct and buy an electic powered hot water heater (use none if possible) and an air cleaner, such as Foust, Martinaire, Allermed or Micronaire, depending upon your sensitivities. Have an air conditioner for the pollen season; take out all rugs, cover the mattress with cotton, and use a cotton pillow. Many times a person's feather pillow or Kapok stuffed couch is the very cause of his symptoms.

The fewer dust catchers and knick-knacks there are, the better. You have to remember that to create an allergy-free oasis in the bedroom, will enable you to wake up feeling refreshed and without symptoms. Then you are more able to deal with the allergic assaults over which you have little control but are confronted with throughout the day. These include symptoms from various perfumes, dusts, smokes, and chemicals which cannot always be managed by injections or medications.

Most wood burning stoves give out a great deal of dust as well as formaldehyde and other gases. Kerosene stoves are a no-no. Humidity is often quite low in the wintertime, especially in the northern states where we require so much heat. The dryness causes our noses to hypersecrete to maintain the normal humidity of our inspired air. Therefore, a humidifier is a necessary adjunct. When you have completed the environmental controls in your bedroom, it should be so comfortable that entering is a delight; it should feel like walking into a cool, clear forest. You should notice the difference immediately as you breathe, and it should even make non-allergic family members more comfortable when they're in it.

Another overlooked area in people who are not improving is that they persist in using highly scented soaps, cosmetics, aftershaves, deodorants, shampoos, hair conditioners and fabric softeners, or they persist in smoking. Unless you remember the concept of total load, your system, which is much like a delicate flower, will be constantly bombarded; and you will never feel better. Many a person, plagued with headaches, cleared only after all scents were removed.

Some people are very lucky and their allergies improve remarkably fast with injections, and they never do any environmental controls. Other people, such as myself, have so many and such diverse allergies that they have to do just about everything possible and environmental controls are a very necessary part of their total allergic management. They should be a necessary part of everyone's, because indeed it would be preferable if we could manage with environmental controls only and never have to give injections. But this situation rarely exists. Environmental controls are also necessary because they will prevent us from developing further allergies at such a rapid pace.

Oftentimes, people with allergies will inquire, "What if I move to Arizona? I hear people are better there." In a 1983, **Wall Street Journal**, there was an article discussing this fact because many people had thought this very same thing and had made the big move only to return. With the genetic ability to become allergic, it is only a matter of time before one develops antibodies to the tumbleweed or sagebrush in their new environment. Also, because many people were moving to those areas, they were importing all of their flowering shrubs and trees that they had liked for landscaping up north and were creating a similar area of pollenosis.

Back on the total load phenomenon, remember Dr. Doris Rapp's fitting analogy: If you had five nails in your shoe and came into the office complaining of a limp and I removed four nails, you would go out thinking I was a terrible doctor and had not helped you. Such is the problem with injections. Some people only need injections. Others must watch the animals, the smoke, the dust precautions, the humidity controls, and a host of other parameters in order to get their allergies all under control.

In the long run, allergies can cause symptoms far more serious than we have discussed above. We will discuss these in the next chapters. They can cause symptoms that defy medical diagnosis, that have left people being told that they should see a psychiatrist, that they have to learn to live with it, that it's all in their heads, or that there is no help at this point in time.

Mold Allergies and the Brain

It has always been a miracle to me why there are not more battered and killed children because the nature of hyperactive children is such that they for no reason lash out and kick and bite their parents and destroy things. It would drive the sanest person criminally insane. Dr. Rapp cleverly calls it the "battered parent syndrome." And when you consider the hereditary nature of allergy and that the mother may have undetected allergies that make her alternate between depression and violence, I really marvel at how these kids have survived. Maternal love is truly a strong force.

Sometimes we have hyperactive children write or draw during mold testing to show the profound affect of mold allergy on the brain.

For Alexander we obtained samples of his writing and drawing. After testing, we could see the results of the allergic reaction that went on in his brain. It appeared as though his IQ level had dropped in half. His writing and his picture drawing were not even close to what they had been just minutes before. And his mood changed for the worse as his hyperactivity flared. When he ingested an apple at home, it took three adults to hold him down. Weeks later in the office, he was sitting happily nestled between his parents working diligently on a workbook. He brought his report card that showed that he was an exceptional student and had indeed scored higher than his grade level. He was getting his first A's. The teacher had noticed marked improvement in him and his parents now had a happier home life because it was like having a mini-adult in their midst instead of a highly unpredictable, destructive child.

Even patients in our testing room would ask the

nurses, "What happened to that little boy? I used to dread coming when he was here and lately he's been so pleasantly calm." Alexander was off all amphetamines within two weeks of completing the testing; and as soon as he discontinued them, he grew, and teeth that had been delayed for two years suddenly erupted. Fortunately for Alexander, he has parents who were more intelligent than the many doctors they consulted. They believed in their son and wouldn't quit until they could find the cause for his abnormal behavior.

Currently, his chronic sinusitis and recurrent colds are controlled because his parents oversee his environmental controls and he receives injections containing his individualized dose of dust, house dust mite, and the newer molds. Using mold plates we discovered what molds were in his home environment; testing showed which dose to use for his treatment. Also, control of his behavior requires his parents to watch his rotated diet and give him his injection of foods as needed. This aspect will be covered more fully in the food chapter.

Months later, I was suspicious that the molds were not crucial to his normal cerebral function and that foods were his biggest problem. so unbeknown to his parents or my allergy nurses, I took the molds out of his injections for three weeks. I was going to call the mother and ask if there had been any difference, but I didn't have to.

She came in wearing a large bruise. Alexander had punched her; his behavior had made a sudden reversal to the "old days" within the last two weeks. His teachers collaborated and asked that he not be returned to school the next year. Also, he had been in the police station twice for discipline. He would call the police, telling them to rush over to the house for a non-existent emergency.

Again, I can't imagine what a life of juvenile detention homes and eventual jail this little guy might have had if his parents hadn't stuck to their very correct convictions that he was a charming, very intelligent boy who was acting under the influence of something that was wrong. That something was a host of inhaled and ingested allergens.

One dear friend and highly allergic individual is one of those human dynamos who works for sun-up to sundown and is often an optimistic delight. She had a few episodes when she would come by the office very depressed, but they always passed.

One day she came in very depressed and also had laryngitis and could barely speak. She ached all over, cried, and felt miserable. She had very good medical judgement, so when she said she needed antibiotics, I was inclined to believe her. But on examining her, I wasn't convinced. We tested her by provocation-neutralization to a mold that happened to be out in extremely heavy amounts that week; and within minutes, she was her old self—smiling, happy, feeling well and no laryngitis. We found she was getting over-exposed to this mold while rototilling her organic garden.

A self-administered injection of this mold kept her normal. She gave it whenever her voice would start becoming hoarse. For when this started we knew the cerebral vessels would soon swell and depression set in. She only requires it sporadically a day or two.

So odd as it may seem, things that we can't even see but breathe in daily, can cause just about any reaction you can think of. Pick a substance, any substance, and you'll probably be able to find somebody who is allergic to it. And it need not cause the same symptoms in any two people who are reactive to it.

Contact Dermatitis and Patch Testing

Some people's allergies are tested with what is known as patch testing. To give you an example, one lady had 40 years of eczema from head to toe. Her skin was all broken out, red and scaly. She had consulted physicians, including dermatologists and allergists, to no avail. My clue to her sensitivity was that she said that even the very creams that they prescribed made her worse and made her skin fiery red and burning.

So we patch tested her to various chemicals that are included in creams. Indeed, she was wildly sensitive to formaldehyde; and, of course, formaldehyde was in all of her clothes and bedding as well. It is in polyester, permanent press, and wrinkle resistant fabrics. Also, it was in the prescribed creams, but it was not required to be included in the list of ingredients so the physicians were not suspicious of it. When we had her use Crisco on her skin for a lubricant and avoid all store bought creams and prescriptions and wear cotton clothes that had tested formaldehyde safe with the formaldehyde spot test, she was indeed clear for the first time.

At one point in time, she accidentally dropped a bit of the formaldehyde spot test on the clothes that she was wearing. Before buying them she had tested the material and found it safe. But now to her amazement the spot turned purple immediately. It was because of this that she discovered that the spray starch she was using to make her cottons look better contained a high amount of formaldehyde. So constant vigilance is necessary in this highly chemicalized society for those with chemical hypersensitivities.

The formaldehyde spot test is a kit that you may purchase through the office. One vial does over 100 tests. Simply take a drop of the solution with a syringe and put it on fabric that you are considering purchasing. If there is over 10 ppm of formaldehyde in it, the drop will turn purple. This is also handy when you are considering purchasing materials for construction, such as ceiling tiles or wallboard. You will be amazed at the number of articles in your closet, home, and on your office desk that contain formaldehyde. Not only is paper currency saturated in it, but most paper products.

In some people their chemical sensitivities are manifested by a dermatitis, and the cause of that dermatitis can be diagnosed by patch testing. In other words, we put patches on their backs or forearms and under these a little dab of the chemical in question is placed. We leave these patches on for 48 hours and then read them. If a dermatitis has been induced under a patch, then we know that there is reactivity. One of the commonest forms of this contact dermatitis is nickel sulphate. Women know they have it when they can't wear earrings, watches, bracelets, or necklaces without breaking out. Or they break out under the places where buttons, zippers, or metal hooks touch their skin. Even coins and keys in the pocket can be the culprits.

I once saw a man who had a dermatitis on his thigh in one little round area and on his right thumb and forefinger. He was sensitive to nickel in coins that he always put in his pocket. Hence he had the dermatitis on his two fingers where he frequently handled his keys, metal key chain and coins. He also had some dermatitis over his right thigh under his coin pocket.

Neomycin sulphate is an antibiotic in many nonprescription antibiotic creams that mothers buy to put on cuts for their children. This is a dangerous antibiotic to have in over-the-counter preparations because broken skin becomes more easily sensitized than does whole skin. It encourages the development of hypersensitivity dermatitis. This means Neomycin is an antibiotic to which it is very easy to develop an allergy called contact dermatitis. Once it has developed, it usually never leaves; and then there can be cross reactivity with other chemicals making life more difficult. Also, many of the vaccines for measles and mumps are processed using Neomycin, and so having an allergy to it can be a contraindication for receiving them; and certainly it is much more important to have the measles, mumps, rubella vaccine than it is to have a topical antibiotic on an open sore. Actually, constant cleansing and soaking is all that is required, and no amount of topical antibiotic is going to make that big a difference. If infection starts in the tissues, a systemic or oral antibiotic is what is necessary.

Another man had over 20 years of severe eczematous dermatitis of his hands. They were so thickened that when he moved them, they would crack and bleed. He was an artificial inseminator or cows and was exposed to many chemicals. He had had the spreading of his dermatitis over his body, and it was indeed getting to a point where it was going to interfere with his livelihood. He had evaluated a number of types of gloves, all to no avail. He got so desperate he stayed in a hotel for a week to see if that would help.

When we tested him, it was found that he was highly sensitive to nitrofurantoin which was part of his daily contact for his work. He spent most of his time traveling in his truck from farm to farm, and he had large containers of it inside the cab of the truck at all times, out-gasing into the air and in constant contact with his skin. He also had multiple dust and mold sensitivities; and when these were all under control, his skin could be clear.

So chemicals by contact or mold in the air are some of the many causes we see of skin diseases and other sneaky symptoms. The point is, there is most likely a cause for every malfunction or symptom in the body.

What Should I Do If I'm Not Better?

If you're having trouble during the pollen season, use this checklist before seeing the doctor.

1. Have I done environmental controls with cotton bedding, no carpet, an air conditioner, and an air cleaner?

111

2. Have I set out a current mold plate to see how much mold there is and how effectively the machines I purchased are working?

3. Did I remember to move my injection interval level to twice a week? Sometimes, this is all that is needed.

4. Am I taking my antihistamine/decongestants and/or nasal and ophthalmic or asthma medicine around the clock?

5. Do I need to test some of the trees or grasses or mold pollens individually as opposed to just the mixes?

6. Have I done the diagnostic diet for two weeks to see if my symptoms are partly due to a hidden food sensitivity?

7. Do I have a hidden chemical sensitivity?

8. Is my total load up because of hidden infection, Candida, nutritional deficiency, too much stress, a pesticide toxicity, heavy metal toxicity, poisoning, EMF radiations, or a hidden cancer?

If you awaken with symptoms, the bedroom is a failure. If you've made the bedroom as clean as possible, you most likely have a hidden chemical, Candida, and/or food sensitivities.

As you whittle away at your total load with injections, the diagnostic diet, environmental controls, the anti-Candida program and so forth, you begin to be able to determine what agent causes what symptoms.

How Can I Have My Yearly Evaluation by Mail?

When you require no medications and are free of all

of your symptoms, you can be evaluated by mail and will not need to be seen in the office for your injections to be continued for another year. Simply use this form as a guide. Mimeograph it and answer every question if you want to avoid a trip to the office.

1. My initial total symptoms that I came for treatment for were:

2. The symptoms I have gotten rid of totally are:
I found these symptoms were due to (diet, environmental molds, chemicals, Candida, nutrient deficiencies, attitude, etc.):

3. The symptoms that are partially better are:

   I suspect they are due to:

4. The symptoms that are no better are:

   I suspect they are due to:

5. I have these new symptoms:

6. I discovered when I started the injections that I also got rid of some symptoms I hadn't been aware I had. These were:

7. I would describe myself as:
   (a) 25% better
   (b) 50% better
   (c) 75% better
   (d) 90% better
   (e) 100% better
   (f) other

8. I take the following medications regularly: (Please

113

include the name, dose, # of times a day, # per week that you take these)

9.   I take for Candida control (Please include the name, dose, # of times a day, and # of times a week):
   (a) Nystatin

   (b) Acidophilus

   (c) Other

   (d) It helps these symptoms:

10. I take these supplements (Please include the name, dose, company, number of times daily, and number of times weekly):

11. I have an air conditioner in the bedroom:

12. I have an air cleaner in the bedroom:
   Type:

13. I clean it once a month or service it regularly:

14. I have removed the carpet:

15. I have changed to cotton bedding and pillows:

16. I take my injections every _____ days.
   They help these symptoms:

17. I take my food injections every _____ days.
   They help these symptoms:

18. Other injections are _____, used every _____ days for these symptoms:

19. I have never had a reaction from my injections.
True/False

20. I have no arm redness, itching or soreness.
True/False

21. I never feel worse with an injection.
True/False

22. If I'm late for an injection I get a fade out (symptoms come back. True/False

23. Comments:

24. I am currently taking medications and/or treatments for additional problems (diabetes, hypothyroidism, hypertension, high cholesterol, etc.):

25. Surgeries and accidents & hospitalization in the last two years:

Name:
Address:
Phone:
Date:
Doctor giving injections:
Address:
Phone:

Note: If you are not clear of symptoms, or if you are not markedly better, or still require great deal of medications, have questions, or do not feel as healthy as you would like; you should not have an evaluation by mail but in-person so we can determine what is missing in your program toward wellness.

Environmental Controls

Since most patients spend at least 1/3 of their time in the bedroom, we want to try to control your environment beginning with the bed. Bedding should be easy to wash and dry, so that it is convenient to change often. Avoid wool blankets. The bedroom should be uncluttered, hopefully as free from dust catchers as possible. The strictness with which you adhere to this should be in proportion to the severity of your symptoms.

The environment of the bedroom sould ideally be controlled as follows:

1. New pillows made of cotton should be obtained. Cotton is preferred for chemically sensitive people. They should be washed monthly and replaced yearly.

2. Mattresses should preferably be cotton. Otherwise, vacuum and encase in cotton zippered covers or several cotton blankets. Do the same to box springs.

3. Blankets and comforters should be made of cotton. They should be washed monthly. Bedspreads should be of cotton or other washable material.

4. A frequently washed cotton sheet/blanket may be used as a mattress pad.

5. Feather, down and kapok filled: pillows, sleeping bags, ski jackets and quilts should be avoided.

6. The bedroom must be completely cleaned with a cloth dampened only with water at least weekly; the floor may be waxed monthly with low fragrance paste wax. The patient should be kept away during these procedures and should stay out of the room for a few hours.

7. The bedroom should be cleared of all sources of dust as well as all dust collectors such as drapes, toys, and book-shelves. If there are shelves, they should be enclosed. Remember to keep in mind that the strictness of this should be in relationship to the patient's symptoms.

8. The bedroom closets should be thoroughly cleaned and used only for clothing in current use. The door should be kept closed. With small children having numerous toys, it would be better to keep the toys in the closet than in the room scattered about. Toys should not be of the stuffed variety.

9. Everything in the room should be dust-proof and washable. Use cotton rugs or preferably none at all. Plain chairs, desks, dressers, chests, and lamps should be used and cleaned frequently with a damp cloth. Curtains may be used (cotton or other natural fibers).

10. Openings for hot air in the floor and wall should be sealed permanently. Several layers of aluminum foil may be placed over the vent and sealed with a wide tape. Install an electrostatic air cleaner or precipitator (Micronaire), or other type air cleaner. Several layers of cheesecloth could be placed over the vent. If the furnace filtration system is adequate, the cheesecloth should remain clean. However, this does not protect against gas fumes from the furnace as a heat exchange system does.

11. For smaller children, encourage play and study in this room and have only wooden or non-allergic type toys.

12. The best bedroom for a pollen-sensitive person has an air conditioner, an air cleaner, and no rugs.

13. A mite is an extremely potent antigen that keeps a lot of

people symptomatic throughout the night or at least awakening with symptoms. These microscopic critters love to live in mattresses and couches. Besides zippered barrier cloth mattress covers to keep them off you, there's an excellent way to kill them: Simply do as the Scandinavian housewife does. Put the mattress outdoors for a day or two in the winter on one of those clear below-zero days and freeze the little buggers to death. Then beat the mattress to clean out dead bodies, dust, and molds.

The rest of the house should also receive consideration if used to any great extent. You may follow these recommendations:

1. Try to prevent the patient from using upholstered furniture or feather pillows in any part of the house. Throw a cotton barrier cover over the couch.

2. Washable scatter rugs are preferred. Otherwise, cotton rugs are recommended. Avoid wool rugs, cow hair, or wool felt pads. Many people are sensitive to rubberized rug pads and any synthetic materials.

3. Do not permit smoking in the house. Post a warning sign "No smoking allowed - allergic!"

4. Whenever possible do not permit the use of anything in the house with a perfume smell or strong odor, expecially aerosols or sprays. The patient should remain out of the house until the odor has disappeared. (Again, you should be keeping in mind the degree of the patient's sensitivity.)

5. Use an exhaust fan in the kitchen while cooking.

6. Dogs, cats, birds, guineas pigs, rabbits, and gerbils should not be permitted in the house.

7. The house temperature should be kept in relationship to the humidity schedule. Generally speaking, the house humidity should be half of the temperature; the temperature should be approximately 70 degrees in the daytime and 65 degrees at night.

Check list of hypoallergenic bedroom:

1. Close heat register and seal off. Substitute a portable electric unit)
2. Remove carpet.
3. Remove as much as possible besides the bed.
4. Cover bed and pillows with zippered cotton covers, use cotton bedding.
5. Wet dust and vacuum biweekly.
6. Air cleaner, preferably electrostatic precipitator or HEPA.
7. No people with scents and no animals allowed.
8. Air conditioner to filter out pollens.

Many people are simply too allergic to ever get better without doing these measures. Your body can only make so much blocking antibody in response to injections. It must have a rest a least eight hours a day with a reduced antigenic load for the best and fastest improvement in symptoms.

Personal Grooming

Many people have reactions to the things they wear. For example, headaches, burning eyes, nasal congestion, and asthma are commonly caused by a person's fragrance, perfume, aftershave, shampoo, conditioners, cosmetics, or hairspray. Don't overlook the antiperspirants, fabric softeners, toothpaste, or polyester clothes. More on this in the chemical section.

Again, bear in mind the allergic person represents a

spectrum of disease. Some people only need to avoid a few things like a cat or the out-of-doors in August through September. Others are more allergic and need injections. Others are even more highly allergic and need to avoid certain exposures; they need injections to produce blocking antibodies, and they need to strictly control their environment to lower their total antigenic load sufficiently to stop triggering symptoms.

For example, you may have thought you were only sensitive to pollens and then were surprised by your test reactions to dusts and molds. This is because once allergies turn on, they tend to spread and the individual rapidly develops sensitivity to many things. It's a rare person who is allergic only to a few things.

Total Antigenic Load

To understand the total antigenic load, imagine you had five nails in your shoe. If you came to a doctor and she removed one nail (that is, she gave you injections for just ragweed) you would go home with the same sore foot and think she was a lousy doctor. She'd have to remove all five nails (injections to the molds out at ragweed time, avoidance of aftershave, etc.) to make you comfortable. That's why you need to understand that many of you will remain symptomatic until you clean up your bedroom and make the environment you are most frequently exposed to as hypoallergenic as possible. You need to reduce the hidden sources of dusts and molds that keep your symptoms smoldering.

Dust filtration for Heating Units

1. Hot air heat with blowers (forced hot air furnaces). Usually these are equipped with a disposable fiberglass filter which must be changed periodically. Filters of this

type will trap large dust particles and also pollen, but they are not of much value for trapping the smaller dust particles which are usually responsible for symptoms in patients sensitive to dust. Even though these fiberglass filters are not very effective for the control of allergy, they can be used to reduce the amount of dust accumulating inside the furnace and for whatever help they may be in keeping the home cleaner. Space guard filters have provided excellent dust and mold control. Your heating man can help you.

The installation of an electrostatic air cleaner in the cold air return of the heating system will remove most of the smaller dust particles and is usually of definite help to patients in whom dust sensitivity is a factor in their allergies. It is important that such a device be satisfactorily installed and that adequate service be available after installation. Electronic air cleaners have the added advantage of reducing maintenance costs in a home since less cleaning and repainting is usually necessary. To operate effectively, electronic air cleaners must be installed so that the furnace blower operates continually. (See paragraph 3 for portable room type air cleaners).

2. Hot air furnaces without blowers (gravity furnaces). Usually these are converted coal furnaces. No central filter can be installed. With this type of furnace 3-4 thicknesses of cheesecloth may be placed under each furnace register which is of help in removing at least some of the larger dust particles. (See paragraph 3 for portable room type air cleaners). Special fiberglass filters may also be of some help and may be made to order to insert in place of or under these registers.

3. Central control of dust is not possible without installation of duct system which is usually extremely expensive. Room type portable electronic dust control devices are

usually of help, providing all the windows and doors are kept closed. If used, it is suggested that a device of this type be placed in the bedroom. Many of the relatively inexpensive widely advertised electronic portable room air cleaners are of insufficient capacity to be helpful even for a small room, so great care must be taken in choosing one. Portable electronic air cleaners are available locally on a rental basis so that their effect may be judged by a patient before final purchase.

In the final analysis, the good objective view of how good any filtration system is can be obtained by exposing before and after mold plates.

Note: The electrostatic precipitator, Micronaire, does an excellent job on dust and mold, filtering down to 0.01 microns. A high speed motor drives air through at a velocity fast enough to overcome closed window use. It cannot filter the great outdoors. The advantage is the filter can be washed, so no replacement filters are necessary. The disadvantage is they redesigned it in a smelly particle board cabinet.

The Foust, Martinaire, Allermed, and Airstar remove some chemicals, but you sacrifice some of the dust and mold efficiency of the Micronaire (which does not remove chemicals). So choose according to your needs and sensitivities. You can smell them and even rent them for a trial from N.E.E.D.S. (1-800-634-1380). We are all different; there are few rules.

Humidification

In recent years great harm has been done to mucous membranes of the nose, throat, and lungs in the winter in the colder parts of our country because of dryness of the air. The mount of moisture in the air measured in terms of the percentage of amount of water vapor actually present as compared with the amount of can actually hold is termed humidity. The Sahara Desert has a relative humidity of 25%. Death Valley, California, the driest area in the U.S. is 23%. However, most American homes in very cold weather have a relative humidity of only 13%. Dry heated air acts as a sponge soaking up moisture, drying out the linings of the nose, throat, and lungs and is particularly injurious in the case of individuals with respiratory allergies.

Relative humidity can be measured by use of an instrument called a hygrometer. Most inexpensive ones rapidly lose their accuracy. Humidity can be measured most accurately with the use of a sling type hygrometer. It can, however, be reasonably assumed that almost any home will have inadequate humidification during the winter heating season without some satisfactory type of added humidity, especially in basements, is often a problem requiring the use of a dehumidifier). Showers, cooking, dishwashers, clothes dryers, and the placing of containers of water about the home do add some humidity to the air, but in insufficient amounts to be of practical help. Condensation on windows on a cold day is not an indication of adequate humidification. As a rule, adequate humidification can be obtained only by the use of a humidifier or sufficient capacity and with a relatively accurate mechanism for automatic control.

The ideal relative humidity in winter is between 40% and 50% when the indoor temperature is 68 to 70 degrees. Most homes, however, cannot tolerate this amount of moisture during the winter months without causing undue condensation and structural problems due to moisture forming between the walls.

The following are the recommended levels of relative humidity:

Outside Temperature (Fahrenheit)	Recommended Relative Humidity
+20 and above	35%
+10	30%
0	25%
-10	20%
-20	15%

Adequate humidification is a necessity and not a luxury. In addition to preventing undue dryness of the respiratory mucous membranes, and reducing dryness of skin, humidification is of economic importance in preventing drying out of furniture (which may ruin pianos, for example). Humidification also prevents brittleness of any woven materials, reduces dust and lint formation, and reduces heating costs since with adequate humidification one feels comfortable at a lower temperature.

Common symptoms produced by overly dry winter homes are bloody noses, dry, irritated nasal and respiratory passages, frequent colds, sore throats, or sinusitis. Be sure to clean the humidifier weekly, or mold growth will worsen any existing allergies.

Mold sensitivity

The data from allergy evaluations indicate that mold sensitivity is part of the problem that you are faced with. Mold spores are a form of plant life; they are microscopic and airborne and very abundant. They do best in dark, damp, and warm areas; and there are high concentrations in the warm months of the year. Freezing temperatures will inhibit their growth on the on the outside; however, they still are very abundant in the homes and offices where there is heat. Species that cause many of the allergic problems are Alternaria, Aspergillus, Hormodendrum, Penicillium, Pullaria, Sporobolomyces, and several others. You cannot get away from all mold spores; however, there are certain things that you can do to help reduce their quantity.

1. Do not go into old barns, granaries, or mulch piles.

2. Do not use organic fertilizers; do not go into musty, damp areas.

3. Mold spores are found in general house dust, so strict dust precautions are necessary.

4. Mattresses, stuffed chairs, furniture, and especially items that are in attics and basements hold many mold spores, also old foam rubber pillows and mattresses can be a source of mold which is why cotton covers are important.

5. If your basement is wet and damp, a dehumidifier in the basement may help reduce mold growth. Good drainage around buildings is also helpful.

6. The following foods have mold antigens:
a) Sour breads, pumpernickel, and foods made with much yeast, such as fresh rolls, pizza.
b) Vinegar and vinegar containing products, pickled and smoked meats and fish, pastrami, corn beef, cider and homemade root beer, wines, beers, liquors, salad dressing, mustard, catsup, and mayonnaise.
c) All cheeses, sour cream, and buttermilk.
d) Dried and candied fruits, raisins, apricots, dates, figs, prunes, coffee, tea, and all chocolate.

e) All alcohols (beer, wine, liquor).

7. Sites that enhance mold growth in the home are refrigerator trays, garbage pails, planters, house plants, laundry areas, shower and bathtub areas, closets with sneakers, dirt floor basements, dark closets, tobacco humidors, vegetable containers, eaves and attics.

8. There are a few chemicals that are capable of reducing molds in the home. Formaldehyde 35% USP (diluted 5 fold) is effective; but it may cause chemical hypersensitivity, so do not use it. Products that are available that do not have as noxious an odor are:
a) Zephiran (roccal 17% concentrate). Mix with 1:5 water and use an old Windex bottle as the sprayer. Atomize the areas that show a high mold growth such as dark closets, cellars, corners and storage areas once a week.
b) Clorox, Borax, vinegar, or washing (bicarbonate) soda and water also make effective cleaners for removing mold, depending upon your sensitivities. Monthly washing of all surfaces and carpet removal are very effective.

9. Patients who are allergic to house dust should stay out of the house during and for several hours after vacuuming. Use a damp or oily mop to dust floors, ceilings, and walls.

Regarding mold spores, cultures will be obtained of your environment and this will be explained to you. There are several chemicals that can be used to control mold in humidifiers and in the room depending on the mold population, but these get aerosolized and breathing them could promote chemical hypersensitivities. Zephiran or Clorox diluted 1:5 can be used to wash down everything. Borax, vinegar or just plain water are suggested for the for the chemically sensitive.

Prevention of mold growth in air conditioners requires frequent cleaning of the coils and replacement of the filters. Central air conditioning systems should also be inspected, especially when symptoms of hypersensitivity worsen after units are turned on.

An electrostatic precipitator (Micronaire) put into the room will remove pollens, dust, and mold spores. The newer Hepafilters have a great efficiency up to 99.99%, but some chemically sensitive people need to smell each unit in use before purchasing. These units can be purchased or rented. It is best to call and compare prices and terms. The following pharmacies carry them:

N.E.E.D.S, Geddes Plaza, 527 Charles Ave 12A, Syracuse, NY 13209, phone 1-800-634-1380 or (315) 488-6312

Rothchilds Pharmacy, 805 East Genesee Street, Syracuse

Ryan's Pharmacy, 1819 West Genesee Street, Syracuse

The Foust units and Allermed units are the only two types at this time that remove dust/mold/pollen, as well as some chemicals. Study the literature from both sources. We all differ in what we can tolerate in terms of machines as well as what we need to remove from the air. For example, HEPA filters do a good job and are used in many surgical operating rooms. However, people like myself do not tolerate the glues used in their construction. So they actually promote symptoms in me even though they clean the dust and mold from the air. See examples of each type of machine in the office before purchasing.

When in doubt, the Micronaire is best. When I had asthma I would walk into a barn and start coughing and wheezing. I would go home and get the Micronaire. To test the Micronaires effectiveness, I slept through the night on a cot in the barn with no symptoms, no medication and just the Micronaire beside me.

Mold Plates

Because we cannot see them, we tend to forget that molds are everywhere. You know if you left a piece of bread where you are right now and returned in a few days, it would be covered with molds. In hundreds of home cultures, we have never seen a house without mold growth nor one without bacteria and yeasts as well.

Allergic diseases manifest themselves by many symptoms:

The antigenicity of molds and fungi has been questioned in the past, but it is now recognized that molds can cause any allergic symptom you can think of. In fact, often other antigens are blamed. Sneezing while dusting is blamed on the house dust. Wheezing in September is blamed on ragweed when it may be due to an Alternaria peak. Nasal congestion or headaches upon ingestion of fruit may really be caused by surface mold resulting from storage. More importantly, mold allergy has been also found to be the cause for many "non allergic" symptoms that have failed to respond to any type of therapy whatsoever.

Mold prevalence, however, changes with time. In the last three years alone, there have been over a dozen new molds discovered in the environment. It is suspected that these get introduced into the atmosphere from a variety of sources, one example being excavation for housing tracts and roads. Once there, they do not disappear when the excavation site is covered over; instead they flourish in their new environment and trigger allergic symptomatology.

Because we provide a Mold Survey Service for allergists/ecologists all over the world, we have had the opportunity of seeing the mycologic flora from a wide number of patients' environments. This data is in the process of being collated and submitted for publication.

So mold is everywhere and in a state of constant change. Molds have seasonal fluctuations in quantity as well as quality. They peak during pollen season, but tightening up the house for winter and turning up the heat and humidifier also encourages the growth of molds.

It is important to determine what molds are present in your environment. Then we can test you to them to determine if they are part of the hidden causes of your symptoms. Our laboratory will supply plates (petri dishes with malt agar) and instructions for their exposure.

Since mold is an extremely important cause of most people's allergies, we need a way to culture the type of mold that is found in the environment and to identify the types and then correlate the findings with allergy test results.

The petri dishes, called mold plates, should have a label on the top which has your name, date the plate was exposed, and location (bedroom, etc.). It is best to culture your bedroom, place of work, and then the place where you spend the most leisure time such as the T.V. room at home. If you do not leave the house to work, it would be a good idea to use one of the plates to culture the basement (a tremendous source of mold for the rest of the house even though you're not there often) or a workshop if a great deal of time is spent there. You should store plates in the refrigerator when you first bring them home and remove them from there at least 1 hour prior to exposure.

When you are ready to expose the plate, remove the top and set the plate in the middle of the room (waist high) to be cultured for one hour. Do not let anyone (animals, children) touch it. After one hour, close the plate, tape it shut all around the edges, and put it in a warm spot where it will not be disturbed until you can bring or mail it back to the office. The top of the refrigerator is such a place, but never place plate in the refrigerator once it has been exposed. When you do bring or mail it in to the office, try not

129

to bounce it around or jar it, and please return it within one week of exposure. Best results occur if returned as soon as exposed.

When it reaches our laboratory, it is inspected daily for six weeks or until it stops growing new molds. At various periods of time when the mold colonies reach certain stages of maturity, slides are made to identify the molds present. Sometimes the mold is an extremely unusual one, and it is subcultured into a special tube where it can grow and develop identifying characteristics which will enable determination of the exact genus and species. All the plates are read by a Ph.D. mycologist (a doctor whose specialty is identifying molds), and two consulting mycologists are available if unusual molds are grown and identification is a problem.

When all the information has been obtained and new molds stop appearing, the plates are discarded. All reports are sent to the patient. We do not have them in the chart until you bring in my copy to discuss. We need to be sure you have been tested to all the molds in your environment. If you have any questions about this, please feel free to ask, since the more you know about any disease or condition that you have, the more comfortable and skilled you will be in handling it, and the fewer symptoms you will have from it eventually.

Because of ongoing research in the mold area, be sure to check back yearly to see if there are newly discovered molds that may benefit you. Remember, they are everywhere; they are inescapable; and they are frequently the cause of symptoms that defy diagnosis. So when in doubt, check it out.

Where Does Mold Come From?

The commonest sources of high mold are dry rot, many house plants or animals, frequently opened doors and windows, heavily wooded areas, farms, greenhouses, nearby excavating, high winds, poor drainage away from house, lack of gutters, wet basement or dirt floors, a tight house that doesn't breathe or exchange air with the outside, or high humidity.

How Can I Best Get Rid of Mold?

Identify the source. Is there dry rot, or high humidity, or unvented bathrooms, etc.? Then do whatever structural changes are required. Install gutters, drainage ditches, cement the floor, install vents with exhaust fans, or install a dehumidifier, check the effectiveness of your action by measuring the humidity and re-exposing mold plates. Remove plants, animals, and carpets. Install an air purification unit in affected rooms or on the entire heating system.

What Do I Clean With?

Baking soda and water, Zephiran, Clorox, Bon Ami, vinegar; whatever you tolerate. The point is cleaning must be done periodically, like every month, since molds are living organisms and tend to recur. Until the source is found and dealt with, the numbers will be excessive. However, even after the source has been rectified, as with housecleaning, molds never truly go away. They require periodic eradication.

Over fifty percent of the time, we have seen marked reduction in molds by the following method: Mix 1 cup each, vinegar and Clorox in a bowl. Do not breathe the fumes and protect your eyes from splatter. Place bowl in center of closed room for 2 days. Do not allow anyone to enter during this time. Many before and after cultures have shown this to be worthwhile. However, it is not universally effective, so be sure to do it before and after cultures to determine its effectiveness in your situation. If it works and you are not sensitive to the ingredients, this will be an effective method to periodically keep the mold in check. Special U-V lights are the most effective, but they can cause eye damage if you forget to turn them off when you enter the room. Discuss this with the doctor. We are researching new methods for reducing mold.

Ragweed Pollinosis (Hayfever)
General Directions

In this locality, the ragweed plant pollinates from the middle of August until about the first of October. The height of the pollination season is generally reached about the last week of August or the first week of September (Labor Day). If possible, you should arrange to take your vacation in a pollen free area, such as the Central Adirondacks, and the last week in August and the first week in September so as to escape the height of the ragweed pollen season. From the middle of August to the end of September the following precautions should be observed:

1. Sleep with your windows closed as much as possible. If it is necessary to have an electric fan going, have it placed so it blows out the window. Filters, which will take the pollen out of the air and at the same time cool the room, are expensive but worth having (air conditioner). As an extra precaution, put two layers of cheesecloth under the plastic grids to filter the air even more.

2. Stay indoors on windy days. Avoid drafts and cross ventilation.

3. Avoid long automobile drives. Do not drive unless absolutely necessary and when you do, drive with the windows closed if possible. If not possible, avoid cross

drafts while driving. If you must take long drives, wear a mask.

4. Avoid members of the ragweed family of plants. Do not smell, pick, or permit these flowers in your house at any season of the year.

Asters,Cosmos,Goldenrod, Bachelor's buttons,Dahlias Marigold, Calendulas, Daisies, Sunflower, Chrysanthemums, Dandelions, Zinnias, Coreopsis and Gaillardias

Pyrethrum is the main ingredient in many insecticides and is derived from the ragweed family of plants.

5. Avoid all strong odors as they act as nonspecific irritants. Especially bad are strong perfumes, fresh paint, gasoline, tobacco smoke, scented deodorants for underarm and room fresheners, and fabric softeners.

6. Do not drink ice cold beverages or eat ice cold foods.

7. All individuals, and particularly allergic individuals, should be immunized against tetanus.

8. The pollen injections should be continued until you have had at least three years free of symptoms and medications and can be on monthly injections You may need to step up the frequency to twice a week during bad seasons, in which case you are obviously not ready to go off injections.

Summary:

So there you have it. Inhalant allergies to pollens, dust, house dust mite, and numerous species of mold can be controlled by allergy injections and intelligent environmental controls. An air conditioner, an air purification machine and removal of the bedroom carpet are a great start. It's like anything else in life; the reward is usually proportional to the effort expended. Since it took many years to develop these allergies, it takes great environmental changes to reverse them in a shorter period of time. You'll know you've arrived when you no longer need any medications, you have no symptoms, and you feel an increase in energy that you haven't felt in years.

Are You Feeling Overwhelmed?

At this point, you may feel confused or lost, so let's try to help you recapitulate and begin to sort things out.

You have a constellation of symptoms, some of which have gone on for years. Piece by piece we are uncovering the many twentieth century causes for breakdown of your immune system. You may already have been surprised with many positive reactions to molds that you never even knew existed. Indeed, once the immune system breaks down it often exhibits a spreading phenomenon. Wouldn't it be great if we were allergic to just one or two things? Instead, many of us are sensitive to pollens, dust, molds, animals, foods, our very own hormones, Candida, and chemicals which we find nearly impossible to escape from.

A logical plan at this point is to start whittling away at your total body burden or toxic overload. You stop whittling when your symptoms are clear and you no longer need medications.

Reducing your total body burden is usually accomplished by:

1. Getting your inhalant injections (pollen, dust, mold) twice a week at the office or from your family doctor. (A

neighborhood nurse is not a suitable substitute). When your symptoms are better and you need no medicine, go to weekly. If your energy level or symptoms are not as good on weekly, go back to twice a week. Usually for the first year or two, you'll need to revert to twice a week when spring and fall come around because of the heavy overload of pollens and molds
.

2. Listen to the environmental control tape. Remove bedroom carpeting, run an air cleaner 24 hours a a day, and install an air conditioner for summer pollens. Be sure you re-expose your mold plate until the report says it's passable.

3. Do the diagnostic diet to see if a hidden food allergy contributes to part of your undiscovered total overload. Be especially watchful for mold foods: bread, cheese, alcohol, vinegar, ketchup, mayonnaise, mustard, coffee, tea, chocolate, and processed foods.

4. Test yourself with glass bottled water for 10 days; then return to tap water to be sure you're not reacting to the many chemicals in it.

5. If it has been prescribed for you, take your Nystatin and avoid mold foods and sweets. Read the Nystatin directions, and read Dr. Crook's book again.

6. Make sure you have a history scheduled with the doctor within one to three months after starting your injections. Bring a spouse or tape recorder, plus a pad and pencil, and all of your questions. At this time, you will want to get all of your questions answered and map out a plan of attack on your remaining allergies. You can get a head start on this by asking yourself these questions after the first month:
1. Which symptoms are better?
2. What do I think my progress is due to?

The inhalant injection?
The environmental controls?
The diet?
The Nystatin?
3. Am I off season for my worst allergen?
4. Which symptoms still persist?
5. What haven't I done that I should have done?

If you have done all of the above and still have symptoms, very likely you may have further undiscovered hypersensitivities or biochemical deficiencies.

By properly preparing yourself, you will enable the doctor to effectively help you in your investigation. Do you have hidden chemical sensitivities and need to test to them? Do you have so many food allergies that avoiding is impossible and you need food injections? Do you have hormone sensitivities? Do you need to test to brain neuro- transmitters (histamine, serotonin, dopamine, acetylcholine, heparin, etc.)? Do you have high levels of toxic chemicals in your blood, such as pesticides and chemicals that outgas from furnishings and plastic? Do you have an undiscovered nutritional deficiency and need levels drawn for certain vitamins, minerals, essential fatty acids, amino acids, or digestive enzymes? Do you have a hidden Candida syndrome? Do you need the special preservative-free extracts? Do you need to go to the ecologically safe unit? Do you have a special diagnostic problem which will require further work- up?

If you have too many pressing questions and cannot wait for your history appointment, you can always call and schedule an evaluation with the Allergy Assistant or the doctor. Bring all of your questions, and she will sit down and go over them with you and help you get further ahead.

Remember, the more you read, the more independent you will become. Our goal is to teach you to be as completely in control of your health as possible. We want you to be symptom-free without having to resort to medications. Then you will be able to tackle the world.

Highlights:

Don't forget to go twice a week in bad seasons if your symptoms start. You're spoiled on weekly or bimonthly injections so it's easy to forget that spring and fall are not only the peak pollen seasons, but also the peak mold seasons. So it's a double whammy for most. There is never a dose change for these changes in intervals between injections, and when you're ready simply go back to weekly.

Never extend beyond a weekly interval if you have to take any symptom medication. You should be off all medication and have no symptoms for one year before you go 10 to 14 days between injections.

If you're having pollen problems, schedule testing of individual pollens rather than the mixes. The individual doses, many of which are quite different from the one dose of the mix, work wonders for many and provide a further fine tuning.

Remember, you'll never give your injections a chance to make antibodies until you awaken with no symptoms. To achieve this, you must have a bedroom oasis: no carpets, no open windows, an air cleaner, air conditioner and cotton mattress and pillow covers. Cover and close off forced air heating vents and install an electric hot water baseboard unit. Get rid of unnecessary clutter. Then no matter how bad your exposure is, you can count on restoring your well-being quickly in your oasis.

If your oasis and twice a week injections don't simmer you down in the winter, you know you have other hidden sensitivities. So do the diagnostic rare food diet or see the doctor about testing chemicals or evaluating the Candida program. Check over the total load section to determine what the most likely culprits could be. Maybe you have a medical problem or nutritional deficiency that slows down your healing. Schedule a full physical or just a consultation with the doctor. Perhaps you require an in depth analysis of vitamins, minerals, amino acids or essential fatty acids.

You are always welcome to use medication and there is an abundance of products, but the goal is to give you total control over your health without foreign chemicals or medications. Sometime they are necessary to tide you over while you get sorted out.

Caution: Whenever a foreign substance enters the body, there is always a remote chance, regardless of how infrequently it may happen, of adverse reaction and even death. This includes all materials used for testing and treating. You must be aware of this before starting and willing to accept this risk and its consequences.

ENVIRONMENTAL CONTROLS
(Transcript of Audio Cassette)

Hello, I'm Sherry Rogers. I'm a diplomat of the American Board of Family Practice, a Fellow of the American College of Allergy and Immunology, and a director, Fellow, and diplomat of the Board of the American Academy of Environmental Medicine.

This tape is on the environmental controls. Simply, the more you do, the sooner you'll clear your symptoms and get on with a happy, energetic and productive life. Mildly allergic people are lucky. They take an over-the-counter sinus pill and get immediate relief. By the very fact that you needed tests and injections, you are not among the mildly allergic and you will also need to do some environmental controls. In other words, as well as receiving your injections, you will have to make your environment friendlier and healthier to you. If you don't, not only won't you get as much relief from your symptoms, but you will not decrease the likelihood of your allergies getting worse. The very fact that your allergies have gotten worse means the governor or the control mechanism of your body is damaged and you can, at any moment, develop much worse allergies.

The control cells are called T suppressor cells and can be damaged most frequently by the very chemicals we are surrounded by every moment. This damage may be the primary reason why there are so many more allergic people now than there ever where before.

There are many environments that contribute to the total load of allergic triggers that are presented to your system and obviously the more triggers there are, the greater the likelihood that your regular old hayfever symptoms can now have added to them food or chemical allergies as well.

This is what happened to me and many other people

139

who are what is called universal reactors. I just had chronic snorting and sinusitis with blinding headaches. My headaches were so bad I didn't even dare tell my husband that I thought I had a brain tumor. Injections cleared my symptoms, but I never did environmental controls. Then shortly after my symptoms were cleared I said, "Ha, who needs these injections anymore?" and I quit them prematurely. Within two years I had asthma. I got back on my injections and got my symptoms cleared. Again I kept pushing my system unmercifully and overloading it with all the monotony of a fermented foods diet and a very dusty, moldy environment. We were constantly building and renovating and I was in barns a great deal of the time.

Then I had multiple food, inhalant and chemical sensitivities and reacted to just about everything. Now my environmental controls are, out of need to survive,excellent. When I gave two lectures at the 9th Advanced Course for Physicians Learning Clinical Ecology Techniques, I had to take my own bedding and foods. I also had to take my own water and food. In Chicago, the month prior where I gave three lectures, I had to rent portable oxygen because I was so sensitive at that point to formaldehyde and natural gas.

As you see, when a person becomes sensitized to chemicals, he reacts at levels that don't bother others. No longer is his life ordinary, even though on the outside he seems to be functioning normally. I'm trying to protect you from becoming this bad. If you are this bad, I'm trying to help you stop from getting worse and also to teach you how to heal your immune system so that you can function again in society.

A clue that you are pushing your immune system too hard and a clue that you may indeed become chemically sensitized is if your neutralizing doses are changing frequently and you require retitration. Normally, unless you are bombarded with a heavy pollen overdose, your neutralizing dose will not change and you will not require retitration. Most people are never retitrated once they are tested. But if you are constantly changing or need retitration, you already have a nutritional deficiency, an emotional or environmental overload somewhere with too much dust or mold, or a hidden food or chemical sensitivity (new furniture, carpeting, construction, stored pesticide overload, etc).

Molds That You Eat Add to Your Inhaled Mold Allergies

So to keep your total load down, what can you do on a practical level? First, think of your internal environment. Remember all of those molds you reacted to? As well as breathing molds you also eat them every day in the form of bread which has yeast in it, cheese which has mold, alcohol, vinegar, soy sauce, ketchup, mayonnaise and mustard. Any food that is aged, pickled or fermented uses mold to make it. Many people get stuffy from cheese or get asthma from beer. That's like drinking moldy ragweed because hops are weeds and then they are fermented. So no wonder many get stuffy or wheeze or break out with these things.

An easy way to tell if you're sensitive to mold foods is to do the ferment-free diet. If you need to determine further food intolerances, obtain the food diet tape or read the section that describes diagnostic diets in detail.

Grooming Aids Can Add to Your Allergies

The next environment is your personal environment. Many people will never get rid of burning eyes, nasal congestion or headaches entirely until they get rid of their deodorant, makeup, shampoo, fabric softener or aftershave. The manual contains lists of hypoallergenic substitutes. A good rule is if you can smell it, pitch it. Although there are odorless lipsticks on the market, every one of them except Almay, Ar- Ex, or Marcelle gives me blinding headaches. I

141

don't know what chemical in them is doing it because I would have to test to each of about 20 ingredients. Since I have a tolerable substitute there doesn't seem to be a good reason to undergo that expensive test.

The same thing with deodorants. It's safer to try the ones we have found safe for many people and have listed in the manual. Remember, we're all unique in our sensitivities so there is no one product that's safe for everyone. Watch out for clothes with old smoke and perfume on them or dry cleaning fluid, or even a purse with old perfume in it.

Another problem is permanent press, polyester, wash and wear clothes. These outgas formaldehyde and give sneaky symptoms.

Create An Allergy-Free Bedroom

After the internal and then the personal environmental controls have been satisfied, we move on to the bedroom. This is the single most important place to control because you spend a third of your life here. Since you're just sleeping you don't need more than a bed. The best bedroom has the least in it possible. If you can put your bed in a room and nothing else and keep your old bedroom as a dressing room and a study, that would be ideal. Then you avoid the smokey polyester clothes from the office with dry cleaning fluid, the plastic bags, the shoes and polish, the closet mold, not to mention formaldehyde-laden papers, books and chemicals from printers ink and carbonless copy paper, all of which cause undue fatigue, burning eyes, headaches and more.

If you remember nothing else from this tape, you should remember one fundamental rule. In order to get better, your bedroom should be clear enough that you always awaken with no symptoms. If you awaken with symptoms, you'll never reduce your total load to your system enough to allow your injections to help you.

The simplest and most direct ways to clean up the bedroom environment are:

1. Remove the carpet. A carpet holds 100-1000 times more dust depending on the pile than a flat floor, and a damp cloth removes dust more effectively on flat surfaces.

2. An air cleaner is a must. It covers a host of sins. The electrostatic precipitator is the best for the money and the best one for most people. It costs more initially, but lasts. I've had many for 17 years and it is easily cleaned by slipping the plate unit into the dishwasher or under the shower and there are no other parts to buy for maintenance. It is an excellent way to remove dust and mold. The Spaceguard can be fitted on the furnace itself. The Foust unit, the Airstar 5 and Allermed remove some chemicals as well if you have a concomitant chemical problem. The Resources Section gives sources for all of these and places to rent them on a trial basis.

3. If you're pollen sensitive you need an air conditioner to filter out pollens and give you cool air in the summer time. All of these machines are tax deductible medical expenses and the allergy nurse can give you a prescription for them.

4. If you have forced air, close the vents and cover with aluminum foil and aluminum tape. Put in an electric hot water baseboard unit in your bedroom. If you cannot afford it, at least put several layers of cheesecloth under the grate and change them monthly.

5. The bed itself is a source of dust, mold and mite as well as a tremendous source of formaldehyde. Dial 1-800-JANICES and ask for a free catalog where you can send for cotton mattress covers and box spring covers. You can also, inexpensively, make cotton pillows. For each pillow desired send for 1 lb of cotton (it's about $5), 1 yard of cotton

muslin (about $2) and in three minutes on the sewing machine you can make yourself a $26 cotton pillow for $7. Gradually replace all the rest of the bedding with cotton. We have a file of catalogs for cotton sheets and cotton blankets that you can look through and choose the ones you would like to send for. One of the very best sources for organic ready made pillows that we have found is KB Cotton Pillows, PO Box 57, DeSoto Texas 75115 (phone 214 223-7193).

6. Obvious things like collectibles, dried flowers, and stuffed toys should be in toy boxes, glass, bookcases or anyplace that will cut down on their out-gasing and keep them from collecting dust. Chemically-sensitive people must get rid of all particleboard drawers and headboards. Many people just plain never get better until they are completely out of a house with any natural gas. With your air cleaner going 24 hours a day you should never allow pets in your room. Never bring barn clothes in there and you should keep the door closed at all times. The rest of your house varies with your sensitivities.

Many dust and mold sensitive people are kept perpetually with symptoms because they're triggered at work and then instead of coming home to clear, they get worse sitting in their favorite old chair by the register watching TV. The dust, mold and kapok in the chair, not to mention the mite, and the dust and mold blowing out of the heating duct, plus the cheese and crackers and alcohol they had before dinner load their systems to the brink. Again, cheesecloth over the ducts, the Spaceguard cleaner on the furnace and a cotton throw over the chair achieves wonders, and have an apple before dinner instead.

What About the Rest of the House?

The classic American family room is a shag carpeted room in the basement and it has paneled walls and contains the family dog. Shag holds up to a 1000 times more dust than a flat surface. Basements collect humidity which fosters mold growth. An air cleaner in your favorite room is an investment that will pay for itself many times over in reduced doctor bills for you and your family.

Obviously, putting a mold plate in the bedroom is a must. It's always better to know the unseen enemy and exactly what you're dealing with. The family room or kitchen would also be worth doing as well as work, or anyplace you know that you have symptoms.

Don't forget, some environments produce delayed symptoms. In other words, you won't have symptoms until 4-6 hours after having been in there, or even after having left. Surprisingly, when we culture work environments and home environments, it's usually the homes that are the moldiest and I think it's the chemicals at work that are the culprits there.

Many React Unknowingly to Everyday Chemicals

While we're on the subject of chemicals I'll elaborate on what the chemically-sensitive patient has to do at home. If you just have hayfever and dust and mold allergies, you don't need to worry about this part, but be aware that many times you're the exact type of person who finally gets that one last bit of chemical exposure that turns him into a universal reactor.

Sandy was a 29 year old janitor. He had headache, dizziness, nausea, inability to concentrate, periods of extreme chest pain, palpitations, muscle spasm and muscle weakness. He saw over a dozen specialists and no one knew what he had because he had the classic symptoms of a brand new disease not in one single medical textbook. He's a classic universal reactor with environmentally-induced illness. He is maladapted to the 20th century. If he had switched jobs he might have had a chance at arresting his disease and turning it about. Instead as he got sicker, he spent more time at home in his parents newly paneled, newly carpeted basement with his hobby of acrylic paints. In other words, he did himself in, unintentionally of course.

By the time we saw him he was extremely ill with no place to go to clear. As well, he had a great deal of denial and resented having to make the changes that I spent hours trying to explain. Mainly because they had just spent a lot of money with the new carpet and paneling and now we were telling them this is what was the cause of their son's symptoms.

He was sent to Dallas where, of course, he did clear and face up to the changes needed. It's ironic that as many people get sicker they resist what needs to be done with more vehemence. We end up sending them to the unit where they spend thousands of dollars to learn the same environmental controls that we're telling you now, only they spend three weeks diminishing any psychological blocks to accomplishing these goals in detail.

Nowadays with phenol-free extracts and better environmental controls, fewer people need to go to the unit to clear. But many still need it to prove to themselves that they have an illness that requires very strict environmental controls in order to survive. It's an expensive educational process.

People who go to the units are usually free of symptoms in one to two weeks. They are stripped of all makeup & toiletries, bathed, dressed in a cotton gown washed in spring water and fasted for several days. The air, bedding, and nurses are all as chemically clean as possible. It is this sudden drop in chemical overload that makes their symptoms disappear. It can be accomplished at home, but

146

instead, human nature being what it is , most try the installment plan. They prefer to do a few controls and see if it's the answer. Then they do a few more and see if that's the answer. The problem is we're all like time-bombs waiting to go off. At anytime we can become much worse. So it's important to get our symptoms shut off as quickly as possible.

So if you're chemically-sensitive, you need to do far more than I just mentioned for the dust and mold sensitive person. First, you need a filter in the bedroom that also removes chemicals and you definitely need an old bed with no particleboard headboard. The mattress should be at least 20 years old or preferably made simply out of layers of cotton blankets washed in baking soda over a box spring. If you must use an old mattress, however, and cannot make your own from layers of blankets, then it should be layered with four layers of extra heavy duty aluminum foil, shiny side up, several cotton mattress pads and then cotton mattress covers as well as cotton box spring covers. Cotton pillows, sheets and blankets are a must as well.

As little synthetic material as possible and only natural fibers, wood and metal should be in your environment. No plastic, no particleboard, no polyester, none of the 20th century products that outgas formaldehyde, toluene, pthalates and hydrocarbons—the very things that made you and me sick to begin with. I know several people who became chemically sensitive and it was initially merely triggered by a new foam headboard on the bed.

As stated, natural gas in ovens, stoves, heating systems, water heaters and clothes dryers sometimes are the cause of many people worsening in spite of everything else they do. Some simply never get better unless they are out of the gas. They are not even better if the gas is merely turned off. The pipes need to be removed from the house.

The more newness in the house such as foam insulation, new paneling, new carpeting, new construction, new furniture, the less intolerable it is. These things often are the cause of most people's symptoms, or the house is tightened with insulation or vinyl siding and the chemicals that are in there are raised to new levels because the house does not exchange air with the outside as frequently anymore as it used to. You have to remember that these chemicals in our environment (there are about a 1000 new chemicals introduced every year) were rarely tested on people. We're the first experimental generation and you, with chemical sensitivities, and myself are the strange people reacting to these first. It seems very bizarre to the medical profession because most have still never heard of this disease.

Even when research laboratories do animal studies on these chemicals they rarely combine the chemicals. They test one chemical at a time. They don't combine many chemicals which is the real way that we are exposed to them in our homes and offices.

Also, there are no animal models that can evaluate the worse symptoms of chemical sensitivity, namely headache, dizziness, inability to concentrate, muscle weakness and nausea. As far as animal studies go, remember, thalidomide did not cause phocomelia, or being born without arms and legs in laboratory rats. It only caused it in humans.

A bedroom of the chemically-sensitive person is spartan. It's not an option, it's an essential to survival, as essential as food. It has no carpet, it has an all cotton mattress or a very old one covered with foil and cotton of many layers. Often it has an oxygen tank for clearing out if you are inadvertently exposed that day. In other words, you must create a mini environmental unit or an allergy-free oasis to which you can escape and clear out. The rest of the house, likewise, must be stripped.

Aluminum foil, several layers of old cotton blankets or spreads washed in borax and baking soda make old foam-stuffed couches tolerable. New ones should be traded for old. don't have Tupperware and other plastics in the kitchen. Have a water filter in the kitchen for drinking and in the shower. These can be purchased from the Foust company or N.E.E.D.S..

One engineer is so mentally confused from chlorine fumes he hardly knows his way to work after shaving.

There are patients you can meet at the HEAL meetings who can go into your home and tell you what's bad and what should go. HEAL stands for Human Ecology Action League and is a national organization of chemical victims working to make their lives better in any way possible. They have a newsletter with articles and tips. We have a local chapter that meets the third Tuesday of every month at 7:00-9:00 p.m. and it's open to all. Generally, every other meeting features a speaker in harmony with ecologic wellness. The alternate meetings feature information and pearls that are shared with members and there is time for an open forum and for members to get to meet one another and gain from their experiences. There's a local newsletter and tape of speakers are available. Call Mrs. Eleanor Hathaway at (315) 492-0091 for information.

None of us achieves our environmental controls overnight, but the speed is proportional to how sick you are. In order to survive many of us have had to strip rooms or buy a $30 cotton cot from the Army surplus store and sleep outdoors, or live in as safe a room as possible until we got our bedroom oasis cleared. Washing walls with borax and baking soda helps and is a necessary monthly chore for many of us to reduce the mold. Periodic assessment of success can be ascertained by exposing a mold plate.

The car is a problem because none of them are airtight and you're surrounded by exhaust fumes, dust and mold from the air conditioning and heating system, not to mention vinyl seats with foam cushions and gasoline, heated oils, carbon monoxide, formaldehyde and sulfur dioxide from the engine.

Some people carry oxygen, others use the charcoal

149

mask that you can get in the office. Foust and Allermed make air cleaners for cars. Don't forget your good old cheesecloth for around the vents, taped with aluminum low out-gasing tape.

Baking soda nasal drops every hour or two hours serve as a great prophylaxis for many. The recipe is 1 tsp. of Arm & Hammer baking soda in 1/2 cup of your tolerated water. Put it in a dropper bottle that you can get at any pharmacy and tip your head back and generously fill each nostril with a few drops whenever you are suddenly going to be in an environment where you want to try to block out the chemical fumes such as traffic, shopping malls, concerts, airports, or indoor sports and games.

What To Do When Overloaded

Now what happens when you do get overloaded? Several things help us more quickly recover. Depending upon the circumstances, the substance and the dose, it may take days or weeks to recover from an environmental overload. Try to get cleared out as quickly as possible so that it lasts only hours at the most. First, fast. Do not eat a thing until your reaction has cleared as you'll only continue to overload an already overloaded system when you eat. Start with 1/2 -2 tsp. buffered sago palm vitamin C which you can get from N.E.E.D.S. (see Resources). Use it every 1-2 hours with at least a quart of water each time. It's a great detoxifier. Some people require very high levels as obtainable only with I.V. or rectal administration. Third, go to your oasis and go on your oxygen if you have some. If your oasis isn't as good as it should be yet, you have no other choice, go outdoors. Others need to see the doctor to get on a customized prescription of nutrients to rev up the detoxification system. And when you get more advanced, you'll learn in our additional books ways to reduce exposure reactions from days to minutes!

Carol spent a year outdoors in Buffalo because she had nowhere else to go while they had their urea formaldehyde foam-insulated house on the market. She slept outdoors until she got too cold and came indoors around 3 a.m. to suffer excruciating headaches that she got from her parent's gas heat and then back outdoors she would go.

Fifth, some people do better with Alka-Seltzer (in gold foil without aspirin), or 4-6 Alka-Aid tablets (N.E.E.D.S.) or Tri-Salts at the first sign of a reaction, then start on their vitamin C., GSH, taurine, selenium, vitamins A, E, and zinc, etc. also help heal ailing immune systems. Others can use their neutralizing doses of mediators that we have found to get them out of trouble. More on these later.

As you can see, this disease entails constant vigilance. Diana was sent to us as a severe asthmatic constantly exhausted and on all medications including prednisone. Within a month, we found she was sensitive to many dusts, molds, foods and chemicals. She did a super job of stripping her bedroom and was feeling years younger since she no longer required any medication. This was within two months of starting. Months later she thought she would put in a nice tile floor in her bedroom to cover the bare floor that was under the new carpet she had removed. She wisely slept with a piece of the tile by her pillow for a few nights to be sure she would tolerate it. She put in the tile and ended up in the hospital with severe asthma. She had forgotten to test the glue. She had to have the tile as well as the subflooring ripped out in order to get rid of the glue smell that so dramatically triggered her asthma.

Linda was sent from New York City and had seen 20 specialists for severe leg phlebitis. She was a universal reactor we found and cleared her for the first time ever in three months. However, on one of her return visits, she stayed in a new section of the Hilton and the next morning her phlebitis was flared from the formaldehyde. It was only a question of getting her a different room and it simmered down.

Tamara had severe rheumatoid arthritis diagnosed by three rheumatologists in Buffalo. She could be neutralized out of pain and stiffness within three minutes with phenol. For her, environmental controls were as tough as for any of us and at first seemed impossible to her and her English professor husband. She managed to gradually do them, because like all of us, she had no choice. Where did she get her phenol sensitivity from? The new furniture, the carpeting, the upholstery, the gas heat and the brand new room that they added in the last five years. Also, they lived near the thruway.

Obviously, it wasn't easy for her to change her environment, but as I say when you're bad enough you have no choice. Because they cannot quickly sell or change the gas heat, the safest and fastest route for her was to create a safe room out of the garage. It can be scrubbed, studs and plasterboard can make new walls, a stone floor above a fiberglass insulated false-floor, electric heat, Foust air cleaner and a cotton cot can get her started fast.

There are some excellent books that will show you how to create products nd a home that is less chemically contaminated. One is Natalie Golas' **Coping with Your Allergies,** another is Debra Lynn Dadd's, **Non-Toxic and Natural**. Books that will help you if you plan on renovating or building a new house for a chemically sensitive person are Bruce Small's **Sunnyhill,** and Rousseaux and Rea's **Your Home, Your Health and Your Well-Being**. Of course, good general books on the spectrum of chemical sensitivity are Theron Randolph's **An Alternative Approach to Allergy,** and Dr. Doris Rapp's **Is This Your Child?**

The Total Load Boat

When you come here, you can think of yourself as in a boat with a hole in it. You are sinking. The boat is loaded with boxes that symbolize your total load. One box has inhalants and new molds in it, another has foods, another chemicals, another Candida, and so forth. You know you have to keep throwing boxes overboard until you raise the height of the boat above the location of it's leak. For some the leak is just below the gunwhales or side and they don't need to do anything or discard boxes. The further down toward the keel the leak is, the more you have to throw out.

Often someone will ask, "How much do I have to do?" The answer is you unload your boat until you stop taking in water and sinking. You keep cleaning up your environment until your symptoms turn off. Human nature being what it is, they still wail, "How soon do I have to do all of this?" Just as soon as you want to feel better. Again, it boils down to **how sick are you of being sick and how soon do you want to feel better?** Then you have your answer.

As you unload your boat, an interesting thing happens. You are able to begin to separate what symptoms are caused by which triggers. For example, a typical finding is after a couple of months of the dust-mold-pollen injections, I'll hear, "I'm not nearly as tired anymore and my congestion and burning eyes are markedly improved. When I fasted I found out my muscle cramps and spasms were gone. When I covered my bed I didn't awaken with back ache and my fuzzy head was due to sugar and wheat." Before they could never tell what was due to what because they were just too overloaded with symptoms.

Some people are so bad, their leak is on the keel and they need to go to dry dock—or an environmental control unit. A poor man's unit would be to fast and go to the mountains or the ocean. For people this bad it's the only way. The boat is too badly damaged and must be pulled from the water for patching.

Mental Stages of E.I.

Many of us with E.I. go through the very same stages of people dying of cancer, as written about by Dr. Elizabeth Kubler-Ross in **On Death and Dying**. The stages of **denial, anger, bargaining, depression** and **acceptance** could last any amount of time, could come in any order, or be skipped entirely. As you recall, the first stage was often **denial**. People may hang out in this stage as I did for years, constantly reassuring themselves, "Well, I'm not bad enough to go through all that! I don't need to rotate—I can feel just as good not rotating".

I was politely sitting in my seat at a Watertown Good Samaritan Hospital staff meeting waiting to be introduced as their main speaker. Just as they were finishing their business meeting an old doc came in and sat behind me, loaded with after-shave. I was too embarrassed to move and decided to tough it out. I made the wrong decision because when I got up to speak, I was as I say, on automatic pilot the first five minutes of my lecture. I knew I was talking and I knew whatever I was saying was not particularly coherent by the puzzled looks on the doctors' faces. I had brain fog from the after-shave. I couldn't think or hear my own voice. I had no idea what I was saying. In 5-10 minutes I cleared out and proceeded with my lecture, but they never referred me a patient! I could have spared myself this agony by not being embarrassed to protect myself when I knew I was going to be in trouble.

If someone had walked into the room coughing with a big sign on his chest reading, "I have contagious TB", you bet a stampede would have occurred. It would have been easier to explain why I had moved, rather than grin and bear it, and come to the platform as a babbling idiot who was no longer capable of explaining.

154

For some there's the stage of **anger** and this one is particularly detrimental to them and the field of clinical ecology or environmental medicine, for they make enemies and instill a bad feeling toward chemical victims. They're the ones who bitch and moan loudly in public places about the things that bother them instead of quietly approaching the restaurant manager with a smile on their faces and advising him they can't return until he has a no smoking section.

Why even entering the world, most babies are already born with detectable levels of pthalates or plasticizers in their blood. It comes from the plastics in I.V. bags and plastic I.V. tubing that was attached to the mothers before delivery. Studies have been done on people who just popped into the drycleaner to pick up clothes. Four hours later they still had measurable blood levels of perchloroethylene as opposed to negative levels in people who hadn't gone. Gassing up your car gives measurable benzene levels, and drinking from a styrofoam cup gives measurable Styrene levels.

So if one is exquisitely chemically sensitive, he is bound to be bombarded frequently without warning. Sure it's enough to make anyone angry, but we can't afford to further damage our immune systems with harmful emotions. Indeed, attitude and emotions have a strong bearing on the total health of the immune system.

A study done on the T cells of men whose wives were in their last months of life with breast cancer, revealed their T cells were at a very unhealthy level. They were ripe for developing cancer, allergies or infection because the guardians of their immune systems were out of commission.

Depression is a phase I find most difficult to deal with. It usually doesn't occur or exists for only a short time if there is a knowledgeable and loving and supportive spouse. Depression robs one of any remaining energy that they could have used to implement their environmental controls and drives away anyone who attempts to help them. Therefore, it's self-defeating in every way and there is no good derived from this stage.

At least in denial you learn that if you go off the diet you feel lousy again. In the anger stage you learn that to most effectively get what you want, you must first work through your anger privately.

Bargaining is a stage we can instantly recognize and have a good laugh on ourselves. But **depression**—it gives us nothing. Perhaps here would be an excellent spot to pick up a paperback copy of Norman Cousins' **Anatomy of An Illness**, or Dr. Anthony Sattilaro's **Recalled By Life**, and see how two men healed incurable conditions.

Or better yet get Beata Bishop's **My Triumph Over Cancer** (Keats Publishing, New Canaan, CT) or read "Rising to the Challenge" in this manual.

The bottom line to depression is the feeling of hopelessness—the giving up because there is nothing more that can be done. Part of the depression can be made worse by your food or chemcial reactions or undiagnosed vitamin deficiencies for sure, but a part of it stems from feeling overwhelmed by the enormity of the task ahead of you. In this case, as Alan Lakein said in his time management book, **How to Get Control of Your Time and Your Life**, when faced with a huge task, whittle away at it:

Conquer small portions at a time and your accomplishments will accumulate.

Don't see the environmental controls as a huge insurmontable task, but chip away daily or weekly at small parts of it until there is nothing left.

In terms of feeling **hopeless**, environmental illness as opposed to many cancers does have hope and lots of it. That's why we have our HEAL groups as proof that you can be devastatingly ill and make a comeback. What a comeback—now they are helping others who were in the same sinking boat. As well, advances are made so rapidly that each year brings new answers and solutions.

Conventional or drug-oriented medicine treats the patient as a child and does everything for him. It frequently has to pronounce, "There's no treatment for this", or "You've just got to learn to live with it", or "It's all in your head".

Health-oriented environmental medicine recognizes the patient has a brain and untapped powers to heal himself. Going one step further, it also realizes that prevention is far more helpful than waiting for the machinery to break down. Responsibility for health is where it belongs—with the possessor.

Environmental medicine goes even further and teaches the victim that all hope lies within himself and is proportional to his involvement. The unjust part is that some have much more to do than others, but few are hopeless. For some we do not have the total answer yet, but the field moves so fast that people we couldn't help three months ago may have answers now. The things I've seen improve that I myself had labeled impossible or hopeless have taught me now that I can never ever be sure of that designation, for there's no reliability in it. Once "hopeless" meets up with the marriage of an ecologic education and a dedicated victim who is eager to take reponsibility for his health and find what it takes to get better, it finds there is no match.

Bargaining is a really easy stage to recognize. "Well if I don't have this on the diet, can I have that?" "If I get rid of this, do I have to get rid of that?" How do I know?!! I don't have a crystal ball and I don't have my head under water to be able to see how far down toward the keel your leak is.

Fourth is **acceptance**, the stage we all strive for. To be able to shlep our foods about in a graceful manner and radiate health and happiness because we are at peace with ourselves and know how to keep ourselves that way. Sure, there are always constant incidents of chemical overload that we didn't ask for, but rather than wasting precious

157

emotions on getting angry, we waste no time in getting cleared out.

So we have a newer approach to allergy, necessitated by newer environmental causes. Our management is necessarily highly comprehensive to match the scope of our exposures. The devastating nature of the symptoms demands immediate action, which ironically enough places proportionately more of a burden on the sicker people. That is, the worse you feel, the more you have to do to feel better; but you're often two sick to do many of the things you need to. This is where you will only be successful if you have a knowledgeable and loving spouse. If not, the environmental unit in Dallas is more feasible.

Beatrice is an example of what all of this is about. She became highly sensitized and she had to go to the unit. She came home on portable oxygen and even came to the office with portable oxygen. She cleaned up her environment to the letter and was healed. It takes us time to get sick or sensitized and it takes us months to heal. It also requires constant vigilance.

Begin Simply

As soon as you are able to tolerate it, try to take 1 Oxy-Guard, Oxyperm, or Anti-Ox and 1 Multi-Mineral two times a day with meals. Schedule a special time with the doctor to get a nutritional program started. Supplements are available at N.E.E.D.S. (1-800-634-1380).

Remember, a clean environment is mandatory or no amount of injections and vitamins can turn the disease around. Many people have tried through multiple injections and vitamins to clear a chemical sensitivity and every single one of them found that until they removed that last relevent chemical from their environment they never got better, and many of them continued to get worse while they were being triggered.

The concept of total load is paramount to conquering this disease. I've gone to medical meetings for years where plagued with sickness, I was nearly unable to deliver my lectures. I remember the first medical meeting I went to in 10 years where I didn't get depressed and didn't get severe back pain from all the chemicals. I had finally arrived and I hadn't even had to rent oxygen. I kept going over and over what I had done trying to figure out what one thing I had done that led to this wonderful state of events that I never thought I would see. Was it my injections? Was it my foil and cotton bedding that I took with me? Was it the food and the water I carted with me? Was it large does of vitamin C every few hours? Was it my other vitamins, the new zinc picolinate, the magnesium, manganese, and molybdenum, the Efamol, the Nizoral, my meditation, my prayers? Then I realized it was all of these. I had finally gotten my total load down to a point where I could again function in a chemically overloaded environment for a temporary amount of time without devastating symptoms. Also, at that time my husband and I had been constantly working at lowering the total chemical load in our work and home environments, which is essential if the immune system is going to heal.

So always remember that the total load is the most important concept to licking this disease and that the first step to getting your allergies under control is to awaken with no symptoms.

HORRAY FOR YOU! You just mastered one of the most boring but essential parts of allergy.

SECTION II
CANDIDA

Remember all those molds we just discussed that can masquerade as just about any symptom? Remember they are everywhere in the air. So to help the immune system heal in spite of a constant on-slaught, we do cultures to see which ones are present. We teach you to make a super mold-free bedroom oasis with no carpeting, air cleaner, cotton bedding, closed heat ducts, avoidance of cross reactive mold derived foods, and getting allergy injections to help build protective antibodies against many types of fungi or molds.

If all of this were not enough, there's one particular mold (or fungus, or yeast, or whatever you prefer to call it) that lives inside the body. In fact, it lives in most animals and humans, and normally does not cause any harm—until this century, that is. You see, this century marks the use of potent antibiotics, birth control pills, and prednisone; and these all foster the overgrowth of Candida.

When you have a strep throat, the penicillin prescribed by your doctor doesn't make a beeline from the stomach through the bloodstream to the throat area; it goes to every cell in your body. It goes to your heart, liver, lungs, and your little toe. In the intestine where this yeast, Candida albicans lives, it is in happy balance with many types of bacteria whose function it is to digest or rot our food so that it is broken down into a form easily absorbed across the intestinal wall into the blood stream. Bacteria are killed by penicillin, but fungi or yeasts, are resistant to it. So the yeast, Candida, has a heyday and grows unhindered. This often does not cause a problem, but is some, there is diarrhea, itchy rectum, groin rash, or vaginitis caused by the overgrowth of Candida.

With the passage of time, some people become allergic to the very yeast they are "wearing" in their guts, or they can also react adversely to the chemical products (acetaldehyde) that the yeast makes. This allergy can be the sneakiest one you've ever experienced. The target organ can be anything imaginable. When the target organ is the brain, as it most commonly is, there is terrific exhaustion, unwarranted depression, inability to concentrate and make decisions, and crying for no reason. Many feel like they are on the outside of themselves helplessly watching this nightmare. Allow me to give you some examples that will show you why this lowly one-celled yeast gets a whole chapter devoted to it.

Anne was a dentist's wife in her early twenties and had been depressed for no reason for ten years. She got even worse mid-cycle until her period came, which means she was bad daily, but half the month she was horrid! Within one month of the yeast program, she became her bubbly happy self and has remained that way for the last ten years.

Don owned a company. He had severe depression, exhaustion, headaches, chronic sinusitis, diarrhea, acne of his face and back, and a groin rash. To look at him he seemed like an average good looking young man, but his life and body were falling apart. After two weeks on the Candida program he described himself as feeling 90 percent improved and better than he had ever remembered feeling.

Seymour was a 51 year old engineer who had been to several medical centers for evaluation of twelve years of weakness and fatigue. As with the rest of these people, he was told it must all be in his head and he'd have to learn to live with it. But after one month of the Candida program, he described himself as 100 percent clear.

So we have a yeast that is in everybody that can grow rampant. Some systems can become sensitive to it or it's metabolic products and it can mimic anything. It can mimic other mold allergies, food allergies, chemical allergies, or nutritional deficiencies.

Randy was a New York City attorney who had a simple hernia operation. Within a month, he had severe headaches and was reacting to foods and chemicals that had never before bothered him. He would burst into tears in a shopping mall. Smoke and perfumes would leave him so dizzy and confused he would have to be helped away from them. On the Candida program he was 90 percent improved.

There is no foolproof diagnostic test for Candida at present. Probably the closest test is the questionnaire in Dr. William Crook's book, **The Yeast Connection**. This book should be devoured by anyone who has the Candida hypersensitivity syndrome. Candida can mimic everything, and the test is actually how you do on the program.

Fortunately, the program is harmless. It consists of a diet temporarily devoid of yeast derived foods (bread, cheese, alcohol, mayonnaise, vinegar, ketchup, mustard, processed foods) and all sweets. Nystatin pure powder with 4 million units per teaspoon is used to reduce the yeast level in the get, and that too is pretty harmless since it is not even absorbed. It just goes down the hatch and out with the stool, never getting into the blood stream.

No one has a crystal ball; we don't know if 20% of your problems are due to pollens, dust, and airborne molds and, 30% is due to Candida, and 40% is due to chemical allergies, and 10% is due to hidden mineral deficiencies. Or maybe 70% of your symptoms are caused by Candida, and 20% by airborne molds. Each person is highly unique. We do know, however, that unless we treat the molds by injection we have very little success in clearing and keeping clear your symptoms. That's why we do the mold plate, environmental controls, and get you tested right away so that you can begin your injections.

For example, one man who owns a printing company and had ulcerative colitis was able to clear his bowel and keep it clear of symptoms as long as he took his pollen/

dust/mold injections and avoided a few foods.

A seventeen year old teenager totally cleared severe cystic acne of his face on the injections alone. It recurs when he goes off and clears when he goes back on.

A New York City orthopedic surgeon had severe weakness and life-threatening cardiac arrhythmias. With the mold injections, his symptoms are 90% improved.

So the logical next step after inhalant testing has been to rule out whether Candida plays a role in your symptoms, if it seems indicated by your history. Most people want to rule it out right away. Others are better off waiting until another stage.

If we gave you Nystatin at your first visit, you're one who's history suggests you may feel markedly improved shortly if you start on the program. To do so, read all Dr. Crook's book, or all this chapter before starting the Nystatin. Then you will minimize any adverse symptoms. We rarely see the severe die off symptoms when people follow our yeast program. When controversy exists, follow our plan as opposed to Dr. Crook's.

Candida is one of many yeasts that can proliferate in the body. Antibiotic use, birth control pills, prednisone, pregnancy and high sugar or junk food diets are the commonest triggers of it's growth.

Some people's immune systems are seriously overburdened by a simple yeast infection or they become "allergic" or sensitive to the toxin (acetaldehyde) produced by the yeast and manifest limitless diagnosis defying symptoms. Sometimes the symptoms are tremendous abdominal gas, bloating, body swelling, rashes, tiredness, irritability, depression, and mood swings for no apparent reason. Sometimes the symptoms exactly mimic those of food or chemical hypersensitivity with headache, dizziness, inability to concentrate, nausea, muscle weakness and flu-like achiness. There are many other symptoms.

A yeast-free, sugar-free diet and Nystatin powder

are the beginning of the program to irradicate the Candida problem. There is no way to diagnose Candida hypersensitivity except to do the Candida eradication program and see what symptoms disappear. The blood test is not yet perfected, but if your symptoms warrant a high degree of suspicion for the problem, you should check out the possibility through a therapeutic trial of ferment-free, sugar-free diet and Nystatin.

Do not confuse your Candida hypersensitivity with the only Candida condition non-ecology physicians are aware of called Candidiasis. Candidiasis usually is fatal and usually only occurs in someone who is immunosuppressed such as on chemotherapy for cancer or someone with AIDS. Their body's defenses are so weak, they are overwhelmed with Candida infection. They are no necessarily hypersensitive to it and do not have the same symptoms. Candida hypersensitivity is not fatal, but most Candidiasis is.

A mold-free diet means absolutely no breads, rolls, cheeses, sour cream, alcohols (wine, beer, liquors), mayonnaise, vinegar, ketchup, mustard, salad dressing, pickles, aged salamies, coffee, tea, chocolate, etc. See ferment or yeast food list in the Food Section.

For a sugar-free diet exclude all cane sugar, honey, maple syrup, chocolate, corn syrup, dates, very sweet fruits, and artificial sugars.

For very yeast sensitive people, all milk and wheat products should be avoided with this diet as well as acids like citrus and tomatos. So what do you really have left when you've eliminated all your favorite daily staples? You're so smart! You're right, the rare-food diet, also known as the diagnostic diet or lazy-bones diet in the next chapter. You have tons of meats, fowl, fish, vegetables, nuts, unlimited water and limited fruits (one or two a day, depending on your tolerance).

164

Nystatin

Nystatin is an anti-fungal agent which works against a wide variety of yeast and yeast-like fungi. It is obtained from a bacterium named Streptomyces noursei. Nystatin is virtually non-toxic and non-sensitizing, and is well tolerated by all age groups even on prolonged administration. Large oral doses have occasionally produced diarrhea, gastrointestinal distress, nausea and vomiting. It is not absorbed from the gut into the blood stream, so quite high levels can be safely used.

Standard Adult Dose for Nystatin Powder:

1/4 tsp. 3 times a day for starters. Some need to start with 1/8 tsp. or even a "dot" on the end of a toothpick. If it provokes symptoms, clean out the bowel with 1 tbs. milk of magnesia or take a Fleets enema.

Build-up Dose:

Day 1-3, take 1/4 tsp three times a day
Day 4-6, take 1/2 tsp. three times a day
Day 7-9, take one tsp. three times a day

If a dot dose is not tolerated, put it in a cup of water and have one drop. An hour later 2 drops, an hour later 3 drops, etc, and get to as high a titrated dose as tolerated and stay at that dose for a few days before attempting to raise it.

Or, buy Capricin at N.E.E.D.S.. It's less potent, but more easily tolerated by many so that they can lower the Candida efficiently to be able to switch back to Nystatin eventually and tolerate it.

Stop anywhere along the way that you feel best and

stay on as long as you need at whatever your best dose is. If no difference at all is noted in 4 weeks, then stop it. If you felt worse with it, this is actually a good sign but too high a dose, so back down and build up gradually to the tolerated dose.

For a white tongue, put powder from finger on tongue and hold it until saliva is absorbed. Then smear paste on tongue and leave, it will be washed away with swallowing. Repeat every 2-3 hours.

Procedure for Mixing Powder:

Mix 1/4 tsp. in 1/4 cup water. Hold this mouthful for 1-2 minutes, then swallow. If you fail to hold it, yeast in the mouth won't be killed. But after one week of this, you can just swallow it. You no longer have to hold it because the oral yeast will have been killed. Coating the tongue works faster and many think it is easier to do.

Procedure for Mixing Douching Solution:

Mix 1 tbsp. Nystatin powder per 1/2 quart of douching solution. Use daily x 1 week. Nystatin vaginal tablets are available in the office, but culture your vagina first on a mold plate. Simply swipe a finger, after a shower, high in vagina behind cervix and smear this on plate. We'll notify you if Candida grows.

Helpful Hints:

1. Nystatin is more effective in an acid medium. Avoid taking salts or antacids within one hour of Nystatin dosage.

2. Nystatin powder should be stored in an air-tight container, either in a refrigerator or cooled area. When traveling it's better to carry it unrefrigerated than not have it at all.

3. Nystatin may alter treatment end points, so usually we will not test Candida and add it to your injections until you have had Nystatin for one to three months. With treatment your skin dose frequently changes, and this will cause you to react to your injections adversely if Candida is in them. So we usually wait until the "history" to schedule a time to test it and add it in. Then it is usually stable after that.

4. If you desire a refill, please stop at the desk. Nystatin is a prescription drug. Many specialty pharmacies will mail Nystatin to you.

5. To be most effective, you should be getting your other mold injections and be on a mold-free diet (no alcohol, bread, cheese, vinegar, mayonnaise, etc.). Also, a sugar-free diet is necessary since yeasts thrive on sugar. Most people can tolerate a small portion of fruit once a day, others cannot until their yeast is gone. Some take months to get rid of theirs.

Everything about Candida hypersensitivity is highly individual and it is recommended that you read the most complete treatise on it, **The Yeast Connection** by William Crook. 1-800-835-1157 toll free phone order number, or purchase from our office. See Dr. Rogers if you need a trial of Nizoral or Diflucan, etc..

If you have a reaction or worsening of symptoms on Nystatin, you may be reacting to the massive release of toxins from many organisms being killed at once, called a die-off reaction. So back way down on the dose, clean out the bowel and start your yeast-free, sugar-free diet for a week before you go to dot doses or dot doses diluted in water or Capricin. Also, start taking Vital-Dophilus or Vital Plex or Probinate-C to restore the normal bacterial gut flora which will compete with Candida. Every day or week try to gradually increase your dose to the top tolerated. Rarely do we see people need more than one teaspoon three times a day.

There are many forms of acidophilus, the good bacteria that is put back in the bowel to compete with Candida. It is important that the best and most viable form be used, for if you use any old brand, the organisms are usually dead, and the Candida will not have adequate competition and will shortly regrow in large numbers again. Klaire Laboratories has the straight Lactobacillus acidophilus in the form of Vital Dophilus and they have another form with three beneficial colon organisms to compete with the yeast called Vital-Plex. Both are good. Some people have a stomach acid that destroys the acidophilus, so Probinate-C is used.

As with other symptoms of E.I., the Candida problem may respond quickly and dramatically to Nystatin or it may take months. After a month on Nystatin you may want to assess Nizoral or ketoconazole, the systemic anti-fungal. As opposed to Nystatin, this does enter the blood stream, goes to every tissue including the brain and can have serious side effects such as liver toxicity. For this reason, anyone taking it must have a blood test to check liver function every six weeks. If there's any suggestion of toxicity we merely stop the drug. You might ask, why would anyone even consider taking it then? The answer is to get better. You see for some it's the missing factor in their total load. Hundreds of patients are on it, we have never seen a serious problem form it because we are super cautious.

Pamela was only 23 and had seen several orthopedists for severe back pain. All the drugs they prescribed made her feel worse. She was also plagued by depression and a host of other miserable systems. These were all very strange to her because she had been an exceedingly bright, bubbly, energetic young woman. She became an ace student of environmental medicine and helped us discover her many pollen, mold and chemical sensitivities. Nizoral, however, provided the missing link. Every time she tried to cut back she got worse so we let her stay on for a year. Her liver enzymes were always okay so we had no worry.

Finally after a year I suggested she cut back to half a pill a day. Within four days she was bedridden with severe back pain and depression. It took four more days of a whole pill a day to return her to her normal pain-free, bubbly, bright self. But when we finally convinced her to test foods to lower her load, she no longer needed the Nizoral.

Angie had severe steroid-dependent asthma and the pulmonologist told her that there was nothing more he could do for her. On a ferment-free diet and Nystatin, she has no asthma and no drugs. Another gal no longer has extremely dry eyes and mouth called Sjogren's syndrome. An attorney no longer had incapacitating headache and extreme exhaustion. A physician lowered his sensitivity to chemicals by treating his yeast.

Many nail and skin diseases that have resisted all treatments are really occult fungal infections. You can be highly suspicious of Candida when you can date the onset of symptoms. There is usually a period of preceding antibiotics, pregnancies, birth control pills, surgery, dental work, or massive chemical exposure (reconstruction or new purchases). Others have a chronic form that has gradually gotten worse very slowly over the years, but originated with childhood antibiotics for ear and throat infections.

We have observed an interesting phenomenon about the Candida problem. If we merely put someone on the yeast-free, sugar-free diet, very few have dramatic improvement. But if we cover the total load with dust-mold-Candida injections, the diet, Nystatin, and often Nizoral as well, dramatic lessening of chemical sensitivity occurs in many. Frequently, the person is 80% better in the first two weeks. But many have reported that the slightest indiscretion consisting of ingestion of sugars or mold foods causes recurrence of their old symptoms. This is in spite of following the rest of the program. I don't know if this means we are feeding the yeasts and making them grow rapidly again or stimulating symptoms with yeast antigen. For some, testing to foods gives them far better tolerance of foods. Persistent vulnerability to Candida simply means your total load is still too high.

Also, many people never can fast or stick to their diet because of cravings. Once you kill the yeast and restore the acidophilus balance, fasting becomes a breeze. I used to eat every three hours. If I missed, I would break out in a sweat, feel faint and would kill for sweets. An Armenian friend would send enough baklava pastries for a small army and I would hoard them in the kitchen, polishing them off in a few hours. I never shared them with the staff. I did a number of disgusting things that only people with horrendous yeast overgrowth can even dream up. As you will learn later, there are many other causes of cravings and ravenous insatiable appetite.

Once you kill your yeast, you will find fasting is a breeze, and when you feel weak, you have a few raw, infrequently eaten veggies like kohlrabi, cabbage, carrots and go back to your fast. Obviously, it is no longer a true fast, but nevertheless an excellent way to detoxify, clear, lose weight, and discover what foods, vitamins, or chemicals you are now reacting to. In other words, it's periodically necessary to sort things out in terms of your having developed any new sensitivities. We aren't dead you know, and living things are in a constant state of change.

It's Not Just Candida

So here we have a generation of people who are so uniquely individual in that they can obtain relief from severe headaches with injections of histamine or serotonin or chlorine or Candida or foods or chemicals such as formaldehyde, and they have to make drastic changes in their eating habits as well as their environmental load of chemicals. The key is individuality.

As Dr. Sidney Baker of New Haven, Connecticut said (at the 1982 Advanced Seminar for Clinical Ecology at Banff), "Mother Nature gave us one assignment and that was to be unique. To be different from any other living individual; and medicine has failed to accept this basic premise because it is easier to assume we are not. People all have their own particular, very delicate and precise balance of nutrients and if your balance is imperfect, it's like standing on one foot. It's easier for me to push you over. You're not quite playing with a full deck, and then when a certain genetic predisposition and chemical or food overload presents itself, we have ecologic illness manifesting as a variety of symptoms". In environmental medicine or ecology we try to restore this balance to the system and create harmony with the environment.

Add to that the fact that we now have a totally different gene pool than we used, comprised of generations of people who would not be here were it not for sophisticated medical technology. And this change in the gene pool changes the way in which we respond to noxious agents. The way in which we transmit disease has changed with increased speed of travel and the change in social morals. Baffling immunodeficiencies such as AIDS appear in epidemic proportions. Extreme chemical overloading of our universe has produced staggering varieties of cancer. I shouldn't see a 31 year old girl with malignant breast cancer. But I did. Our milieux has changed abruptly and many human organisms cannot adapt well to these assaults.

So all bets are off that something as simple as pneumoccocal infection will present the same way in the future as it has in the past. It too could present as environmental illness. Likewise, Candida, was once thought of as a seemingly simple and innocuous yeast infection, now causes death in people who are immunosuppressed. People who are on cancer chemotherapy, for example, do not have a normal mechanism for fighting disease, they can become overwhelmed by a simple Candida infection and even die. Likewise, people with immune dysfunction triggered by a mal-adaptation to environmental chemicals and toxins, can react differently to Candida, with serious symptoms.

At a recent Candida Symposium in Dallas, attended by many of the top thinkers around the country, they shared their fund of knowledge in order to show the broad base of symptomatology this one organism alone could produce. In treating it, they had been able to clear a variety of symptoms and diseases. Of course, any of these symptoms or diseases could have been accompanied by chemical and food sensitivities. Candida symptoms can mimic just about anything. The treatment of Candida: mold injections, low carbohydrate diet, a low yeast diet, (see mold-derived foods list in Food Allergy Chapter) and extraordinarily large doses of raw Nystatin powder—1 million units per 1/4 tsp. The powder is obtained from the chemical manufacturer so that the coating with a dozen chemicals, the corn-derived excipient, and the high cost of the tablets are avoided. It is in a concentrated form so higher doses can be used less expensively.

The dose is highly individualized since a person can get markedly worse if it's not done correctly. Nystatin is an anti-Candida, anti-fungal agent, that is not absorbed from the intestine, and is one of those rare drugs that has had no serious side effects seen. Some require ketoconazole, a systemic anti-fungal that can have potent serious side effects in the form of liver damage. Because we are so cautious to check the liver every six weeks, hundreds of patients have seen no serious problem. Among the patients thus tested, marked relief has been seen in depression, total lethargy, uterine hemorrhaging, vaginitis, urethritis, prostatitis, psoriasis, chronic otitis, rheumatoid arthritis, multiple sclerosis, chronic diarrhea and cramps, Crohn's disease, intense sugar cravings, migraines, constipation, lymphoma, colitis, distorted thought process, myasthenia gravis, auto-immune hemolytic anemia, Sjogren's syndrome, systemic lupus, emotional and behavioral problems, urticaria, Sarcoidosis, and other dermatoses.

These people were already on an allergy program and the addition of this anti-Candida program provided the last boost that markedly brought relief. They could turn on and off the symptoms by varying the program. Others with diseases seemingly unrelated to Candida such as psoriasis of skin or nails had marked improvement or total clearing after a course of Nizoral. Of course, there are many people with these same conditions who had absolutely no difference with Nystatin. That's what is meant by the tremendous individual variation. Your best bet is to give yourself every benefit of doubt and do a therapeutic trial.

As Dr. Baker says, "We need a fresh look at disease. We need to look at illness and see the individuality of people". There's new information appearing, for example, that perhaps the reason some people become sensitive is that their cell membranes do not have the normal integrity to keep chemicals out. Linseed or flax oil replacement and primrose or borage oil have provided missing essential fatty acids for cell membrane integrity in many.

You might wonder how a yeast like Candida can have become so important and so prevalent and be responsible for such a wide variety of symptoms. First, you must remember that yeasts in general are extremely prevalent in the air. Out studies in the **Annals of Allergy** of molds in the air, shed invariably the number one most prevalent organism was not a bacteria, not one of the common molds to which allergists test, but they were yeasts. Sometimes, you can even smell a yeast when you're in a crowd of people. It's that rather fishy odor, and of course, there is increasingly more yeast in the air we breath because we're in retrofited or tightened, poorly ventilated buildings.

Yeast is present in all of our bodies, it colonizes the 23 feet of bowel, and we even augment it with antibiotics. We also eat yeast, in the form of ferments or in mold-derived foods. Yeast thrives on sugar and we sure do like our soft drinks, candies, desserts, and excess fruits. It also is probably an even more prevalent antigen even in the foods that we eat because of the treatment with antibiotics. Eggs, chicken, pork, beef, and even many vegetables and fruits are fed, dusted or sprayed with antibiotics to control bacterial overgrowth. More money is spent on prophylactic antibiotics for livestock each year than for people.

Some people with arthritis, migraines, eczema, sinusitis or psoriasis can be totally clear with just elimination of all yeast-containing foods for several weeks. When they get clear, all they need to do to prove whether Candida is involved is to challenge themselves and reintroduce these foods to the diet and see what happens.

Bear in mind that the intestinal tract has the surface area of a tennis court. In other words, it's the largest surface area of the body that is exposed to antigens, our food chain, and because of the tremendous use of antibiotic shifts the flora toward yeast so that we are surrounded by and ingesting more yeast all the time. This leaves the intestinal tract exposed to this antigen much more prevalently than in the past, and once present in the bowel the yeast grows and multiples.

Janice recently had two years of face, hand and feet swelling. She also had daily headaches. Friends didn't recognize her because of the swelling. She had seen seven doctors without so much as a diagnosis. She was markedly clear in four weeks on a yeast-free diet and on injections of molds which she was found to be allergic.

174

The commonest symptoms that are cleared or simmered down with a yeast-free, sugar-free diet and Nystatin are fatigue, depression, general allergies, asthma, eczema, diarrhea, poor memory, and constipation. The only way one knows if they have a Candida problem is to jump in and try the treatment. There is no sure-fire diagnostic test yet, although, many are being developed and marketed. I have tried several of the diagnostic antigen blood tests for Candida on people with known Candida and they came out negative, but they cleared on a therapeutic trial. The questionnaire in "The Yeast Connection" is the closest guide you'll find to helping you decide whether you should try it.

R.T. was a 39 year old businessman whose world was falling apart and try as he might he couldn't stop it. He was depressed, exhausted, couldn't force himself to send out bills to clients who owed him tens of thousands of dollars. He had headaches nearly daily, chronic sinus problems (which were the very least of his concern), inability to concentrate and a failing memory. He had seen innumerable specialists with a record number of blood tests, x-rays, drugs and finally the eventual and predictable recommendation to see a psychiatrist.

In spite of his years of symptoms, we had him 90% better in three days and it was all uphill improvement thereafter.

On exam, he had the classic white furry tongue, acne- like lesions on his back, shoulders and buttocks, and a groin rash. You're getting so smart! You guessed what dozens of doctors never heard of—Candida hypersensitivity syndrome.

The primary factor which predisposes to developing the Candida Hypersensitivity Syndrome (C.H.S.) is having an antibiotic. For people who have felt lousy all of their lives, it stems form childhood. Often, we can ask "When do you last remember feeling well?" When they can give us a

175

date, they can invariably recall a preceding antibiotic.

Other factors which predispose are a high sugar or junk food diet, oral contraceptives, pregnancy, prednisone, diabetes, anesthesia, immunosuppressant drugs, or undiagnosed nutritional deficiencies.

Common signs that these people display are a white coated tongue, sweet cravings, vaginitis, heartburn, constipation, groin rash, hives, adult acne, ridged nails or rectal itching. However, they are usually too sick to complain of these minor things because their lives are being devastated by one or more of the classic symptoms: depression, exhaustion, headaches, severe sinusitis, muscle or joint pain, abdominal pain, failing memory and concentration, mental spaciness, autoimmune disease, psoriasis, or food and/or chemical hypersensitivity. Some women have recurrent vaginitis, pelvic infections, endometrosis, infertility, or cystitis. Men have impotence, prostatitis, and infertility.

Key questions to ask yourself are "when was I last well? When was my last antibiotic? When did I start getting worse? What antibiotic or new exposure was commensurate with that?"

The goal is to reduce the body yeast and then do all in your power to keep from feeding those yeasts that never leave, so they never again get the upper hand. The program outlined will be for someone who is super sensitive to yeast and does not want to trigger a duplication of all their worst symptoms by killing off vast numbers of toxin-releasing organisms at once. They have to carefully ease on into treatment and almost sneak up on the yeasts. Others are not as sensitive and can accelerate the course to their own choosing.

The commonest cause for failure or inability to become totally clear, in spite of being yeast sensitive, is failure to address the total load. In other words, you most likely need to test to yeasts and molds, and have injections to these to increase your tolerance. Also, you need to

address your food and chemical sensitivities and environmental controls. Nutritional deficiencies must be taken
care of, in particular, borage oil (one tsp.), flax oil (1-3 tsp/
day), Anti-Ox (3 a day), and Super B Complex, yeast free (2
a day), and Multi-Min (3 a day) are a good start. Others
need to see the doctor for a special program of
proacanthocyanidins, manganese, magnesium, molybdenum, taurine and liquid A-C-E, selenium, and whatever
was found to be low on blood testing

The best supplementation is by assessing what your
levels of vitamins and minerals are at first. Then I know
what areas of your biochemistry are the most stressed.
There are certain key nutrients that are required in higher
amounts when Candida is present. Each person has an
over-riding, exquisitely unique biochemistry.

As you improve, it's important to schedule to see the
doctor, so the rest of your program can be tailor made.
Frequently, your Candida dose is changed so retitration of
it is needed. If you have done all of the above and two
months of the total program produces no difference, you
most likely do not have a Candida problem. But beware, the
commonest reason for failure or for regression after you
have gotten well is cheating on the diet. Many people have
experience marked worsening of symptoms when they
cheat the diet. The mount of cheating necessary is individual, but is not tolerated until you are totally healed.
Sometimes, the person does not produce enough gastric
acid to keep Candida down, but that can be assessed and
treated.

If you have the disease, you need a thorough education in the intricacies of it's management. The most thorough treatise is Dr. Crook's book, **The Yeast Connection**.
Answers not found in Crook's or here, reflect that no one
knows the answer and it's a matter of individual trial and
error.

How does yeast damage our systems? There are a

dozen mechanisms, found in **TIRED OR TOXIC?** and **WELLNESS AGAINST ALL ODDS**. Dr. Truss has found that the yeasts produce acetaldehyde. This disrupts cell membrane function, collagen production, synapses, the citric acid cycle, and alters protein synthesis. It also is a close cousin to formaldehyde and is also one of the breakdown products of chemicals. Hence, all the crazy symptoms as well as chemical intolerance.

Red cell membranes have to be very soft and pliable to squeeze through small capillaries. When acetaldehyde damages and stiffens them, they can't scrunch up to squeeze into to small capillaries in the hands, feet, or brain. Hence, cold extremities, irritability, and mood swings.

Dr. Horrobin also found a marked change in amino acid and fatty acid synthesis (major components of cell walls). Dr. Iwata found a substance produced that suppresses T cells (the same cells that are depressed E.I., which Candida mimics, interestingly). Dr. Witkin found lymphocytes are paralyzed by a serum factor produced by Candida. In spite of this, it remains disputed.

It's ironic that at this writing, conventional allergists limit their practices to IgE reactions. This antibody attaches to cell membranes that govern the release of histamine. What they are not aware of (and yet you the "unknowledgeable" patient is) is that allergy is really any adverse reaction that occurs. So chemical, food, Candida, toxicity reactions, and nutritional deficiencies all have a role in affecting cell chemistry and are within the scope of allergy. Candida, for example, puts out chemicals that derange cell membrane function. Fifty percent of the adult populous is already deficient in the enzyme D6D so they can't make gamma linolenic acid, crucial to the function of cell membranes and need borage oil.

Studies show that Candida can cause disrupted cell function. There are over 4,000 references in the literature on how chemicals disrupt cell function. With deficient knowl-

178

edge of these mechanisms, doubters have the audacity to say there is no such thing as a chemical or Candida sensitivity reaction!

In 1986 the American Academy of Allergy stated there was no such thing as the Candida Hypersensitivity Syndrome. They assessed their 3,000 plus members $100 each for a nationwide television, radio, and magazine campaign to stamp out and discredit Candida and ecology. Wouldn't it have been grand it they had used that money to learn more about it? As they stated in the spring A.C.A. newsletter, these treatments were cutting into their share of the allergy marketplace! For Pete's sake, come to our courses and learn!

Candida can mimic everything from undiagnosable symptoms to autoimmune disorders or even food and chemical allergies, it behooves anyone suffering to rule it out.

If you still have many questions about the Candida problem, after reading the following pages; or if it still seems too much for you, then you are right. It is and you should not explore it.

Many people have allergy or hypersensitivity to airborne molds. Molds can cause any symptom imaginable, from depression to diarrhea. We can skin test to these molds, culture them from the environment, learn how to reduce their numbers in their environment, and even receive injections to reduce one's sensitivity and resultant symptoms.

Many people are also sensitive to far more elusive sources of molds the ones they ingest daily and the ones that are actually growing in their bodies.

Remember that molds are synonymous with fungus, yeast, or ferments, so they are found in foods that utilize the fermentation, aging, or pickling process. They are found in foods that contain yeasts. In other words; breads, cheeses, alcohols, vinegars, salad dressing, mayonnaise, ketchup, mustard, chocolate, coffee, and tea are common sources of mold antigens, as are most processed foods with chemicals such as citric acid. Many other acids, enzymes, added B and E vitamins, stabilizers, anti-oxidants, and flavorings are commonly the by-products of fungal fermentation. They're used in fruit drinks and sodas, and nearly all packaged foods.

About the only foods that do not contain mold antigens are fresh vegetables, beans, meats, some fruits and seeds and nuts, chicken, fish, and glass bottled water.

Besides ingesting yeast, we can also grow them in our bodies. Common places are in the mouth a white tongue often has yeast on it, a normal tongue is pink. It is also found under the nails (ridged, peeling, thickened, or deformed nails), in the vagina (itchy vaginal discharge), and on the skin (tiny pinpoint water blisters along the fingers, redness, burning, itching, or peeling the hands, feet, groin, or under the breasts).

The commonest place for yeast to be hiding though,

is in the gut. The surface area of the gut is comparable to a tennis court, so if a gut is colonized by yeast it can have a tremendous impact on the victim and cause a multitude of symptoms. Burning esophagitis or burning stomach, frequent indigestion, much bad smelling gas, cramps, bloating, diarrhea, but more commonly constipation and rectal itching are common complaints.

More importantly, yeast can cause other symptoms by merely adding to the total antigenic or allergic overload to any one system. We find this out easily by observing what symptoms disappear when only the yeast is treated. Treatment of yeast has resulted in dramatic improvement in a variety of symptoms. Common ones are chronic unwarranted depression, extreme fatigue, severe PMS, dizziness, weakness, inability to concentrate, headaches, migraine, sinusitis, asthma, colitis, endometriosis, hypoglycemia, prostatitis, constipation, and arthritis. Surprisingly, in many people, it dramatically reduces the total load so that they are markedly less sensitive to foods or chemicals than previously.

Why does yeast grow in the body? First, it is a normal inhabitant of the bowel. When something disturbs that normal balance between yeast and all the other bugs or microbes in the gut, the yeast can grow in enormous amounts. The host can even become allergic to it. Antibiotics, prednisone, pregnancies, birth control pills, anesthetics, ulcer medicines, and high junk food and sugar diets are all capable of disrupting this balance.

Some people develop overgrowth of yeast very slowly. Maybe they haven't had an antibiotic since they were a child and now have yeast symptoms as an adult. In other people, the yeast takes over very quickly. They're the ones who can date the exact onset of their downfall and undiagnosable symptoms to after the delivery of a baby, after a root canal, after years of tetracycline for acne, or after a particular hospitalization or auto accident.

So here we have a yeast that is a normal inhabitant in all bodies, but is capable of growing out of control and/or fostering an allergic response toward it. On top of that, it can manifest itself as just abut any symptom one can think of, but more commonly as vague, nebulous, life robbing symptoms such as depression and extreme exhaustion.

There are, as yet, no reliable diagnostic test to determine whether someone is a yeast victim. Many people are potential candidates, especially those with any form of allergy. Therefore, we're left with only one alternative, a therapeutic trial. Simply put, it means try the treatment. If it works, you'll know you have it because you'll be demonstrably better. If it doesn't work, you probably didn't have it.

Now, in some people, the treatment can be worse than the disease, unless it's done carefully. You see, if you have millions of organisms in the gut that you're allergic to, and they are metabolizing and producing a set amount of toxins daily, your symptoms will be fairly constant. If we kill off thousands of these yeasts suddenly, you'll release more toxins all at once than you normally do, and you're liable to have a severe flare of your worst symptoms. This is called a die off reaction. To avoid this, we have worked out a pyramid program with a stepwise, cumulative approach to the diagnosis and treatment of yeast related diseases.

1. The first step and base of the pyramid for eliminating yeast overgrowth is to stop antibiotics, sugars, mold foods, or ferments. In other words, nothing with sugar, corn syrup, maple sugar, date sugar, beet sugar, honey, cakes, pies, cookies, processed or packaged foods, chocolate, soft drinks, or tonic water, etc. No bread, cheese, alcohol, vinegar, coffee, or tea, etc.

If you suspect you're a universal reactor or just plain are able to handle a more restricted diet and want to rule out other commonly hidden food allergies, eliminate all milk and wheat products as well. Some people are just not creative enough to restrict as much as they need and so be it. There is much written in the food chapter and other references. However, what these people want is someone to plan, chop, cook, and serve it, and then they'd probably cheat in between meals! All of us with important food allergies had to do it the hard way, and unless you're independently wealthy, you will too. If you can't figure out a way, then I guess you're either not sick enough or resourceful enough.

2. The next stage is to empty out the bowel with 1-2 tablespoons of milk of magnesia. This will help to eliminate a severe die off. If you can fast one to two days as well, it will speed you along. It's not absolutely vital to do this stage. If you're at the other end of the spectrum where you're very sick or anticipate a severe die off, then do it.

Each step or stage of the pyramid can last a few days to a few weeks depending on the severity of anticipated die off reaction. If you do not anticipate one, the stages can be short. If you are suspicious of a potential one, it's smarter to spend a week or longer at each step to evaluate it and get the maximum control of your yeast with each stage before moving on the next stage.

3. Next, start half a teaspoon of Vital-Plex or Vital Dophilus, twice a day. This contains the most viable form of acidophilus we can find to restore the normal bugs to the bowel flora. Many forms of acidophilus found in health food stores are dead and contain no viable organisms. Once the flora has been restored, these helpful bowel bacteria can now compete with the yeast and help keep you clear longer once you are off your treatment. It can also be used as a vaginal douche to normalize vaginal flora.

4. The next stage, and remember they are additive, you do

not drop any stages but keep adding new ones, is Nystatin. Nystatin is a pure powder with about a million units of activity per quarter teaspoon. It is purchased from American Cyanamid.

Other pharmacies do carry Lederle's Nystatin or Mycostatin powder, which is for topical use only, it is only 50,000 units and is cut with talc powder. It is not to be ingested, and it is too weak a strength with other chemical additives that may be deleterious to our patients. Only knowledgeable people know this, and many doctors and pharmacists will insist they have what you want. You can always compare with the product available through NE.E.D.S.. When in doubt, get some of this Nystatin and smell it, feel it, dissolve it in water, and taste it raw on the tongue. In other words, compare with all your senses because if you are wrong, you may never clear Candida.

For the average person, start with 1/8 teaspoon of Nystatin dissolved in water with meals, twice a day. Gradually, every other day or slower, increase that amount to 1/4 teaspoon twice a day, in water, with meals, and then to one teaspoon twice a day. The amount of water can be a cup or a glass. Most do not require higher doses. One teaspoon twice a day is a good top dose for many to stay at. You can go higher to 1-2 teaspoons, three times a day, if you need. If at any time you get nausea, diarrhea, or any other symptom, merely back off to a better dose for you. Stay at this lower dose as many days or weeks as you need before proceeding to try a higher dose again. Maybe you will never be able to tolerate a higher dose. You can only do what you can do.

If you're very sensitive, dissolve a dot dose (the amount on the end of a toothpick) in a glass of water. Have one teaspoon of the mixture twice a day, the next day two teaspoons of the mixture twice a day, the next day three teaspoons twice a day until you finally get up to a full dot dose twice a day, then proceed to two dots, etc.

Remember, any symptoms other than nausea are probably due to die off, since Nystatin is not absorbed. It only goes in the mouth and out with the stool. It does not go into the blood stream. It can only kill yeast in the gut. Nystatin depends on stomach acid to be effective, so always have it with meals. Also, Tagamet (cimetadine), Zantac (ranitidine) and antacids will decrease it's effectiveness. These agents that decrease stomach acid, also foster the growth of yeast in the stomach.

5. Stay on your top dose of Nystatin with the diet and Vital Dophilus for one to three months.

6. Then begin the descending side of the pyramid. Cut down the Nystatin, cut it out. Cut out the acidophilus and then resume your normal diet. The purpose of the descending side is to be able to determine what you need to do to stay as clear of symptoms as you have become at the top of the pyramid. Obviously, if after a month at the top of the pyramid you have no change, you don't have yeast problems and you can stop it all at once.

I However, if any symptom is better, or you just plain have more energy or an enhanced feeling of well being, you want to see if you need to stay on Nystatin or stay on the diet to keep that feeling. So you drop the Nystatin for a week and see how you feel. Then drop the Vital Dophilus for a week and evaluate, then drop the diet.

7. Through all of this, I assume you already are receiving allergy injections for your molds, since in many this program won't work unless they are receiving allergy injections. Another point we have found, is a person can do the diet alone and have no change, he can do the Nystatin alone and have no change, he can do the diet and Nystatin and have marked relief of the symptoms, but cheating on the diet with the slightest amount of sweets or mold foods and

many have reported recurrence of all his prior symptoms. Therefore, since we can only go so long being good, it's better to have one junk day a week, for example on the weekend, rather than a little cheating every day. Then you know if you caused your symptoms and you know what to do to get them straightened around again. I repeat: Nystatin doesn't do a darn thing for most if you're not also on the yeast-free, sugar-free diet.

8. Occasionally the last block in the pyramid is a trial of Nizoral (ketoconazole). This is a systemic anti-fungal. It goes into all tissues but the bowel, which is why you still must be on your pyramid with the diet and Nystatin to facilitate it's effectiveness. Some people never get rid of yeast until they use this drug for a while. Because it has the potential for being toxic to the liver, we are overly cautious and demand a blood test for the liver enzymes every six weeks when someone is on the drug. In this way, we've been able to avoid anyone ever having a problem from it. If you are on the drug and want a refill because your symptoms get worse without it, you must schedule a blood test before you will receive another prescription. If you're from out of town, you can send a copy of your recent liver profile or chemical profile with your self-addressed, stamped envelope and request another prescription. You need to also state what symptoms the Nizoral relieves and what happens when you go off of it.

Also, for the first two weeks of a Nizoral trial, all women should be on a vaginal anti-fungal medication. This will make sense when you realize you must kill as much yeast at one time as possible. Nizoral only goes into the tissues, but cavities such as the vagina and intestines do not get a high enough level. Hence, a three-pronged approach is needed vaginal, bowel, and tissue.

Nystatin powder does not require blood tests and can be mailed to patients whenever they need more.

It's important to bear in mind that for many of us the yeast problem is only one part of the total load on our immune systems, but we never know how important a part it will play. It is crucial to keep our load as good as possible, including the correct nutrients to enable our chemistry to perform at it's maximum.

Some people, like myself, never cleared Candida until we used Nizoral and corrected multiple severe nutritional deficiencies. If you suspect you are among these, schedule to see the doctor to get it straightened out. If you improved on the program, be sure to schedule testing to Candida and get it added in to your injections.

Here are some examples of what we have seen. O.J. was told by the pulmonary specialist, "We've done all we can for you." She was on prednisone and all asthma drugs. On the Candida program she had no asthma and needed no medication within two weeks. She got worse if she went off.

R.D. had severe weakness and chemical hypersensitivity. On Nystatin he had marked relief. Off Nystatin his symptoms recurred.

T.T. had multiple food and chemical intolerances. On the Candida program, she reduced her sensitivity by 50 percent. She could then tolerate many foods and chemicals that prior caused reactions. When she cheated on the diet, all her symptoms recurred.

A.J. said, "I can stand the twenty years of rheumatoid arthritis, but not the last three years of Sjogren's syndrome" extremely dry eyes requiring artificial tears every fifteen minutes). With mold and food shots she no longer needed pain medicine for her arthritis. With the Candida program, she no longer needed the artificial tears.

D.M. was on the maximum pyramid program for over a year. Every time we tried to take her off Nizoral and reduce the dosage, she as bedridden in four days with severe recurrence of her back pain and depression.

Most people with severe yeast problems have so

many symptoms that they have never told all of them to one doctor at once for fear of being labeled neurotic or hypochondriacal. Multiple symptoms are the rule, but examples of single symptoms are easier to comprehend.

There are so many symptoms we have seen to vanish with the Candida program, that I find it mind boggling. But when you remember that antibiotics are one of the most potent and frequently used tools in medicine, you can understand how we've created this monster. For many people, when they were first searching for the answers to their symptoms, they would go from specialist to specialist. When all else failed, they were prescribed an antibiotic. This just added fuel to the fire.

Weight loss usually accompanies the program. If you do not need to reduce your weight, do not lose weight. Eat plenty of beans, squash with cold pressed oils, nuts, and meats. You may even have to have yeast-free rice bread available at the organic bakery, On The Rise, Walton Street, Syracuse. You may have to bend a little and cheat on some other foods.

If you have trouble losing too much weight and have not chosen to schedule a diet consultation with the doctor or allergy assistant, then stop the diet and the yeast program.

If you are overweight, as you kill off your yeast, you will find you no longer have your hypoglycemia and cravings. Once you cheat again, you encourage the growth of more yeast and they start screaming for sweets. So don't feed them and they will go away leaving you not hungry and able to shed those unwanted pounds, as well as do a little detoxifying in the process.

If you have any questions, save it for your visit and devour **The Yeast Connection**, by William Crook available at our office. You must become an active partner in your disease control and read. If you have a question, it probably doesn't have an answer or we would have put it in here. We have heard every question.

The most resented questions are "Can I eat such and such?" Dr. Crook outlines all the foods so well that if you still can't decide, don't eat it. When you're better, then you can find the answer out for yourself. Eat it and see if you tolerate it. One exception I take with Dr. Crook, however, is that I would have you eat one or two fruits a day, as soon as you feel improved If it makes you worse, then hold off a few more months.

For individual problems, see the doctor. There is a great deal of individual variation that can only be worked out one on one. Don't forget much of the diagnosis of this disease is by trial.

Keep a careful diary, because at your periodic meetings with the doctor, she will want to know the highlights of your Candida program. Predominantly, what adverse affect did you have, how did you conquer it, what symptoms are better on the program, what do you have to do to maintain a clear state? Also, a dairy is useful for many reasons. It helps you see what you did wrong as you get more sophisticated. When you're feeling great there's a tremendous tendency to cheat. If you get worse, it's very handy to read exactly what you were doing when you felt great.

If you absolutely cannot take the Nystatin, it comes in capsules. But remember they don't dissolve in the esophagus so you don't kill yeast there. You may have a chronic source of it that never gets cleared. If you still can't even take a small sip from a dot dose in eight ounces of water, you could try Capricin (Neesby), available at N.E.E.D.S.. Use the directions on the bottle. We know it is tolerated by many, but effectiveness is highly individual. Some people take Mycostatin tablets, but we tend to frown on these because they have over a dozen chemicals, including a chocolate covering, and are not tolerated by highly chemically sensitive people. Also, each tablet is only half a million units, whereas a teaspoon of the powder is four million units or eight times stronger. The tablets are much more expensive also, and do not kill yeast above the stomach.

The doctor is always appreciative of notes from patients describing what the Candida program did for them. Eventually, we will have a diagnostic test, and this information may be useful in developing one. It is truly fascinating that a disease such as this could be the by-product of man's medical technology.

The Most Frequently Asked Questions:

1. What's the worst thing that can happen? The worst thing, because Nystatin is not even absorbed, is that you will have nausea or diarrhea from the powder, or severe depression from die-off. Some people have been suicidal because their die- off depression was so severe. This, of course, is only possible if suicidal feelings were one of your symptoms to begin with. So, as with anything that you try, have someone responsible with you to be of help.

2. What about Taheebo tea? It helps some. But be sure yours comes for Argentina. The ones from Brazil are reportedly contaminated with Agent Orange and dead not living bark is harvested.

3. What's the best that can happen? The best that can happen is that you will be rid of a host of symptoms that have plagued you for years and have been elusive sources of discomfort, not creating positive blood tests, x-rays, or any diagnostic phenomenon that doctors are accustomed to relying on.

4. How can I tell if anything is happening? What do I look for? If you can't tell anything is happening, just spend two to seven days at each stage and move on to the next stage.

When people have a response to the Candida program, it is quite dramatic and noticeable. You will know if you are getting better. If you have any doubt at any stage, back off a little or stay there a little longer. If you notice nothing, progress forward. Maybe you don't even have it. But it certainly won't hurt to kill off over abundant yeasts in a diagnostic trial. Who knows...it may prevent you from getting the yeast problem.

5. Does it mean that I can have absolutely no fruit? That's a tough one to live with, so we often have to modify it according to each individual person. If you have a severe yeast problem, you should not have any fruit until you can determine how good can you feel on the program. Then go ahead and put in the fruit and find out if it causes any problems. If you're underweight, go ahead and have bananas daily for some bulk. Sometimes apples are tolerated as well as pears, but not real sweet things such as grapes, citrus and watermelon. If not having fruit is a tremendous problem for you for any reason, then you will have to modify it and have a fruit each day. Also, how strict you need to be with carbohydrates will need to be is individually determined once you get better. I prefer not to have anyone on a high meat diet. So the sooner you can tolerate grains, beans, potatoes, Jerusalem artichokes, and other starches and some fruits, the more balanced your diet will be.

6. Which diet should I be on? The rare food diet or Dr. Crook's diet? Actually, both of them are quite similar. All we basically want to find out is how good can you feel when you're not on the foods you normally eat? Obviously, you normally eat sweets and ferments, so they're out on Crook's diet and to go one step further, if you go on a truly rare food diet, you will find even more information out about yourself. It's simply a fact that some people cannot do as much

as others, so if you can only handle the sugar-free, ferment-free diet, fine. It's better than no diet.

7. How strict should I be? This question is probably asked more often than any other question. The fact is that our crystal ball is broken this week. No one knows exactly how allergic you are. Therefore, we don't know how perfect you have to be. If we knew how allergic you were and could say, "Oh, don't worry, you can have all the fruit you want on the diet," then we wouldn't have to do the diet in the first place. Obviously, the more strict you are on the diet the more information you will get out of it, the more hidden food sensitivities you will uncover.

Remember, the five nails in their shoe analogy. If you go on the diet half way and are not better, you're going to assume you don't have food allergies. Likewise, if you do the diet only half way you're never going to know whether or not you really had severe yeast or Candida problems since many people never clear until they strictly adhere to the diet. How much you can do is an individual thing. How much you should do is to go all the way.

We realize, however, many people for a variety of reasons are not capable of this. We can all only do the best job that we can do. We can't be angry at you for having done the best job you can do. We can be angry for asking a lame question such as, How strict should I be?

8. How long do I stay at any particular stage? Until you are sure you have a good idea of what that stage is all about. Is it producing any change in you? Are you stable? Are you getting better? Are you getting better every day? Is it producing nothing? When you're sure you have the answer, then go to the next stage.

9. Is it necessary to taper off the Nystatin? No, if you had no difference on Nystatin and the whole pyramid, then just

abruptly stop it and resume your normal life.

10. Does Nystatin come in a pill form? The pill form of Nystatin in the pharmacy has over a dozen chemicals and it is only half a million units. It is not acceptable for people with chemical problems and capsules don't treat esophageal Candida.

11. Should I stop the Nystatin when I'm on the Nizoral? Absolutely not. Nizoral goes into the tissues, Nystatin goes into the bowel. We need to kill yeast in both places (as well as the vagina).

12. How high should I go with the Nystatin? One teaspoon three times a day is probably maximum. If there's no difference after that I wouldn't go higher. In fact, I would recommend for most people to only go to one teaspoon twice a day and if after a month there's no difference, I would discontinue it. Only occasionally people might have to go to two teaspoons. That would be someone who knows they absolutely have a yeast problem, but they're not better on one teaspoon two or three times a day.

13. How long should I stay at the top dose? If after three or four weeks there is no difference, then obviously you should discontinue it. If, on the other hand, you feel great why be in a hurry to go off? But you can see what the effect of going off is at any time.

14. Can I cut back once I get established? Sure. Once you have established how good you can be, then you can cut back to see what the minimum of medication is that is required to keep you that good.

15. Are there special foods and vitamins? Yes, there are many ancillary treatments that have helped. Biotin 300

mcq, and a tablespoon of flax oil, and 250 mg pantothenic acid 3 times a day are just some of many. The doctor would have to help you individualize these.

16. Should my spouse take Nystatin? I don't know without examining your spouse. We do not know if it is sexually transmitted. I cannot treat people that I have not examined.

17. Do mold plates show Candida? Yes, sometimes we culture people's tongues, the vaginas, their stools, their sputum, skin, and their bedroom. We occasionally grow Candida from all of these sources.

18. What if I can't do the diet? Then probably it's a waste of time to do the Nystatin. Usually, if someone is on sugars and ferments, they will not improve even though they're on Nystatin, but you might be an exception.

19. What if my symptoms are worse? You're probably having a die off. You should cut back your dose to a point where the symptoms are not occurring. Stay there for a few days or weeks until you're able to advance the dose. Some can't do so until after a year. Some people have too high a total load and should see the doctor.

20. What should I do if I'm worried and want to call the office? Reread Crook's book and all of this material so that you have a very firm grasp. All the information is at your fingertips. The urge to "reach out and touch someone" is frowned upon. Several hundred people call our office each day. Therefore, we are very appreciative of patients who learn a great deal about their illnesses by reading and do not ask questions that we have gone to a great deal of effort to explain in this manual and in the books provided. We have expended untold time and effort to keep track of all of the questions asked over the years and to make sure they are

answered in here. If it's not in here, it's because it's too individual. You have to find it out for yourself in your own system or schedule to see the doctor. The nurses cannot possibly be all things to all people. There's an epidemic of E.I. and not enough trained physicians. We have two choices. Treat only a few people and coddle them and not require that they exert much on their part, or help a larger number by taking those interested in having an active part in their illness and wellness.

Some people do not have the make-up to be treated here and require spoon feeding. We are not a spoon feeding office. The doctor is equipped to answer any questions you throw her way, but the nursing staff are at various levels of training. Therefore, many of your questions cannot be answered by them and that's precisely why we've made such exhaustive printed materials available. Where can we get more trained staff when there isn't even a medical school course to train doctors in this new field? This takes time and tremendous effort and we're paddling as fast as we can. Bring your questions with you to each appointment so you can get them answered.

This is a different medical specialty because it requires total re-education of a patient. Some do not belong here because they want to be led, not educated. They want to have it easy. Others are eager to help themselves to wellness. They read and re-read, keep diaries, come to the doctor prepared with notes and have a sense of organization and control over their lives and health. We want to help them all, but because there are so many ill people from all over the country, we can only help those motivated enough to read and study all the material first.

The most important reason for insisting you become totally involved in your care is that studies of cancer and chronic illness victims show that those who take an active part in their treatment and feel they have control over getting well have a much higher success rate than passive people. Commitment, control and optimistic acceptance of the challenge are wellness ingredients. Wellness in the face of seemingly insurmountable odds is what this is all about.

Warning

Candida albicans is the commonest species of yeast to affect people. It is killed in the gut by Nystatin pure powder. Candida tropicalis is the second commonest Candida yeast form and is resistant to Nystatin. In other words, it is not affected by it at all. Therefore, you can see that after several months of Nystatin, one could conceivably kill off sufficient numbers of Candida albicans and develop an overgrowth of Candida tropicalis that does not respond to treatment.

Therefore, if you need Nystatin beyond three to six months, you had best stop it and schedule to see the doctor. There are other ways to handle your problem. In the meantime, you want to look at the obvious and make sure you have not skimped on the following:

1. Soak 15 minutes and wash fresh vegetables and fruits in Clorox, one tsp to a quart of water. Rinse in water or Shaklee Basic H. Diluted peroxide can also be used but requires individual instruction.

2. Drink no prepared fruit juices, only freshly made.

3. Eat no gross sugars and processed foods or mold foods.

4. Be sure you've recolonized the bowel with Vital Dophilus; see if you need a digestive, HCI, or pancreatin.

5. Be sure your nutrient program contains vitamins A, C, E, selenium, magnesium, and zinc, manganese, chromium, and more. Avoid supplements derived from yeast or con-

taining sugars, mold antigens or cysteine. The latter can cause a more aggressive form of Candida to grow.

6. Consider garlic, sorbic acid and other adjuncts written in Crook's. Sorbic acid douches have helped many cases of resistant vaginitis (from Ecologic Formulas in Resource Section).

7. Get a mold plate and do a stool or vaginal culture for Candida, or check your tongue and culture it if it is white or furry.

To do a stool culture, you take a fresh warm piece of stool. Put one level tsp of it (use table knife and tsp.) in one teaspoon of water. Gently mash to dissolve stool evenly. Then take 1/4 tsp of this liquid and pour it into the petri dish. Seal, label, incubate 1-2 weeks on top of refrigerator, then take the plate plus a prescription from us (instructions for the lab) to your local lab.

8. See the doctor. Your total load is too high and you are missing something in your biochemistry to allow you to proceed to a higher stage of wellness.

Many people are afraid to take future antibiotics for fear of reactivating their Candida. We can always treat your yeast providing you're not dead because you failed to take penicillin for your pneumonia. The fact is, there are still antibiotic indications we can't live without. Just stop your Nystatin and Nizoral while on the antibiotics, get cured, and restart the Candida treatment after. Again, we have to maintain a logical balance of what's best for the body in the short and long-term scheme of things.

There is tremendous research going on and new things are being learned all the while. Check back yearly to see what may pertain to you. Also, this may be a surprise to many, but once you get clear the diet is not a lifetime sentence. You can eat goodies and sweets with no symptoms. The trick is most of us wouldn't do it everyday, more like once or twice a week.

I taught the Candida course in 1986 as part of the advanced course for physicians learning clinical ecology techniques. I was glad to see a host of new books come out on Candida. Top among them were, **Back to Health. A Comprehensive Medical and Nutritional Yeast Control Program** by Dennis Remmington, M.D. and Barbara Higa, R.D. (Vitality House International, Inc., 3707 North Canyon Road #8C, Provo, Utah 84064) and **The Yeast Syndrome** by John Trowbridge, M.D. and Morton Walker (Bantam Books, Inc., 414 East Golf Road, Des Plaines, IL 60016).

Even though you will gain a few tidbits from each, you run the risk of further confusion because many contradictions exist. This merely further points up the individuality and the reason we cannot spoon feed you as in other medical specialties. Our apparent "toughness" is a necessity in the first medical specialty that demands total patient education for patient success. This idea is so foreign to medicine that insurance companies will frequently not pay one dime for educational materials or time spent. For failing to do so, they show that they believe that patient education is totally irrelevant to getting better (or patients are not teachable!). Only drugs and surgery are reimbursed and sometimes psychotherapy.

Highlights

Candida is thought of as a harmless yeast that causes vaginitis. In a compromised host such as someone with AIDS or on cancer chemotherapy, it can kill by massive infection. Very few physicians are aware of the Candida Hypersensitivity Syndrome as discovered and described by Dr. Orion Truss and popularized by Dr. William Crook.

The Candida Hypersensitivity Syndrome (C.H.S.) can mimic any disease. Commonly it mimics chemical hypersensitivity in that chemicals previously unnoticed now cause symptoms. The commonest C.H.S. symptoms are depression and exhaustion for no known reason and chronic bowel problems. The second commonest symptom is that difficult to describe, foggy head. C.H.S. can also keep chemical hypersensitivity and PMS from getting better by acting as a major (hidden) load to the total system.

The worst victims have to do everything: the yeast-sugar-milk-wheat-free diet, have food, mold and Candida injections, lower their chemical overload, especially at home and work, use Nystatin, Vital Dophilus, and Nizoral to get better (universal reactors).

The commonest causes are birth control pills, antibiotics (sometimes they were 20 years ago in childhood), prednisone, general or local anesthesia, a high sugar or junk food diet.

WARNING: Do not stay on Nystatin longer than four to six months without consulting the doctor. To do so puts you in great risk of promoting the growth of the second commonest type of Candida, Candida tropicalis. Unlike Candida albicans, Candida tropicalis is resistant to Nystatin and there is not yet any antifungal to kill it without harmful side effects. The point is you want to lower Candida albicans numbers in as short a treatment time as possible and then learn to keep it controlled by means other than chronic Nystatin use, which will only foster the overgrowth of resistant species for which we have no treatment currently.

Remember if you need Nystatin more than six months you're "not playing with a full deck." Candida is harmless to normal people. so see the doctor so you can figure out what's keeping you from being healthy.

HOORAY FOR YOU! You have just succeeded in teaching yourself about a new medical problem. And now when you test yourself to see if you have it, you may have one of the happiest surprises of your life — new clear headedness, energy, and optimism that you haven't seen for years.

20th Century Decision: To medicate or educate.

Addendum: If you do not pass a sweet-smelling, easy bowel movement at least once a day, first be sure at least 50% of your diet is raw vegetables. If still not successful, see the doctor, for constipation and bad-smelling gas and stools will delay total wellness. Colitis patients have special problems and will not be able to gradually eat 50 percent raw veggies. See the doctor.

SECTION III
FOOD ALLERGY

By now if you've started on injections for your inhalants, done your bedroom and personal environmental controls and ruled out whether or not you have Candida. Things should be changing. If you're starting to feel better you're unloading some of your sensitivities. But what if you're not feeling as symptom-free or energetic as you know your capable of? Or what if you're not any better at all? You may have a hidden food allergy and the most accurate and inexpensive way to determine, not only if you do, but which foods are the culprits is to do the rare food rotation diet.

If you turn out to have a few sensitivities to foods, avoid them for three to forty-eight months and a tolerance often returns. In other words, it's not a life sentence.

If, on the other hand, you only feel good when you don't eat, or you're a universal reactor, or you have so many bad foods that there's very little to eat, you'll need to test foods and learn to give yourself injections to them. For example, I had about 50 foods that gave me facial eczema. On food injections I was clear and able to eat most of these foods. Also, like many others, I found that food allergies were a sneaky part of the cause of depression and exhaustion that I had never been able to find a cause for (chemical sensitivities Section V). Again, most of the work is going to be done by, you guessed it, YOU. Do you recall the reasons why?

1. If there were a pill to make this go away you'd already be on it.

2. Allergies are so highly individual, no one knows what you're going to be allergic to. Therefore, you need "the doctor" to go home with you to map out the diagnostic trial,

shop for, prepare, and serve the food. It's best to train you as the doctor, since:

    a.   you know the patient better than anyone else in the world.

    b.   you'll be with the patient 24 hours a day for total observation.

    c.   you cost less.

    d.   since you have allergies you want to know as much as possible about the field.

3. There are too few trained specialists or consultants in environmental medicine at this point in history and too many people suffering from E.I. Therefore, it makes sense to teach you to become the family practitioner or doctor, and we will remain your consultants. The only problem with this arrangement is you will, when you finish with this program, know more about the specialty of Environmental Medicine than any "real" doctor you meet.

This tends to make some of them react peculiarly. If it threatens their egos they'll get angry or hostile or deny its worth and tell you it's hogwash. After all, if you know something they don't, it must be worthless, right? Beware of this type for he is dishonest. He has no qualms about registering an authoritative opinion on something he knows nothing about in attempt to maintain an all-knowing facade. Eventually, you'll meet one who is knowledgeable and who is honest and has a healthy ego. He'll be able to say "I don't know much about this, but I'd like to learn, especially when you tell me it is helping you."

As with most life endeavors, the reward is proportional to the effort. If you need to do the rare food rotation diet, it's because you have a dead end or undiagnosable condition that medicine has given up on. If we hadn't seen so many astounding results over the years with this trial, we would not have the enthusiasm and conviction to go through all the effort to teach a lay person how to be a doctor in a new medical specialty.

For most of us, as difficult as the diet was initially, we have been rewarded a thousandfold over. For we now possess total control over how we're going to feel. No more guessing, "Is tomorrow going to be a bummer or a winner?" I can create my tomorrow by how I choose to eat today. Once you have that kind of control you'll never want to go back. You'll just plain get hooked on feeling good.

David had spent thousands of dollars on psychiatrists and medical doctors for his depression and headaches. Without giving him a single injection, we started him on the diet. In two weeks, he was happily clear of depression and headaches for the first time in twenty years. He was even able to stop his antidepressant medication, Elavil, that he had been taking for eight years.

There are hundreds of examples of baffling symptoms that have been found to be caused by certain foods.

Monica had severe asthma that three allergists could not clear. She was ecstatic when she called to report that wheat (really it was yeast as well) elimination allowed her to stop her dangerous steroids.

Karen was a math professor who had severe chemical sensitivities. When she learned to give herself injections of her food allergies and rotate her diet, she dramatically unloaded her system and made her chemical sensitivities better.

Introduction

We have two basic diets:
1. The Lazy-bone Diet, which is a two to three week diagnostic diet, for novices, and
2. the Rarefood 4-Day Rotation for severely sensitive individuals.

Read through all of the material several times before

203

starting your diet. If you have questions, do not ask the staff, but read it again. There is a limit to our tolerance of laziness.

Then buy your notebook, write out your diet, go to the grocery, shop for it, and then begin. If you don't do it correctly the first time, that's only human. Reread the material, read the references, modify, and dig in again. Do not hound the staff for help. Everything we can teach you is contained in this manual. If the answer isn't in the material, then there's a good reason; there is no answer. This a highly individual disease, you have to try it to find out the answer for your system. If you still have a problem, schedule to see the allergy assistant or the doctor (but you'd better have done your homework). If you can't fit a two week Lazy-bone Diet into your life, don't expect to be better.

Remember a diagnostic diet is not a life sentence. It's a temporary change to infrequently or rarely eaten foods to see how good you can feel. Aren't you worth a two week change in lifestyle?

Food Allergy I
How to Diagnose Food Allergy: Step One

Food allergies have been found to be the cause of many people's miseries. Unfortunately, these people have been to many specialists and spent a great deal of money only to have a fancy label applied. Food allergy is not among the diagnostic possibilities offered by most physicians and the full scope of this disease is still not taught in medical school.

The biggest reason we develop food allergies is that we eat the same foods day after day.

The second reason is that there is not a dramatic flare of symptoms after eating the food to make one think of a cause and effect relationship. On the contrary, many people feel better for a few hours after they have had their allergenic food, much the way a drug addict temporarily feels better after a fix. Likewise, the food addict feels worse when his "fix" wears off; he has a recurrence of his symptoms. He knows if he eats again he'll feel better, and so the cycle goes. Then when an allergist comes along and prescribes a diet devoid of this craved allergenic food, he feels worse and thinks of any excuse to stop the diet or to cheat and eat his craved food. For when he is off that food, he goes through a withdrawal phase with a worsening of symptoms. This phase may last up to five days. Actually, it is a good sign to feel worse, for it tells him that he has stopped a food that was a major cause of his symptoms.

Once the five days are over, there is generally a relief of all symptoms that were caused by the foods being avoided. If you are only partially relieved, then there are other unidentified causes: food, chemical, hormonal, nutritional deficiency, pesticides, lack of environmental controls, etc. Perhaps, you have inhalant or chemical allergies that have not yet been addressed. You may be still eating a food which contributes to these symptoms, or you may be one of the rare individuals (like myself) who need food injections for total control of their food allergies.

Arthur had severe headaches every Saturday for five years. These headaches left him bed-ridden all day. Although he lived in three different houses during these five years, he still had these severe headaches every Saturday. He worked in the same job. He thought I was crazy when I suggested that the cause of his headaches could be coffee. He told me, "I have coffee every day at work and never get a headache there." But he left work early on Fridays and never had coffee while at home. On Saturday he would awaken with a screaming (withdrawal) headache, and on Sunday he would recover. Then on Monday, he would return to work and resume his coffee allergy/addiction/ withdrawal cycle. Now you can see how easily food allergies become "masked" or hidden from our suspicion. If he stayed off coffee for four to seven days, he found that when he returned to it the headaches would return also. In fact, an unmasked food allergy usually returns in a dramatically exacerbated form. But by now he was too smart to try that.

Where Do I Start?

Since no one knows how sensitive you are nor how many hidden food allergies you have, let's get all your symptoms cleared first. Then we can find out how many different foods you can tolerate in a day. The longer you avoid certain foods and give your system a rest, the more chance you will have of regaining some tolerance. After some time, you may find that you can have it produce symptoms. Remember, the diet is not a life sentence, only a trial.

Just as people vary in the types of symptoms that foods can produce, they also vary in the types and numbers of foods that cause their symptoms. Some people are so sick that the quickest way for them to get relief of food-caused symptoms is to fast with glass-bottled spring water for five days. It may even be necessary to stay home with a medical excuse due to weakness, withdrawal, or hypoglycemia. After this they should try to find one tolerated food. Obviously, the foods that should be tried first are those that are rarely eaten; that is, not eaten more than once a week. It's the frequently eaten foods that are the causes of chronic symptoms.

Others are lucky, they take a shotgun approach. That is they stop only those foods which are statistically the top four common causes of allergy, and find relief of their symptoms. This is done by simply omitting all foods that have any milk, wheat, or corn. Corn is a sneaky antigen because most people think they only eat it in August, but they eat it every day. Corn syrup and corn sugar are in nearly every food and beverage. Corn oil is in almost all fried foods and in those containing "hydrogenated vegetable oil". The fourth food to be avoided with this approach is all foods derived from yeasts or molds. These are called ferments and include cheeses, breads, alcohols, vinegars, malts, mayonnaise, salad dressing, catsup, mustard, mushrooms, foods fortified with B vitamins (yeast-derived), canned or frozen fruit juices, coffee, tea, chocolate, and more.

Remember that mold is one of the commonest and least suspected causes of allergy symptoms. These symptoms can mimic many diseases. For example, a woman had consulted nine physicians over three years for recurrent depression and swelling of her face, hands, and abdomen. Testing her to molds, giving injections to these, and having her follow a mold-free or ferment-free diet made her totally clear in two weeks.

Obviously, people who first fast and then rotate rarely or infrequently eaten (less than once a week) foods get better quicker than those who try the shotgun approach.

The diet should consist of pure, unadulterated veg etables, fruits, meats, fish and poultry. Nuts and oatmeal with fresh fruit juice, rice cakes, beans and many more foods make good bread substitutes. When your symptoms are clear, add back one food every one to two days and observe which symptoms reappear. But, be aware that many symptoms such as eczema, colitis, adult acne, phlebitis, or arthritis may take up to forty-eight hours to occur (commonly ten to twenty-four hours). By then you will have eaten other foods and may incriminate the wrong one. Therefore, a diary is essential. In some cases of delayed reappearance of food symptoms, it would be best to add back a food for two days in a row rather than one.

Most cerebral reactions, for example, depression, hyperactivity, migraine and tiredness, are more immediate and usually occur within minutes to hours of ingestion. If you do not clear, then look for other common causes, such as can sugar, peanut butter, coffee, chocolate, citrus, tomato, beef, eggs, potatos, apples, or even preservatives or insecticides and omit foods that you can now see should have been eliminated to begin with. Also, make sure a spouse or friend helps you keep track of your diary in case you have cerebral symptoms.

The majority of people are sensitive to many foods. Once they find the causes for their symptoms, they can effectively eliminate the incriminating food. Later, after several months of avoidance, they may find that they can tolerate it once a week in modest amounts. Other are not so lucky. They can only eat one to five single foods a day, or they overload their systems and have symptoms. Usually, these rare individuals need injections of foods as well to increase their tolerance. They can only tolerate rare or unusual foods that they eat less than once a week. If they eat these new foods too frequently, they will, with time, lose their tolerance to them also. Therefore, they must limit themselves to eating each food only once in every four days. This is called a rotation diet.

As you can see, just as there is a wide variation among people in the magnitude and severity of food allergens, there also is a variety of possible diets that are capable of clearing symptoms. Statistically, most people can get clear on a one week diet of infrequently eaten foods. Such a diet could include unlimited amounts of bananas, almonds, (breakfast) sliced Jerusalem artichokes fried in cold pressed safflower oil, sweet (not white) potato, avocado, rice cakes, and sardines in water, (lunch) zucchini, sole, lamb, turkey, cabbage, carrots, turnips, (dinner) and water—preferably bottled. If you crave a sweet then have dates or figs. Have winter squash with cold pressed almond oil or pure maple syrup. If you need more substance in the form of starch, then cook lentils in water with salt, onion, carrots, garlic and bay leaf. You can eat it as a soup (cold or hot) or as a salad with a bit of almond oil. Have cashews, almonds, poppy seeds, sunflower seeds, or Brazil nuts to snack on.

You should live on this diet for a week in order to see how many symptoms are relieved. If you are a mildly sensitive person and have cleared your symptoms, then you may add back foods at the rate of one a day to assess tolerance. Start with the foods that you ate less than once a week. Of course, do not add a food that you already know give you symptoms. Once you have built a sizeable reper-toire of foods that keeps you symptom-free, then you can start testing the common foods containing milk, wheat, corn, or ferments. Only one new food should be added every day or every other day.

If you have trouble, you most likely need to return to only one to three oddball or rarely eaten foods a day and learn to rotate. You probably need food injections because you're much too allergic.

Points to Remember

The trial diet should not contain any foods made with milk, wheat, corn, or ferments. It should consist of only rare foods and single pure foods. Nothing should be eaten that has to have a list of ingredients stamped on its container. In fact, nothing should be eaten that contains anything you normally eat at least once a week, such as sugar, coffee, orange juice, tomato, potato, and beef.

Watch out for hidden antigens. Milk is in creamed dishes and soups, cheeses, ice cream, breads, donuts, scrambled eggs, dressings, mashed potatoes, gravies, but-ter, margarine, salad dressings, and sherbet.

Wheat is in breads, crackers, cereal, pretzels, whis-key, breaded fish, gravies, hamburgs, hot dogs, cookies, candy, macaroni, and even spaghetti that says "made from

Jerusalem artichoke hearts". You must learn to read all labels.

Corn comes in many forms, such as flour, cereal, oil (vegetable oil), starch or thickener, margarine, or sugar. Sugar alone may just be designated in a label as "dextrose," "glucose," "sweetener," or "sugar." It's in most alcohols, nearly all packaged foods, and even processed foods like cold cuts, bologna, and sausage. It's even in your vitamin pills and other medicines, it is the binder that holds the pill together. If you cheat and have a food with an ingredients list, at least read it and be sure you know what you are eating.

The ferments are breads, cheeses, alcohols, vinegar,s pickles, salad dressings, mayonnaise, mustard, catsup, coffee, tea, fruit juices, chocolate, and more. (See complete list of ferments.)

It's best to eat only pure and chemically uncontaminated foods. You only want to take a week to identify the culprits. If you cheat, it may take a great deal longer. You have your whole lifetime to be sick if you choose; so why not take one week to get well?

This diet is temporary, and it lasts only seven to fourteen days. (However, three to four weeks are necessary for severe cases of eczema, and colitis and for universal reactors). You only want to see how free of symptoms you can get by manipulating your foods. It is not a life sentence. If you can't take one week out of your life to see how good you can fee, then you really don't feel that bad to begin with.

Write down everything you eat. Then if you have a problem, you can figure it out. Also, write down every symptom; you will learn thta foods cause more than what you initially thought. For example, most of us, regardless of whether we tested foods to clear eczema, adult acne, asthma, colitis, arthritis, fluid retention, abdominal gas, diarrhea, headache, sinusitis, or whatever, found much to our surpirse that other symptoms were also cleared. For instance, the commonest symptoms were periodic tiredness and depression for which there had been no reasonable cause. Most people also experience increased energy and the loss of many body aches. So what are you waiting for? Start now.

Remember the concept of bipolarity: the same food that makes you feel wonderful when you eat it (that's why you crave it), also makes you feel lousy when you don't have it, causing withdrawal symptoms. The alcoholic craves alcohol and feels lousy when he's not high, and even though he appears adapted to alcohol, he is gradually destroying his body organs (liver, brain, blood vessels, etc.). Adaptation, being able to tolerate something that is really harming you, has its price. It causes deterioration, or degenerative disease, and adds to the body's total load thereby dragging you down and making you increasingly vulnerable to acquiring further chemical, food, mold, or hormone sensitivities. In this way, you develop nutritional deficiencies that further weaken your immune system because your biochemistry has the chronic stress of trying to adapt to this food and mask an acute response to it.

The commonest form of food allergy is not the acute type, such as hives caused by strawberries. Rather, it is the masked type where you have a chronic symptom that does not seem related to food. There appears to be no reason for it. In fact, the very food sometimes even makes you feel better. But after four days of unmasking (being off the food) either through fasting or eating rarely eaten foods (foods not eaten every week), reintroduction of this food can cause symptoms, sometimes even exaggerated or unrelated symptoms.

A morphine addict can work himself up to needing 2 grams of morphine a day. Take him totally off for a month; then give him 2 grams and you'll kill him. Or have him abstain from smoking for a whole month. Then give him an I.V. nicotine dose that is equivalent to a pack of cigarettes, and you will kill him.

I Need Something Spelled Out

So many people say, "Just tell me what to eat"; they don't want to go through the work of figuring it out. Then as we offer suggestions they say, "Oh, I don't eat that" or "I don't like that" or "I'm a vegetarian" or "I don't have time to shop and prepare that!"

Now you know why so many people have hidden food allergies. We only eat what we like or what's convenient because we prefer vegetarianism. Remember, the causes of your hidden food allergies are probably the very foods you crave.

I was shocked to find I could turn off years of unwarranted depression and exhaustion by simply eliminating wheat and sugar. Mike was delighted when ten years of headaches disappeared after just three days without coffee. He lived on twelve cups a day to help him through a high pressure job and a type A personality.

A nurse with severe hypoglycemia was relieved to find that milk (cheese!) and eggs caused her hypoglycemic symptoms. These were the very foods she carried with her to treat her "hypoglycemia."

The first few days weren't very easy for any of us, but our lives are very different now that we have control over our symptoms. We can now have small amounts, occasionally, of our allergenic foods.

So what's wrong with a breakfast of almonds, carrots, sweet potatoes, broccoli, or turkey. It's not a life sentence; only a diagnostic tool.

Remember, after years of doing this, we have heard every question, every excuse. If your question is not answered in here, do not ask the nurses. Their crystal balls are broken. If it's not answered in here, there is no answer. There is tremendous individual variation in this disease, and no one knows the answer for you. Just jump in and do the diet and find your own answer. When in doubt about a food, do not eat it.

If you have too many reasons why you could not possibly do the diet without extensive modification, then don't. But don't monopolize the nurse's time with questions related to diet. They are much too busy. We see desperately ill people from all over the country who must get better as soon as possible. There isn't anything they won't do to be better. To them a dietary change sounds so astoundingly simple; they can't believe answers to their health problems could come so easily.

Remember this is not a spoon-fed specialty. You must work hard and study and know as much about this disease as possible. There are no universal answers about the diet. How much food do you add back? How often? Every meal? Can you eat the same food each meal on the rarefood diet? Can you stay on the same food for two weeks? No one knows. Follow our guidelines and find out by listening to your body.

The most perfect way of testing it is the rarefood rotation diet. Here you eat one to three different foods each meal rotating your days. Add back one food (three times a day if each addition fails to cause a reaction) every one to two days. Then go on to another food. If you get bad, go back to a diet you know was safe and stay there until you clear again before further testing of additional foods.

BEWARE: Unknowledgeable people will always be trying to thwart your efforts. There will always be someone who says, "What are you eating like that for? It's crazy. Surely you could have a little spaghetti, a little can't hurt you." You can ask this person if they would like to be a little pregnant. There is no such thing as a little, you are either pregnant or not. You're either on the diet or you're not. You either have wheat antigens in your body or you don't.

The Lazy-Bones Diet

For those who are not ready to learn how to rotate, but must discover which hidden foods are contributing to their misery, we have the non-rotated rarefood diet or Lazy-bones Diet.

Many patients have hidden food sensitivities that need discovering, but they are not severely enough afflicted to necessitate rotating. You may be among these people who do not need to rotate. In other words, for a trial period you don't need to worry about varying your diet from day-to-day as discussed in Dr. Mandell's book.

It's more important for you to have infrequently eaten foods, for it seems that the culprit causing your symptoms may indeed be something that you eat every week. Not having to rotate makes it much easier on you. Just be sure you avoid all ferments: cheese, bread, alcohol, mayonnaise, ketchup, mustard, vinegar, salad dressing, etc. See the list in the manual. Also, avoid all acids: chocolate, coffee, tomatos, sauces, oranges and other citrus, soft drinks, tea and anything that has the slightest acidic taste. Finally, avoid any other food that you have at least once a week: milk, wheat, egg, corn, cane sugar, beef, pork, etc.

Stay on this rare food diet for two weeks and then evaluate if any of your symptoms have improved. Then you can add back one food in large amounts each day to see which food causes which symptoms. However, if you are not overwhelmed by the idea of rotating, go ahead as suggested because the results are even better. But for the average person who finds rotation to be beyond his capabilities, he should make all four of the following days into one and he should just be sure that the foods selected were never formerly eaten more than once a week.

Summary:

So there are only two types of diet and one is the Lazy-bones Diet. This is the rare-food diet, but it is not rotated. You can eat any of the rarely eaten foods on any day, and you can eat as much as you want. Your only rule is that anything you put in your mouth is not ingested (nor is any ingredient contained in it ingested) at least once a week. If you are wondering if you can have a certain food, **DO NOT ASK THE NURSES**. The answer is no. If you're not absolutely sure a food qualifies as a rare food, then simply do not eat it. When in doubt (don't ask, just) leave it out.

Rules for Lazy-bones Diet:

1. Xerox the Four Day Rare Food Diet.
2. Cross off the words "Day 1, 2, 3, 4"
3. Go through the foods listed and cross out any foods that you eat once a week or more often. Be sure you know about hidden antigens.
4. The foods that remain are your diet for two weeks in any amount as often as you like. But do not eat anything that is not on your list.
5. Take your list to the grocery store and shop.
6. Make up your diet, start your notebook and start the diet.
7. After two weeks, assess which symptoms are better because you're not eating the foods that cause them. Also, assess which ones are only partially better; for these you may need food injections, or you may have to be tested for chemicals, Candida, and / or other causes.
8. Select one new food each day and test by eating it three times a day. See directions for adding foods.

4 Day Rare Food Rotation Diet

The purpose of this diet is to remove the commonest

antigens, such as milk, wheat, corn, eggs, beef, ferments, potato, tomato, oranges, coffee, peanut butter, alcohols, highly acidic foods, etc. No two patients are exactly alike. There are certain rules you will want to remember when following this diet:

1. There is no one diet for everyone.

2. Omit all things that you normally have once a week or more frequently. With every food you write into your diet plan ask yourself "Do I have this in anyway, shape or form at least once a week?" If yes, do not include it in your trial diet.

3. Omit anything that you know or suspect bothers you.

4. When it names a food that you can have, it means that food is only allowed in a pure, unadulterated form, not one packed in sugar, swimming in butter and salt, etc. It means that food in as pure and fresh a form as you can feasibly obtain. In other words, if it says tuna, try to pick one packed in water, not in oil; and if it says avocado, it means just that, not one swimming in salad dressing. Obviously, cooked things are better broiled or steamed, so that you do not have to use oils unless they are included in that day's diet. Uncooked is best if you can tolerate them, such as raw vegetables.

5. If you follow this diet for two weeks without any cheating, that is without resorting to pills, vitamins, smoking, coffee, alcohol, aspirins or goodies. If you do not have any improvement, then you most likely do not have a food allergy. You most probably have an inhalant or chemical problem or possibly a hidden nutritional deficiency.

Remember, that the first five days you may feel worse and you may crave certain foods. You are actually going through a "withdrawal" from the foods to which you are highly addicted. If your withdrawal symptoms are bad enough, you may find any excuse to give up and get your food. Make a note of the food you crave the most. That food is probably one of your main addictions. If you feel better in any way, then you most likely do have a hidden food allergy contributing to your symptoms.

A food allergy can cause any symptom that you can think of. If you are only slightly better, then you should consult the doctor or the nurse; either you still have foods in your diet that bother you, or you may need injections to help you manage your food allergy. If you are better on the diet, then you can gradually, add foods back one food a day. This way you can have a greater variety of foods and at the same time discover the incriminating foods. Rotate these four individual days over a two week period to see how symptom-free you can become without any injections.

Also, be sure to write out what you eat each day along with your symptoms. If you are a very food sensitive person or a universal reactor, you must know the food families and look them up when in doubt. Single simple foods three or less a day are best while you're testing for one to two weeks to see if food is your problem. Cheese is not a simple food. It has mold and milk and dyes and preservatives. Store-bought milk is not a simple food, but it is a compromise that many must use because not many people have access to raw milk. Raw milk is a simple food because it doesn't have the waxed carton or plastic jug outgasing into the contents and it hasn't had processing and the addition of vitamins. Nor has it had nature's original vitamins destroyed through pasteurization and homogenization.

Bread is not a simple food, but many who do not have severe allergies test with it. Just be aware that you are actually testing baker's yeast, sugar, egg, salt, water and a variety of chemicals. If you really wanted to test wheat you would test organic cracked wheat with a known safe fruit juice or honey added, providing it was a compatible day on

217

which to have that juice.

So when adding foods back, add one new food a day. The severity of your symptoms determine how simple your food has to be. Besides, if you react to bread, you can always go back to the diet that cleared you. Then break down the components to see if it's really wheat that you react to. It must always be borne in mind, there are those so chemically sensitive that they are not reacting to the food; but rather the chemical fertilizers, insecticides and fungicides used in growing, transporting, and storing.

For example, a woman had numbness in her face and tongue from eating grapes. Organic grapes produced no symptoms. She was reacting to the chemicals.

It's Easy

Just remember, if you wonder whether you should have a food in your initial test diet, just ask yourself, "Do I have this food antigen in some form at least once a week?" If the answer is "yes", don't have it. If you rarely have it once a week, then use it in your initial test diet; it would be unusual for it to be the cause of your chronic symptoms.

Some suggestions to help you in planning your rare food rotation diet:

School lunches are a problem. See Dr. Rapp's and Ruth Shattuck's books for kid's party ideas.

Meats - cold chicken, cold pork chops, sardines, hard boiled eggs

Nuts - sunflower seeds, cashews, almonds, pistachios

fruits - apples, bananas, kiwi, coconut, pineapple, dates, pears, melon, watermelon, cherries, plums, peas, peaches, papaya

veggies - carrot sticks, celery sticks, raw broccoli or cauliflower, anise, yam (cold, sliced), kohlrabi, cabbage, turnips,

collard greens, Jerusalem artichokes
beverage - Mt Valley, glass-bottles spring water
grains - brown rice, millet, oats, buckwheat, guinoa
beans - lentil, split pea, navy,

Since the Earl of Sandwich reigns supreme, let's try these combos:

Foods to replace bread:
>Rye bread—wheat-free at On The Rise Bakery
>Rice cakes
>Buckwheat pancake
>Non-wheat flour muffins—oat, soy, amaranth
>Celery, carrot sticks, green pepper halves
>Lettuce boats, cucumber slices

Spreads: Chopped meats and eggs with homemade mayonnaise with fresh squeezed lime in place of vinegar
>Tahini, cashew butter, honey, maple syrup
>Mashed avocado with cold pressed almond oil, garlic, mashed baked beans, or lentils
>Nearly any vegetable sliced or mashed tuna, salmon, sardines (in water), shrimp, crab
>Cucumber slices, cabbage, mashed chicken livers, sprouts

Also, the food manual from Dr. Rea's unit is available:
>Rotational Bon Appetite!
>WJR & Associates, Inc
>8345 Walnut Hill Lane, Suite 205
>Dallas, TX 75231

Four Day Rare Food Rotation Diet

This is for the more allergic, more organized, more intelligent and for all universal reactors:

Day #1

Select any of the following foods. Be sure it's a rare food for you.

Shrimp, cod, haddock, crab, herring, sardine, lamb, sweet pepper, avocado, apple, raisin, grape, pecan, walnut, oats, rice, basil, paprika, mint, cinnamon.

For example, for breakfast you could have oats cooked in apple juice. For lunch you could buy rice cakes at Wegman's and have sardines on top of them. This is easily taken to work. In the evening you could have lamb and sliced avocado, and for desert, some pecans, grapes, or an apple. Or have all of these if you're hungry.

Day #2

Tuna, mackerel, turkey, spinach, olive, cucumber, squash, zucchini, apricot, cherry, peach, plum, melon, almond, olive oil, tapioca, banana, honey.

For example, you could cook up three tablespoons tapioca in one and a half cups of water with one or two slices of banana and a couple of tablespoons of honey for a breakfast treat. You could have almonds, a can of tuna (packed in water) with olive oil or cold pressed almond oil added, and sliced cucumbers for lunch. For dinner you could have a spinach salad with olive oil, sea salt, turkey and either a peach, an apricot or a melon. Again, you're free to eat all of these.

Day #3

Clam, oyster, scallop, snail, abalone, bass, perch, trout, salmon, rabbit, pork, carrot, sweet potato, artichoke, lettuce, date, pineapple, rhubarb, raspberry, coconut, sunflower seed, safflower oil, buckwheat, nutmeg, dill, tarragon.

For example, you could have dates and pineapple and sunflower seeds for breakfast; lettuce with safflower or sunflower oil, tarragon and dill for lunch; and sweet potato, trout or pork, and artichokes or steamed or (preferably) raw carrots for dinner. Again, all if you wish.

Day #4

Swordfish, flounder, halibut, sole, turbot, chicken, asparagus, garlic, onion, broccoli, brussel sprouts, cabbage, cauliflower, collards, watercress, radish, green beans, lentils, split pea, soybean oil, fig, cashew, pistachio, tahini, garlic, mustard.

For example, you could have figs and cashews, sesame seed, or pistachios for breakfast; chicken with cold lentil salad with garlic for lunch; sole, asparagus and broccoli for dinner. Again, all if you wish.

Remember: This diet will not be successful unless you plan your menu beforehand and make a specific shopping list and be sure that you have all of these things on hand for the two week period.

Attention all Lazy-bones:
You can eat any of the above foods as many times as you like on any day and on as many days as you like regardless of their families. You do not have to rotate if you are not capable of sophisticated rotating. Just be absolutely sure that you put no food or beverage in your mouth that is normally eaten at least once a week. In other words, eat rare foods ONLY.

Hidden Food Antigens

Besides knowing the food families (see Choices), you must be aware of hidden food antigens. This is the only way you can successfully determine what foods cause your symptoms. For example, you may be attempting to avoid wheat because you are testing yourself on the rare food or avoidance diet or you or you may have already determined it causes symptoms and are eliminating or rotating it, depending upon the severity of the allergy.

Then obviously, you need to know what foods contain wheat. The diet will not be worth doing unless wheat in any form is avoided. If there is any question regarding a prepared food, check the ingredients listed on the label.

For instance, all of the following contain **wheat**:

Breads, cakes, cookies, crackers, pretzels

Breakfast cereals, bran

Flour and flour products such as macaroni, spaghetti, noodles, vermicelli and ravioli's
Pastries, pies, bread crumbs, batters (waffles and pancakes), and cones. Breaded fried fish, chicken, etc.

Postum, ovaltine, malted milk, beer, ale, and canned soups such as Campbell's chicken soup.

Whiskeys contain wheat, but you should never be having alcohol anyway on a rotation diet if you have severe allergies.

Sauces, chowders, soups, gravies, or any other food prepared with flour or a thickener or containing noodles. Rice flour, potato flour, kuzu, flaxseed, or apricot paste, corn starch, arrowroot, or tapioca may be used to thicken soups, gravies or sauces.

Sausage, hamburger, meatloaf unless ground at home without wheat filler, croquettes, fish rolled in crackers, wiener schnitzel, chili con carne, or canned baked beans. sometimes these things contain soy instead. As a substitute for hot wheat cereal, you may use cornmeal mush, oatmeal, or cream of rice. As a dry cereal, you could use corn flakes, rice krispies, puffed rice, oatmeal, or rice flakes.

Although rye mixes contain wheat, they can be eaten if you are not extremely sensitive to wheat because rye mixes contain wheat contaminant. If desired, rice cookies or coconut macaroons or wheat-free soybean bread may be used. Also, you can make buckwheat pancakes as a bread substitute to send kids to school with "sandwiches".

You must read all ingredients carefully, but in the first two week test period you shouldn't even be having foods that are complicated enough to have a list of ingredients. A whole meal may be just squash, period!

If you're very wheat sensitive, you should avoid rye, barley and oat products because these products can be contaminated with wheat and are all gluten-containing which could be your nemisis. In fact, if you're very, very sensitive you may not tolerate any of the grain family, such as rice or corn. Some people are mildly sensitive and can even tolerate other members of the same family every second day, but this should only be attempted after you are totally clear of symptoms. Barley and graham flour are wheat. Substitutes for wheat flour could be lima bean flour, soy flour (both of the legume family), potato flour, or tapioca flour. Other hidden sources of wheat may be bouillon cubes, chocolate, gravies, sauces, bologna, and MSG.

Likewise, in avoiding **milk** you must be aware of the common sources. The following contain milk:

Most baked goods, bologna, butter, cheese, sauces, creamed soups, escalloped or au gratin dishes, scrambled eggs, hamburgs, ice cream, mashed potatoes, sausage, margarines, pancakes, salad dressings, sherbets and crackers.

Corn, egg, soy and cane sugar are likewise hidden antigens. You must read ingredients and even then you can go wrong. For example, ice cream doesn't require a list of its ingredients, so you have no way of knowing that it contains formaldehyde, glycerine, derivatives, corn syrup, etc.

Corn is probably the sneakiest because of its addition to even non-food items such as adhesives for envelopes and stamps, and because of its use as an excipient (vehicle) in aspirin, vitamins, prescription and non-prescription tablets, capsules, and suppositories. It is also in paper cups and plates, plastic food wrappers, MSG, talcum and other powders, toothpaste, hairsprays, and ironing starch. The edible list containing corn could fill a book.

Soy is in the oil of many fried foods, such as French fries and doughnuts. It is a filler in burgers, and it is in hydrogenated vegetable oil. Oil is sneaky for it could be cottonseed, corn, soy, peanut, olive, safflower, sesame, walnut, etc.

A good rule is not to have processed foods, then you avoid chemical additives as well as hidden antigens.

Ferments
Yeasts, Malts Mold Containing Foods

People with airborne mold allergies and Candida hypersensitivities are often worse when they eat foods related to these molds and yeasts that they already know bother them. Therefore, they will feel much better avoiding all ferments, yeasts, malts, and mold containing foods for a few weeks or months until they get entirely clear of symptoms. Then the foods can be tried once a week for tolerance to determine if it's time for them to be able to have them again.

Aside from the obvious mold (aged cheese, fermented alcohol, bread yeast), nearly every processed food has yeast antigens hidden in it. If a food isn't whole or fresh (apple, carrots, chicken, etc.), it has to have things done to it to make it last until it gets to your house. First, important vitamins are removed so the bacteria and mold will not attack the food so quickly. This is done, for example, in bleaching and refining of white flour and sugar. Then chemicals synthesized from mold and yeast extracts are used as stabilizers, flavor enhancers, and preservatives. These are all those chemical names in the list of ingredients that you can't readily define, like citric acid in soda pop, alka seltzer, soups, baked goods, and boxed easy to prepare goods.

So basically, if it comes in a box, a bag, a jar, or a wrapper, you don't want it because the nutrition has been processed out and mold derived preservatives have been added.

The following foods contain yeast as an additive in preparation, often called leavening or baker's **yeast**:

Breads, light bread, hamburger buns, hotdog buns, rolls (homemade or canned), canned icebox biscuits.

Pastries, cookies, crackers, pretzels, cakes, cake mixes, donuts, croissants, Danish.

Flour enriched with vitamins from yeast. This includes pasta, spaghetti, and noodles.

Milk fortified with vitamins from yeast (the B vitamins).

225

Meat fried in cracker crumbs and flour.

The following contain yeast or yeast-like substances because of their nature or the nature of their manufacture or preparation (including brewer's and distiller's yeast and malt):

Vinegars (apple, pear, grape, and distilled) and the foods using vinegar, such as catsup mayonnaise, French dressing, salad dressing, barbecue sauce, tomato sauce, horseradish, pickles, olives, condiments, spices (pepper, cinnamon), mince pie, Gerber's oatmeal, barley cereal, soy sauce, steak sauce, and sauerkraut. Tomatos and citrus fruits are not ferments, but their highly acidic nature makes them antigenic to many people; so they should also be avoided.

Fermented beverages, such as Whiskey, wine, brandy, gin, rum, vodka, beer, root beer, gingerale, coffee, tea, and chocolate. Cocoa beans are fermented before chocolate is produced.

Fruit juices, all juices canned or frozen. Only home squeezed are yeast free and allowable.

The following contain substances that are derived from yeast or yeast-like substances:

Dried fruits—prunes, raisins, figs, apricots.

Vitamin B capsules or tablets. Any vitamins with B vitamins in it. Unless it specifies yeast-free.

Flours that are enriched contain vitamins derived from yeast. Includes enriched or fortified pastas, cereals, chips, breads.

Malt products: Cereal, candy, and milk drinks that have been malted and some fermented beverages; also some bakery products.

Edible Molds: Mushrooms, truffles, morels.

Mold containing foods: Cheeses of all kinds, including cottage cheese, buttermilk, cream cheese, sour cream, and sour cream butter. All chocolate, coffee, tea.
Foods which acquire mold growth during processing or after exposure to air, even when refrigerated, such as ham, bacon, butter, preserves, jams, jellies, syrups, all chocolate, molasses, canned fruit and vegetables, and breads.

Mold derivative: Antibiotics or oral drugs which contain antibiotics, meats prepared from animals fed antibiotics, or milk that contains penicillin or other antibiotics.

Instructions: Pancakes, waffles, muffins, cornbread, biscuits, etc. made with baking powder or soda may be substituted for yeast breads. Freshly squeezed lemon juice may be used in place of vinegar in mayonnaise. New Hope Mills has stone-ground, unbleached, unenriched flour (Skaneateles Stores) or write: RD 2, Rt 41A, Moravia, NY 13118. On the Rise Bakery on Walton Street, Syracuse has organic breads which are yeast-free and a rye bread which is wheat-free.

More Hidden Antigens

Milk

Milk is found in these foods: Baking powder biscuits, baker's breads, Bavarian cream, bisques, blanc mange, boiled salad dressings, bologna, butter, buttermilk and butter sauces.

Cakes, candies (except hard or home made), chocolate or cocoa drinks or mixtures, chowders, cookies, cream, creamed food, cream sauces, cheeses of every description, curd and custards, doughnuts.

Eggs, scrambled and escalloped dishes.
Foods prepared au gratin, flour mixtures (prepared and fritters), foods fried in butter, such as fish, poultry, beef, and pork.

Gravies

Hamburgers, hash, hard sauces and hot cakes.

Ice creams, yogurts, cheeses, margarine, butter

Junket

Mashed potatoes, malted milk Ovaltine, Ovamalt, meat loaf, cooked sausages, milk chocolate, and milk which includes condensed, dried, evaporated, fresh, goat's, malted milk, and powdered milk.

Omelets, oleomargarines, pie crust made with milk products, popcorn, popovers, prepared flour mixtures, such as biscuits, cakes, cookies, doughnuts, muffins, pancakes, pie crusts, waffles, and puddings.

Rarebits

Salad dressings, sherbets, soda crackers, souffles, soups, milk or cream, Spanish cream and spumoni.

Whey and waffles

Wheat

Wheat is found in the following foods:

Beverages such as cocomalt, beer, gin or any drink containing grain neutral spirits, malted milk, Ovaltine, Postum, and Whiskey.
Biscuits, crackers, muffins, popovers, pretzels, rolls and the following kinds of breads—corn, glutin, graham, pumpernickel, rye, soy, and white bread.

Bran flakes, corn flakes, cream of wheat, crackers, farina, grapenuts, Krumbles, Muffets, Pep, Pettijohn's Puffed Wheat, Ralston's Wheat Cereal, Rice Krispies, Shredded Wheat, Triscuits, Wheatena, and other malted cereals.

Buckwheat flour, corn flour, gluten Patent flour, rice flour, rye flour, white flour, graham flour, and lima bean flour are often contaminated with wheat.

Miscellaneous foods, such as bouillon cubes, chocolate candy and chocolate, cooked mixed meat dishes, fats used for frying foods rolled in flour, gravies, griddle cakes, hot cakes, ice cream cones, malt products or foods containing malt, meat rolled in flour, do not overlook meat fried in frying fat which has already been used to fry meats rolled in flour— particularly in restaurants!, most cooked sausages, wieners, bologna, liverwurst, lunch ham, hamburger, etc., matzos, mayonnaise, pancake mixtures, sauces, synthetic pepper, some yeasts, thickening in ice creams, waffles, wheat cakes, and wheat germ.

Pastries and desserts, such as cakes, cookies, doughnuts, frozen pies, chocolate candy, candy bars, and puddings.

Wheat products, such as bread and cracker crumbs, dumplings, hamburger mix, macaroni, noodles, rusk, spaghetti, vermicelli and zwieback. Even pasta that says "made from Jerusalem artichoke" contains wheat.

Egg

Egg is found in the following foods:

Baked eggs, baking powders, batters for French frying, Bavarian Cream, boiled dressings, bouillons, breads, and breaded foods.

Cakes, cake flours, candies, coffee if cleared with egg, consommes, coddled eggs, cookies, creamed eggs, creamed pies, croquettes, and custards.

Deviled eggs, dessert powders, doughnuts, dried eggs, dried eggs in prepared foods and dumplings.

Egg albumin and escalloped eggs.

Fried eggs, fritters, frostings and French toast, griddle cakes and glazed rolls.

Hard-cooked eggs, hamburger mix, and Hollandaise sauce.

Ices, ice cream, icings, glazes on breads and rolls.

Laxatives

Macaroons, malted cocoa drinks, macaroni, meat load, meat jellies, marshmallows, pates and meringues (Torte).

Noodles

Omelets, Ovaltine, and Ovomalt

Pastas, pancakes, pancake flours, patties, poached eggs, puddings, and pretzels.

Salad dressings, sauces, sausages, sherbets, shirred eggs, soft cooked eggs, souffles, soups, spaghetti, and Spanish creams.

Tartar sauce and timbales.

Waffles, waffle mixes, whips, and wines. Many wines are cleared with egg white.

You must determine if egg is used in your own brands of pastries, puddings, and ice creams. Dried or powdered eggs are often overlooked when inquiry is made! Egg wash often coats breads and pastries.

Corn

Common sources are:

Fruits, canned or frozen and sweetened with corn syrup
Ice creams
Meats, processed and/or canned
Containers for packaging of foods
Cooking oils
Sugar, frozen, processed, canned foods
Vegetables, frozen, canned, packaged
Medications, tablets, capsules, liquids
Pressed make-up powders
Envelope glues
Refined forms: flour, flakes, oil, sugar, syrup, glucose, dextrose, meal, starch, grits, popped, succotash

Modes of Exposure

Inhalant exposure: fumes from cooking corn, ironing starched clothes, body powders and bath powders

Contact exposure: Starched clothing, corn adhesives (stamps, envelopes)

Ingestant exposure: as oils, flours, thickeners, sweeteners, fillers, and alcohols

When a corn sensitivity is suspected and some form of elimination diet is introduced for either diagnostic or therapeutic purposes, the following list of corn contacts will be a necessary reference in achieving total elimination. It should be borne in mind that present labeling requirements permit the addition of small amounts of corn without notification or identification. Should it be necessary to continue a corn-free diet for a longer period of time, additional foods can be added or substituted from the list given of corn-free products. Any dietary additions or deviations from the enclosed lists should be checked with the manufacturer to ascertain the possible presence of corn derived ingredients. This is particularly applicable where any medication, tablet, capsule, or liquid is being used.

Further Instructions for Avoiding Corn

Corn-free cooking can be accomplished by using only fresh, non-packaged fruits, vegetables, meats, or the use of home canned foods where only beet or can sugar have been used. Water packed foods may be used. Arrow root or kuzu (see **Macro Mellow**) may be substituted in equal parts in recipes calling for cornstarch. Many cardboard containers are powdered with cornstarch, as are also many milk cartons; glass-bottled milk avoids this problem. All medications are to be avoided unless it has been determined they are corn-free. Regarding newer medications, contact the manufacturer for such information.

Foods and other items which may contain refined corn & other corn products:

Adhesives
Deep fat frying mixtures
Ale
Aspirin & other tablets
Envelopes (gum for sealing)
Excipients (diluents) in
capsules, lozenges, ointments,
suppositories, vitamins

Baking powders
Bourbon & other whiskies
Breads & pastries
Breath sprays & drops
Cakes
Candy
Candy bars, commercial,
box candies, all grades
Carbonated beverages
Catsups
Cereal, many processed
Cheeses
Cheerios
Chili, all forms
Chop Suey
Chow Mein
Coffee, instant
Colas
Cookies
Confectioner's sugar
Corn flakes

Dates, confection
Dentifrices
Dextrose
Egg Nog
Bacon
Baking mixes
Batters for frying
Fish,prepared/processed
Flour, bleached "
Foods, fried
French dressing
Fritos
Frostings
Fruits, canned/frozen
Fruit juices
Fruit pies
Frying fats
Gelatin capsules
Gelatin dessert
Glucose products
Grape juice
Gravies
Grits
Gums, chewing
Gummed papers
Gin
Ginger Ale
Hams
Holiday type stickers

233

Corn Soya
Corn Toasties
Cream pies, puffs
Cough syrups
Cream O Soy
Bath powders
Body powders
Cooking fumes of fresh corn
Hair sprays
Popcorn
Starch while ironing
Starch on clothing
Talcums
Ketchup
Jellies
Laxatives*
Leavening agents baking
powder, yeasts
Lemonade
Linit
Life Savers
Liquors

Bacon
Ham, cured/tenderized
Meat pies
Sausages, cooked
Weiners (Frankfurters)
Metrecal cookies/wafers
Milk in paper cartons
Mono-sodium glutamate
Mull-Soy, Sobee, Pablum
Noodles*
Soups
Soy bean milks

Ice creams *
Cups (paper)
Paper containers, boxes,
cups, plates—only when
foods have a moist phase
in contact with these.
Pastries, cakes, cupcakes
Peanut butters
Peas (canned)
Pickles
Pies, creamed
Plastic food wrappers
Pork & beans
Post Toasties
Powdered sugar
Preserves
Puddings
Blanc Mange, Custards
Royal puddings
Ravioli
Rice, coated
Margarines & root Beer
shortening Meats, pro-
cessed Salt
Salt cellars in restaurant
A & P Four Seasons Salt
Salad dressings*
Sandwich spreads
Sauces sundaes, meats,
fish, vegetables
Sherbets
Similac
Soft drinks
Spaghetti
Zest
Syrups, commercially

Sugar, powdered
Teas

club soda
Tortillas, waffles
Vanilla

prepared: Cartose,
Glucose, Karo,
Puretose, Toothpaste
Sweetose. Tonic Water,
Vinegar, distilled
Vitamins, tablets

*Some brands are corn-free

Common Symptoms of Hidden Food Allergy

Name:
Date:

Circle any of the symptoms below which bothered you in
the last year.

1. Eyes/ears/nose/throat:

headache
dizzy
vertigo
unsteadiness
floating
lightheaded
blurred vision
itching, burning eyes
photo-phobia
itching palate
postnasal drip
sneezing

ear noises
deafness
blocked ears
itching ears
crusting ears
draining ears
watering eyes
seeing spots
edema of eyelids
rhinorrhea
blocked nose
sores in nose

frequent sore throats or swollen glands
other _____

2. Respiratory:

dyspnea
laryngeal edema
sore throat
wheezing
sinusitis
shortness of breath excess phlegm
other_____

hoarseness
dry cough
recurrent laryngitis
recurrent respiratory infection
tightness of chest

3. Cardiovascular:

rapid heart beat
skipped beats
chest pain
hypertension
numbness
flushing
sweating spells
recurrent phlebitis
other _____

palpitations
extra beats
hypotension
fainting spells
tingling
chilling
Raynaud's

4. Gastrointestinal:

nausea
indigestion
abdominal cramps
pain
nervous stomach
mucous colitis
constipation
canker sores
other _____

vomiting
gas
diarrhea
rectal bleeding
irritable bowel
ulcerative colitis
bloating
spastic colon

5. Skin:

urticaria

eczema

rash	hives
acne	itching
red	scaly
flaky	dermatitis
seborrhea	psoriasis
other_____	

6. Muscle/Joint:

muscle cramps	weakness
stiff joints	leg aches
arthritis	fibrositis
other ___ _____	

7. Neurological:

restless	nervous
mental confusion	depression
irritability	brain fog
poor concentration	spacey
unreal feeling	hyperactive
lethargy	undue fatigue
abnormal sleepiness	poor memory
insomnia	amnesia
learning disability	behavior problem
mood swings	weakness
numbness	tingling
irrational outbursts	lapses of consciousness
paralysis	undue anger
other_____	

8. Genito-urinary:

mid-cycle pain or depression
| premenstrual tension | menstrual cramps |
| hemorrhage | heavy flow |

scant flow   irregular menses
vaginal itch/burn   vaginal discharge
frigidity   impotence
bed-wetting   incontinence
recurrent herpes   frequency of urination
burning of urination   prostatitis
burning penis
other_____

9. Metabolic/endocrine:

fluid retentionbloating
swelling   edema
finger/toe   numbness
fingers/toes   get cold easily
fingers/toes   turning white
fingers/toes   turning blue
chill easily
sick after chilling
compulsive eating   binges
uncontrolled bursts of anxiety
depression for no reason
cry for no reason
flushing
sweats
other_____

      If any of this seems repetitious, you're right, it is. We have found that the diet is the most confusing task for most people. So we've explained it in as many ways as we possibly can think of.

Important: Don't forget to think of chlorine sensitivity; over 30% of E.I. victims have it. The only way you'll know for sure is to get off city water and go on glass-bottled spring water. Boiling city water removes only some of the chemicals. Mountain Valley is tolerated by most and is available (delivered to door) from George Luttman (See section on Resources or phone book yellow pages). Other glass bottled spring waters are available at Wegman's. Never buy plastic bottles since the plastic leaches into the water. If there's a handy spring or waterfall, be sure to check out what industries or sprayed croplands are nearby or even miles upstream. You may have to avoid it during May and June, or whenever you know the spraying occurs.

Often chlorine and other water-borne chemical sensitivities are the reason a person doesn't clear with fasting. It's the last box in their total load boat.

Highlights

Foods that are rarely eaten are unlikely causes of symptoms; whereas, frequently eaten and craved foods are common causes.

Worsening can occur in the first five days because you are actually going through a withdrawal period. This is a good sign. Afterwards you should feel much better.

Add back one new antigen every one to three days to determine which symptom is produced and the amount of the antigen needed to produce the symptom.

If you are not successful with one rare-food diet and still suspect you have a food problem, you should try another diet of unrelated foods or just fast to see if the symptoms lighten up.

Don't forget that a common reason for not clearing on the diet is an unsuspected chlorine sensitivity. This can be overcome with glass-bottled spring water. If this is unaffordable, boil the city water to get rid of as much chlorine as possible. Water filters have many draw-backs, none are perfect.

If you have far too many food problems or react to every food you eat, you should rotate safe foods and get tested for food injections. Testing is not used to tell you what foods you are allergic to. It is used to tell me what does of that food should go into your injection to help you tolerate more foods.

At first we tended to be apologetic for repetition in our manual and attempted to edit it out. Then we realized, the repetition was proportional to the questions and misunderstandings people had in trying to master this difficult area of medicine. Therefore, we elected to leave in the repetition for those who need it and we offer our humble apologies to those who do not.

The following rare food diet is not rotated and hence, equivalent to the Lazy-Bones Diet. Go for it!

Note: Anywhere that rice is recommended, we mean brown rice and organic if possible which is available at many health stores, not the grocer. Likewise all wheat should be whole wheat when eaten.

Rare Food Diet
Audio Cassette Transcript

Hello, I'm Sherry Rogers. I'm a diplomat of the American Board of Family Practice, a Fellow of the American College of Allergists, and a member of the Board of Directors, Diplomat of the American Board of Environmental Medicine and Fellow of the Academy.

This tape involves the rare food diet. We've devised the rare food diet as a diagnostic tool to see if hidden food allergies cause any of you symptoms. If you are about 80% better after having inhalant injections for asthma, head-aches, chronic sinusitis, or depression, then there is a good chance that you have a hidden food allergy causing the rest of your symptoms.

Many people have an immune system gone haywire. Many have been bombarded by 20th century chemicals by nutritionally inferior diets, and now they have immune systems overloaded by sensitivities to molds, chemicals, foods, and many other triggers. To see if food is one of your hidden sensitivities, the only way to know for sure is to go on the diet.

Food testing is done in the office, it's not for purposes of telling you what foods to avoid. It is reserved for highly food allergic people who need injections. The testing tells us the dose of the food to put in your injections to help you tolerate ingesting more foods.

You most surely have hidden food sensitivities if you are a universal reactor or if you have eczema, colitis, hyperactivity, or chronic headache. Since your symptoms are every day or at least every week, you need to eliminate all the foods you eat at least once a week during your ten day trial. You want to eat only infrequently eaten or rarely eaten foods to see how good you can feel off the foods that are causing your symptoms.

The trick is to eat strange foods for ten days and see how good you can feel; then add back one food a day to find the culprit. You could just as easily fast for ten days and get the same information, but most prefer to eat. If you could fast, for even one to four days, you would get a headstart in finding your hidden food allergies.

Some people are too rigid in their lifestyle, or they're not sick enough yet to try the diet. They offer a multitude of excuses. Just remember, if you're sick enough, you'll figure out a way to make it work. for in the end, it's not the inconvenience that's the real difficulty. Heck, I've shown up at a steak dinner carrying a can of mackerel, a bag of pistachios and a bottle of Perrier; and I had a marvelous time. I've been on a dinner cruise with nothing more than a head of raw cabbage and three apples. I've been to a board of directors dinner meeting (at a hotel out-of-state) and brought along my own raw carrots, raisins, organic hard boiled eggs, organic almonds, and Mt. Valley water.

If you're feeling good for the first time in years, nothing can make you go off your diet. The inconvenience is nothing; inconvenience is the excuse of procrastinators. However, their procrastination says something about their condition. Their symptoms must not be that bad. If your symptoms are bad enough and you've been around the horn to every specialist and been referred to shrinks and told to learn to live with your symptoms, you'll do anything to get better. A simple diet change would be a welcome remedy.

The worst problem is getting past the cravings and withdrawal symptoms. Those can be tough. Withdrawal may give you symptoms worse than the ones you're complaining of now. But they will be over with by the fifth day and sometimes even sooner. Usually, you'll need to enlist the emotional support of a loved one and structure your days to keep you super busy so you don't get a chance to cheat. However, if you get a monster mash withdrawal headache, you can always go back to your coffee or whatever else caused it and get out of your withdrawal and into your addicted phase for a little rest. But sooner or later you'll have to tough it out and go through the withdrawal. Sometimes it takes a couple of unsuccessful plunges into the diet before you get through.

It may be easier to wean rather than to go cold turkey. Or maybe you would rather take away all the other foods except your toughest one. Save it for last after you've been on the rare food diet a week or so. In order to be successful, you must plan and write out your ten day diet. Shop for it and get a note book in which you record the foods that you eat, the symptoms that you experience, and the medications that you need. Don't wait for a two week period when nothing is going on or your foods will rot.

There's always an excuse to go off the diet—an invitation somewhere or a holiday. If you want to go out to dinner and not take your foods, then order something simple like a steamed sole, a boiled potato, a salad with no dressing and no tomato, and plain water. If you're a universal reactor you may still become overloaded because of the natural gas from the kitchen, the perfumes, the chlorinated water, the cigarette smoke, and the formaldehyde. If you have arthritis, of course, the potato most likely will flare your symptoms.

No system is perfect for everyone because our allergies are so uniquely individual. But there are good guidelines. There are special problems like the person with colitis and weight loss who should not attempt to fast and usually can't tolerate roughage in nuts and raw vegetables. Some people have an extreme aversion, or even a life-threatening reaction called anaphylaxis, to fish. Some kids are extremely fussy and make dieting difficult; summer vacation may be the only time for them to try the diet. If that's the case, something is always better than nothing.

You might, instead of the rare food diet, try to be lucky and guess what foods are the culprits and just eliminate those. A good guess would be all milk and wheat products since they're the commonest antigens (things that we eat every day). Omit those for two weeks and then reintroduce them, one a day, and see what happens. Now eliminate all processed foods with dyes, additives, preservatives, and lists of ingredients for two weeks; then reintroduce them. Or try the ferment-free diet with no cheese, bread, alcohol, vinegar, ketchup, mayonnaise, or mustard. However, if your child is sensitive to something in every category, he's never going to get totally well because the remaining culprits will still be causing symptoms. But it's worth a try if it means either this or nothing until summer.

There's a handy paperback by Ruth Shattuck called **The Allergy Cookbook, A Milk-Free, Wheat-Free, Egg-Free, Corn-Free Cookbook**. It's written especially with kids in mind. It has ideas for school parties, picnics, and lunches. Don't forget that many mothers throughout the United States have suffered through multiple food allergies with their children and they've written innumerable books to help other mothers out. **Allergies and the Hyperactive Child** by Dr. Doris Rapp is also helpful.

A common question is what can I drink? Glass bottled spring water is best. Mountain Valley has a distributor listed in the yellow pages? If too costly, you can boil city water and at least get rid of the chlorine. Coffee, tea, alcohol, sodas, and milk are out for obvious reasons; and one glass of apple juice is like having half a dozen apples and it threatens to overload your system. It's healthier to eat raw food or fruit; you consume less and are more satiated from the bulk, and you don't get as much mold and fungicide residue.

Soy and lamb based baby formula, or soy milk or rice milk from the health food stores can be used on buckwheat or oatmeal cereals if peach juice is intolerable. Be sure there is no corn syrup in the juice. A banana mixed with water in a blender is a great milk substitute; grated almonds or fresh coconut mixed with water in a blender is another. After blending, run it through a sieve. If it's chilled, your kids will probably like it better than milk. But remember, it's only for small amounts like cereal or cooking, it's not for drinking.

So how do you start the rare food diet? First, you'll want to flip off the recorder while you go get a paper and pencil and then we'll be ready to start. First, we're going to have you write down a list of all the foods you cannot have. You can turn off the recorder as you need to catch up with your writing list. Under no circumstances should you have your writing list. Under no circumstances should you have any of the following foods. Let's start writing.

Bread or anything such as wheat, pasta, rolls muffins, cookies, cakes, pies.

Milk, cheese, or anything with milk in it, such as cream sauces, butter, yogurt, or ice cream.

Any alcohols (beer, wine), any vinegars, or anything pickled.

Corn. You'll have to read the ingredients and usually if a food has a list of ingredients, you don't want it anyway. Corn is the cheapest form of sugar. It's a sweetener that is in almost all packaged foods. It's in liquors. Corn starch is a thickener for sauces and gravies. Corn syrup is the cheapest sweetener, and corn flour is in chips and tacos.

Eggs, tomatos, chocolate, coffee, peanut butter, cane sugar, oranges, lemons, grapefruit, apples or their juices. No packaged foods with an ingredients list on them and no cigarettes.

Don't bother calling the office to ask, "On the diet, can I have such and such a food?" Just don't have it.

Now the following foods you can have. However, as you go through the list be sure to ask yourself, "Do I have any of these foods at least once a week?" If you do, or if you have a known allergy to any of them, then you cannot include those on your "have" list.

The following is a list of foods you can choose from:

buckwheat grouts	glass bottled spring water
boiled city water	cashews, almonds, pecans

sweet potatoes	tapioca made with honey & water
rice cakes	lentils, oatmeal, teff
brown rice	quinoa, barley,
Brazil nuts	macademia nuts
sesame seeds	
sunflower seeds	lamb

any fish not breaded including swordfish, cod, soul, perch, halibut, sardines in water, tuna in water, lobster, clam, crab, shrimp, salmon, scallops

turkey	duck
rabbit	celery
squash	avocados
cucumbers	spinach
green beans	collards, kale
beets	artichokes
bamboo shoots	asparagus
onion	cabbage
broccoli	brussel sprouts
cauliflower	green peppers
carrots	parsnips, turnips

fried sliced Jerusalem artichokes in sesame oil (tastes like potatoes)

kohlrabi	sprouts
bananas	cherries
watermelon	kiwi
mangos	pears
plums	melons
pears	raspberries
blueberries	coconuts
dates	papaya
pineapple	

Most any bean that requires soaking prior to cooking, and most any green vegetable
any sea vegetable (see **Macro Mellow**)

For **oils**, make sure they are all cold-pressed including sesame, sunflower, safflower, olive, or apricot kernel.

For other **sweeteners** use maple syrup or honey.

For **spices** use nutmeg, basil, and sea salt.

For a **spread** on rice cakes Tahini, which is ground sesame seeds, or mashed sardines, mashed avocado, safflower margarine, cashew butter, etc. Be creative.

For a **milk substitute** on cereal use soy or lamb-based baby formula, rice milk, soy milk, banana blended with water, or almond or coconut milk (blend with water and strain).

Now, how do you prepare a diet trial for a week at a time? All the foods that I've just listed that you can have, or rather that you've just listed, are available at grocers or through catalog ordering from Walnut Acres or Mountain Ark Foods (see **Macro Mellow**). Many of the foods, such as the cold-pressed oils are only found in the health food section since all the oils in the regular grocery section are heat-processed and contain the dangerous trans form of oils that potentiate arteriosclerosis.

Right now we'll write a list of fourteen different breakfasts that you can have.

1. You could steam or bake seven to fourteen sweet potatoes, wrap them in aluminum foil (shiny side inside) and store in the refrigerator. They're ready to peel, slice, and eat cold in the morning for an entire week.

2. Buckwheat grouts in home-frozen, no sugar added, peach juice (with the peaches as well), or with honey, or rice milk (amasake) or real maple syrup.

3. Baked beans. Don't snub your American nose at this!

3. Baked beans. Don't snub your American nose at this! This is a legitimate, first-class British breakfast. You could cook the beans with lamb bones and your safe water with sea salt, onion, carrot and basil. Cook up a batch of it at the beginning of the week and just plunk it in the freezer or refrigerator to have when you're hungry.

4. Cashews, raw carrots, and dates. This is one of my favorites; don't laugh at it.

5. Brown rice cooked with sea salt, safe water, and date pieces if you need some sweetening in it, or you could saute it later in apricot kernel oil. Freshly pan roasted (salted) sunflower seeds are good sprinkled over it.

6. Lentils cooked in water, sea salt, garlic, and olive oil.

7. Tapioca, cooked in your safe water with sea salt and honey. You can put in apricots as an egg substitute to give it more body. You mash them and blend the apricots in water. It's a trick used as an egg substitute that is found in many allergy cookbooks.

8. Lamb, roasted on Sunday for the entire week.

9. Any fish.

10. Turkey, again roasted on Sunday for the week.

11. Tahini, which is ground sesame seeds, on rice cakes. Tahini is a substitute for peanut butter.

12. Bananas

13. Apples, pears, pumpkin, squash

Now here you have enough breakfasts for fourteen days. All of them can be prepared in advance, and you can combine any of them if you're hungrier. They contain much more nourishment than any box of junk cereal you can buy in the grocer.

If you're mildly food sensitive and really have a great deal of mental difficulty handling the diet, you can eat the same rare food breakfast every day. Heck, cook up a turkey and eat it all week. If you can handle more, then try to vary your diet every other day by having an unrelated food on alternate days. Of course, if you're an ace, you can do a four day rotation diet.

If you're a universal reactor like myself, you have no choice. You need to start with one to three odd foods a day; eat one food at each meal and build by rotating and adding one to three new foods each day. Soon you'll have more foods than you can possibly eat in a day. When you're beginning, it seems as though you're going to starve.

Now, start writing what you can have for lunch. These lunches have been designed so that you can take them to work or school; they're things that can be packed and carried.

Glass Bottled Mountain Valley water

cold lamb	cashews/almonds/pecans
cold turkey slices	tuna in water, sardines in water
tahini on rice cakes	buckwheat pancakes (a bread substitute)
celery	sesame & sunflower seeds
avocado	cabbage
carrot	green pepper
bananas	peaches
plums	melons
pears	coconut
dates	pineapple

249

dates   pineapple
                               brown rice

Now, I think you get the picture for dinner. Just look at your list of unlimited foods; and if you can't think of anything to have and you're ten pounds overweight, pass it up. You could treat yourself to a handful of almonds and dates.

It's best to eat different foods at all three meals and rotate, but if you can't, eat the same food all day and try to vary your days. If you can vary both your meals and rotate your days, you're an ace. If you can't, do the best you can, it's better than nothing. The sicker you are or the more eager you are to get clear, the more perfect you will need to be.

We've given you enough ideas to enable you to have a different diet every day of the week. All we ask is that you try to vary it every other day at least. If you could do a three or four rotation, all the better.

An alternative is to have the same diet daily for one week and then pick a totally different diet for the next week. You'll find having them every other day is much more enjoyable than the monotony of a week at a time.

Remember, this is not a diet to live by. This isn't a life sentence. It's only a two week diagnostic trial. It may even be less than two weeks if you clear your symptoms sooner. Of course, the universal reactor is an exception; he will be on it for quite a while because there's nothing more that he can tolerate.

There are many problems with this diet. It's not balanced, it's not practical; there are not things in it that you could go out and get easily in a restaurant; but that's exactly why it works as a diagnostic tool.

If you're a person with arthritis you definitely want to leave out all the beef, pork, lamb, green peppers, white potato, chili, paprika, tomatos, wheat, and milk. Most fruits should be eliminated if you have colitis and eczema because most people with these diseases are intolerant of anything with the slightest acidity. This includes tomatos, vinegar, blue cheese, coffee, chocolate, citrus fruits, sodas, and alcohols. The nuts would have to be eliminated for someone with colitis unless they were ground in a blender with water and used as a nut butter on sliced bananas or rice cakes. Many of the foods would be better pureed for these people too.

Rice and oatmeal may not be tolerated by someone who is very wheat sensitive since they are in the same family. These same people tend to retain fluids and to be depressed for no reason. Certainly, the heat-processed margarine made of safflower is not something I would even recommend for daily consumption. Many foods have been treated with insecticides and sprays, the bananas have been gas-ripened in box cars, the meats may have been gas-broiled and have had hormones added as well as antibiotics.

So there are still many problems with this type of diet, but it clears so many people that it's definitely worth your investigating. In other words, there is no perfect diet for everyone except fasting. But because you have to work and eat, we're eliminating the commonest causes to see what symptoms can be alleviated. Since your symptoms are frequent, we remove the frequently ingested foods and just let you live on oddball foods that could not possibly be a cause of your symptoms because you don't have them that frequently.

You probably realize by now that there is a whole spectrum of patients and their symptoms. There is a large degree of variability in the severity of the illness that people have. At one end of the scale there is the person who can only have one food a day and has no other choices because he has such severe symptoms to everything he eats. On the other end of the scale is the person who is functioning perfectly well and would just like to feel a lot better.

Then there's a tremendous variability in the ability to carry out the diet. A lot of kids are very finicky eaters, so summer is the only time that they could possibly try the diet. Some people react as though it's an insult to suggest they alter their eating habits for only two weeks, but this only tells me that they are just not that sick.

There is tremendous variability in willpower, and that's why it's very important to plan a diet and get in a proper mind set. Attitude is crucial, especially with kids. We need to instill a feeling in them of a new adventure; that it's more fun crunching on rice cakes than soggy standard white bread.

Many times it's helpful to have the rest of the family go on the diet for several reasons. First, it helps the cook; second, it may uncover hidden allergies in other family members. Many times a patient will come back and say, "Hey, we found my brother was hyperactive from sugar, additives, grape, or cinnamon", or "my sister's eczema cleared when we took her off the mold foods and the acids," or "my father's stuffiness cleared when he couldn't have any milk and my mother's backache disappeared when she stopped eating beef."

Now Monica was another case. She was ostensibly a person who should have every reason to get better as fast as possible. She was a very attractive young gal with severe asthma; it was so bad she could hardly speak. She was breathless just from talking. She had been on steroids for many years and she knew the many dangers. I could never get her to go on the diet until about nine months after she had been on inhalant injections. When she did go on the diet, she called from a few hundred miles away and excitedly told me, "You were right, I'm off the steroids for the first time in years, and I have found that it was the wheat and yeast in bread that were giving me the additional asthma."

So we all have a certain time at which we finally get

ready to try the diet. On the low end of the sensitivity scale is the average person who can work up two different days of the diet and then rotate those. If there's no difference in ten days, he probably doesn't have a food allergy. The only way to be sure is to fast or to follow the legitimate four day rare food rotation diet. He may be able to handle it by the, after he has had a little practice with a two day rotation.

On the highly sensitive end of the scale is the universal reactor, this is the person who has to start with one to three foods a day and then gradually build from there. This is admittedly much more difficult, but he has no choice because he is so sensitive.

You must never, and I emphatically say never, call the office ask, "On the diet is it okay if I eat such and such?" The mere fact that you are asking shows several misunderstandings on your part. In asking for a particular food you're telling me that the diet would be more manageable if you could eat that food. This puts up a red flag that makes me ask, "Are you addicted to this food or a component of it?" In terms of manageability I can only add that the purer the diet, the more accurate the results. If you feel your compliance would be much better with that food, then try it. If there's no difference in symptoms after ten days on the diet and you are highly suspicious of a hidden food sensitivity, then it behooves you to try a diet of different rare foods omitting this one as well.

Also, by asking if you can eat a certain food you appear to be seeking special permission, a child's trick, or maybe you are thinking that we have some special powers. We do not have a crystal ball and we do not know which foods you will be allergic to. The whole point of the diagnostic diet trial is to have only infrequently eaten or oddball foods to unload your system of the allergic reactions being caused by the foods you normally eat.

Another good test of whether you can have a particular food is this: Does it have a list of ingredients or constituents? If so, write them all out on a piece of paper. Now, for each ingredient, determine what family it is in. Dr. Mandell's book is excellent for this, and there are dozens of other books about the rotation diet that also list the food families (also see next chapter). Then determine whether that ingredient is related to any food you eat at least once a week. Obviously, if the ingredient is a chemical, you should not have that food. If any of the other ingredients are eaten once a week or in the families you eat once a week, then those foods should not be eaten either.

A great simple rule is when in doubt, don't eat it. If you have to ask if you can have a food, don't have it. Remember, the rare food diet is not a life sentence. It's only a ten day diagnostic trial. Remember, during the first five days you may have withdrawal symptoms that make you feel even worse. Many people will use this as an excuse to say to themselves, "There, I knew I shouldn't try this diet; I feel even worse on it." If you feel even worse, then that's a good sign because in a few days you're going to feel better than you have in years.

If the diet still seems impossible, your only recourse is to buy Natalie Golas' book, **If It's Tuesday, It Must be Chicken**. This book is available through Dickey Enterprises (Resources), or you can order it from the Economy Book Store. She has color-coded the four days, rotated every food in existence, and provided shopping lists, menus and recipes. No more could be done. But you must go through the book first and cross out every food that you eat at least once a week. So all you do is omit every food that you have more than once a week. You then have rare foods spelled out for you, and they're automatically rotated for you on the four day schedule. Who could ask for anything more?

Admittedly, the diet is difficult because it puts all the work on your shoulders. As you've discovered already, this 20th century disease changes all the rules. It makes you (the patient) a partner in the treatment; and you must in gies than the average doctor. Many of us have developed food sensitivities because chemicals in our 20th century environment have damaged our immune system and caused our antibodies to recognize as foreign, things that never before were recognized as foreign.

These chemicals have damaged cells called the T suppressor cells which normally control how much antibody is made against beef, milk or wheat. Now that these cells are damaged, our immune systems have gone haywire, and we have developed symptoms to foods that normally we tolerated for years. This 20th century disease changes all the rules of medicine. It turns the patient from an unknowledgeable creature of pill popping passivity (one for whom everything is done) into the dietitian, the prescriber and the physician. Yes, you actually become the physician. I'm just your consultant. That's exactly why we can only take the most intelligent and motivated patients. This is not a disease like tuberculosis, where we can take all comers and all you need to remember is to take a pill each day.

When you start on the rare food diagnostic diet, you are showing that you already know more about 20th century medicine than the average physician because you know one of the diagnostic tools and one of the treatments.

With all my sarcasm, don't let me lead you to believe it's easy. It took me two years to figure out how to incorporate the rotation diet into a family lifestyle, then a working wife lifestyle, then last a traveling lifestyle. Oh yes, I had so many food sensitivities that when I went to Dallas or Chicago to St. Louis to lecture, I took my own food, water, air cleaner, and bedding for years.

Most of you don't have that severe a problem. You'll maybe have half a dozen foods to avoid, and you'll probably not even need food injections. You will find that within two months of total avoidance and rotation, you'll soon be able to tolerate the forbidden food once a week in moderate able to tolerate the forbidden food once a week in moderate quantities. Then a few months later, you'll probably be able to have it twice a week. I wouldn't push it more than that because human nature being what it is, your rotation will have gotten pretty sloppy by then. The more you push or repeat certain antigens, the greater the chance of losing tolerance to them. If it's a tolerance that you've already lost but were lucky enough to get back, don't push your luck. You could lose tolerance for that food forever.

Once you've done your ten to fourteen day diet, observe from your record book what symptoms are better and what ones are gone. Now to test milk, choose one day and add back all the milk, cheese, butter, ice cream you want. Of course, the more knowledgeable of you will recognize that you're also testing mold in the cheese, cane sugar in the ice cream and so forth. See what happens. Do you get congested, sleepy, moody, or headachy? Do you have a stomach ache? If so, leave milk products out of your diet for now and go on to testing wheat. So all breads and pasta (ah, now you can have macaroni and cheese if milk was okay) can be added. This helps the sandwich department immensely.

If you reacted to the milk group, then back up and clear again before starting to retest again. Only now, you should just test milk on day one. Then cheese the next day. So if you're okay on day one but not okay on day two, you know milk is okay but the mold in cheese is not. You might do okay with yogurt or cottage cheese which one is moldy, but it does have added antigens. So test those another day.

Of course, if you had symptoms with bread, then you want to break it down to see if it's the yeast or the wheat. So you could have wheat (Essene bread) or bran cereal three times a day. If it's the yeast, the fresher the bread, generally, the worse the symptoms will be. Then add another food.

Generally, add back whatever will make life easier for you, so you can expand your dietary repertoire. Coffee

256

is not even good for you; so (since you've been off it for ten days) why not stay off it? No sense wasting a test day on that.

You'll want to start each test day with a small amount of the substance; then in an hour try a larger amount; then at noon and dinner try even larger amounts. This way if any reactions occur you will be warned in time to halt the test at that point.

There was an asthmatic who foolishly jumped into testing eight eggs all at once; she died that day. She knew a small amount of egg caused severe asthma, but she wanted to see what an overload would do.

Never test anything that you think could be dangerous. If you're dying to have a food that you suspect makes you suicidal or depressed, closes your throat, or causes asthma, you should schedule to eat it in the office where you can get first-hand emergency treatment if necessary. We've had more than one person testing shrimp cocktail in the office. (You just have to bring enough for the nurse and me, too).

If your symptom is asthma, purchase a peak flow meter at the office so you can measure your lung output as you test foods. Some symptoms like colitis and eczema require two days of adding a food before they appear again. With my eczema it only takes a day of testing the food, but the sneaky thing is that some foods make me break out within minutes or hours and others take twenty-four hours. That's why a diary is crucial.

When in doubt about the cause of your symptoms, go back and eliminate everything you had in the last twenty-four hours. Then stay on that diet until you are clear before testing foods again. Now proceed at a slower pace and test the foods in a different order. In other words, if you get into trouble and have symptoms you can't figure out the cause, go back to a diet day where your diary says you felt fine. Stay there a few days until you're sure you're okay;

257

then begin a test trial of a food.

Universal Reactors

Now, some of you like myself, are what we call universal reactors. You know who you are because you have so many food allergies, you don't know what to eat to stay alive. You obviously need food injections. You should get tested as soon as possible. In the meantime, you may be able to tolerate only one food a day; then later two a day and so forth. Because you're trying to build a life-sustaining list of foods before you dwindle away to 98 pounds, you want to stay on the oddball foods as long as you can. In other words, when you're ready to add another foods to your list, you won't start with common things like milk, wheat, eggs, corn, packaged foods and ferments because these are the commonest causes of food allergy. You don't want to provoke any symptoms. You're too busy trying not to have symptoms. So you should test something from the rare food list like turkey, and hope that you don't react to the hormones and injected preservatives. You should give commercial broccoli a mild chlorine bath followed by a baking soda rinse (or a Shaklee Basic H bath) and hope the insecticides don't make you react.

When you're at this stage (a universal reactor), you know it will be months before you'll dare test any conventional foods; and you'll probably never test a processed one with a list of ingredients. It's people like you and me who can tell if a food is organic or not because we're abnormally sensitive to chemicals as well as foods.

How do you know if you need food injections? That's pretty easy. If you find that you only have six or less foods that cause symptoms, then you can avoid them. You don't need food injections for that. Oftentimes after a few months, you can tolerate the forbidden food once a week. Some foods, however, are fixed food allergies, and they will never be tolerated. For example, I would never eat a tomato or an orange even if you paid me, and no amount of food injections can help me tolerate them. On the other hand, if your symptoms are better when you don't eat (and it seems like everything you eat causes symptoms), then you need injections.

Some have the erroneous idea that food injections enable you to eat any food you want; that's not true. But they do greatly expand their repertoire if you rotate. If they're not willing to rotate, then food injections definitely will not help.

For example, with my eczema, I was best but not great if I didn't eat at all. Within two weeks of food injections I was clearer than I had been in six years; and I continued to get progressively better the longer I was on them. Without such shots, a bite of a pear would cause me to break out within an hour. The first year, I was able to eat a couple of pears if I had a shot on that day. The second year, I could eat a couple of pears and not even need a shot that day. Now, six years later, I can eat a dozen pears and not break out and not need an extra shot. I could stay on my every four to five day injections and not require an extra shot for that indiscretion. If I get sloppy with my rotation then I need a shot every day. If I'm late for a shot, I start breaking out within hours (Of course nowadays, I no longer need any shots, as I no longer rotate or eat special foods. That's what getting well is all about.)

What does my shot contain? It's a phenol-free extract of the neutralizing dose for eighty-five foods. They were all tested individually. Is it a drag for me to eat cashews and dates for breakfast, or sweet potatoes and cold steak? That's nothing when you compare it with the misery I suffered with my face a bloody mess and being chronically tired and depressed for no blasted reason.

You see, a lucky thing happens when you identify the bad foods for you. You get hooked on feeling good, and

259

there isn't any food that will tempt you sufficiently to be willing to return to your old symptoms.

If you are hooked on processed foods and think organic foods are unnecessary for you, read Beatrice Trum Hunter's, **Consumer Beware**. It tells what has been done to food before you get it. Much of your success depends on repetition of the teaching tools that we've provided. It never came easily to any of us. How much you learn from the diet now depends solely on your resources of intelligence, perseverance, and motivation.

Remember, you have your whole lifetime to continue the way you currently eat and continue your symptoms. Aren't you worth a two-week trial to see how good you can really feel? Bon apetit!

You are to be commended. Pause and congratulate yourself for having persevered this far toward your total wellness goal. Admittedly the diet is a drag. But yearly when hundreds of patients flock back to the office I ask, "Of all the things you have done so far, what single factor do you think has made the biggest difference in your getting rid of years of symptoms that prior were resistant to all treatments?"

The majority of the time the answer will be, "No question, it was the diet."

Caution: Five times in my life I saw people unmask severely. When they went off pizza and Pepsi and on the wholesome rare food diet, they brought out their chemical sensitivities. Suddenly they were smelling and reacting to everything. it's frightening and perplexing, but a blessing in disguise, for now they know what they are reacting to.

Can I Give My Own Injections?

Anyone giving their own injections (foods, neuro-transmitters, hormones, miscellaneous mediators) must declare inability to receive injections from physicians at the times the injections are needed, as well as willingness to accept the possibility of death as a possible reaction.

As far as giving one's inhalant injections at home, we do not advise it. Anyone can be taught to give an injection, we have even taught seven years old, but few can treat a reaction. I've treated reactions where a person needed injections every 12 minutes for 4 hours. The only reason she is still alive is the timing of all the other drugs I gave intravenously. There is no neighborhood nurse or para-medic relative who has that type of facility or skill.

The next argument we hear is they live so close to the hospital or ambulance. But let me tell you, the worse a reaction is, the quicker it must be treated. There is a point that occurs within seconds, beyond which the most sophis-ticated medical treatment is powerless. Timing as well as training are of the utmost importance.

Foods are less potent and must be given by the patient. If you are giving injections, you will have passed the oral and written exams in the office, even if you are a nurse, dentist, or physician. The inhalants are pollens, dusts and molds potentially much more reactive than the food antigens, so we really are not eager for those to be given at home. Asthmatics are too precarious and should always have their inhalant injections in a doctor's office. You never know how overloaded you might be on injection day that could tip the scales.

Anaphylaxis

Sudden life-threatening symptoms to a food or injec-tion are termed anaphylaxis. If this is a possibility for you, it is assumed you have scheduled your training and examination in recognition of symptoms and use of medication. A brief synopsis follows for fast reference only. It is up to you to memorize and periodically review the separate written instructions you received and keep yourself and the person who will treat you well versed. You have the responsibility for your life and death.

1. 0.3-0.5cc adrenalin injected directly into the muscle under the tongue.

2. Tourniquet above the site of injection.

3. 0.3cc adrenalin into the site of injection.

4. 50mg Benadryl in a vessel, or muscle if untrained in intravenous injections.

5. 2 vials of Luffylin in muscle if asthmatic.

6. Repeat 1 and 4 on way to hospital, if no response in 3-5 minutes. Also, may be needed if symptoms recur as medications wear off in 5-20 minutes.

It is your responsibility to be sure your emergency medications are not outdated and that you schedule periodic (minimum yearly) re-examinations of your knowledge of this protocol.

Leaky Gut Syndrome

If you have an escalting food allergy, where you keep becoming more and more sensitive to a greater number of foods, you probably have the hyperpermeable or leaky gut syndrome **(see WELLNESS AGAINST ALL ODDS).** We need to fix that.

SECTION IV
ROTATION

Who Needs to Rotate?

Only highly sensitive people, highly chemically sensitive people, universal reactors and those on food injections need to rotate! However, if you have been asked to evaluate a diet of any level, you will obtain better results by familiarizing yourself with this material even though your presumed food allergy isn't bad enough to require rotation yet.

The severity of food allergies varies widely. Anyone who cannot control his symptoms by avoiding a few foods, and needs injections to help control his food symptoms has severe food problems. But even in the severe food allergic category, there is a spectrum of severity; no two people are alike. If you need food injections, you also need to rotate for two reasons.

1. Your body will not tolerate foods even with injections if you overload it by having a repetitious diet of the same antigens day in and day out. It's like romping through a ragweed field for eight hours a day when you know you're allergic to ragweed.

2. The more you abuse a particular food by eating it too frequently, the more you increase your chance of losing your tolerance to that food and becoming allergic to it also.

"Abuse it, you lose it". By the very fact that you have so many allergies already, we know your genetic structure is like a time bomb waiting to go off. There have already been certain events in your life that have triggered the onset of your allergies. Now we want to minimize your chances of developing more.

263

How Do I Begin to Rotate?

First, you must familiarize yourself with the food families (see Choices I). Every food on the same line is in the same family. So they can be eaten on the same day, but you don't have to eat them all. But do not eat any of the foods on that line for four days.

Then choose four unrelated (not in same family) and rarely eaten foods. If you have the severest form of food allergy, you'll need to start at stage zero. This name is appropriate because it stands for what you can eat—zero. The more highly sensitive people fast on glass bottled spring water for five days to turn off their symptoms. Then proceed to stage one. Less severely sensitive people can start at stage one.

So start at Stage One. Choose four unrelated and infrequently eaten foods like banana, sweet potato, sole, and squash. Have one food a day until your symptoms clear (three to six days is usual). Remember you may get worse before you get better. That is a good sign of withdrawal, and it shows you have effectively eliminated a food that was causing symptoms. The worsening of symptoms (withdrawal) usually only lasts two to five days.

Then proceed to Stage Two. Now you can have two unrelated rarely eaten foods a day. As long as you stay clear, you can add one new food a day, providing the previous cycle left you free of symptoms. So you might add cashews, oysters, broccoli, or pineapple. Remember, you are eating to live—not living to eat! You just keep building your diet and eliminating those foods which cause symptoms. Shortly, you'll have a list of foods that are safe. However, remember if you eat a safe food more frequently than once every four days, you can at any time turn it into a symptom-producing food. By the very fact that you have food allergies, we know that you have the genetics to go on and develop further food sensitivities at any time.

Stage IV

After you have about sixteen (safe, unrelated, infrequently-eaten, and tolerated) foods, you're home free. This means that you can eat four different foods each day and rotate them on a four day cycle. Regardless of what you test, you always know what diet to go back to in order to get clear. Now you are in control; and you are the master of your destiny. You can test any foods and make up recipes; if you have symptoms, you know how to turn them off. If you get really bad and want to clear the fastest (pardon the pun!) way possible, just fast (Stage 0).

Lest I make it sound so easy, it took me two years to learn to rotate well and comfortably. So go easy on yourself. I bribed myself with one "junk day" (Saturday) a week. But you will soon outgrow your need for that too, as you begin to realize that the choice is between pigging out and wasting your day having symptoms or eating well and having tons of energy.

You have really arrived when you manage to incorporate more organic or chemically less contaminated foods into your rotated scheme. This is the ultimate; although realized by few, it is well worth the effort. Admittedly, I could never have handled this plus the rotation initially. But every few months, we keep expanding our shared resources to make this more attainable by those who require it in order to live symptom free.

How do you know if you are chemically sensitive and would feel better on organic or chemically less contaminated foods? You guessed it. Try it for a few weeks; then pig out on store-bought and restaurant foods for a few days and compare. As always, your body will give you the answer if you are willing to test and listen to it.

Most people who do this test expect one of their food symptoms. On the contrary, most of us get chemical symptoms which are more subtle or mimic "non-allergic diseases". For example, inhalants (dust, molds, pollens) give me migraines, sinusitis, burning itchy eyes, and asthma. Some medicinal allergies give me laryngitis. Mold an food allergies give me itchy ears, water blisters in the back of my throat, and severe facial eczema. Various chemical exposures give asthma, burning eyes, mental confusion, irritability and severe back pain. Formaldehyde exposure of an hour an a half in a shopping mall gives me severe back pain in the site of an old injury. Even narcotics won't relieve it, but two hours in normal air will. Insecticide exposure (a chemical contaminant of all restaurant and grocery items) in the quantity that would normally be consumed in three days of regular eating gives me tiredness (to the point where I conk out for a two hour nap), back pain, and large tender breast cysts. Do I subject myself to needless irradiation for a back x-ray and mammogram? Not when I can turn off every symptom within forty-eight hours by just a day of fasting and then resuming my diet.

I share this with you to help you understand the scope of just one person's allergic response to the environment so with your increased awareness, you can learn to respect your body's responses to your environment.

Most people that have to rotate in stages have so many food allergies that they need food injections. Be sure you read this whole chapter thoroughly before attempting to test foods.

But What Can I Eat?

After several weeks or months, you may reach Stage V. You will have found at least twenty safe, unrelated foods, five for each of four days.) Now you will be eager for more sophisticated combinations. But although it is more fun and gives greater variety, it takes more planning and thorough familiarity with the food families. Many people choose not to go this far and are happy with simple unadulterated pure foods. Some people are so sensitive that they cannot proceed this far.

But for the adventuresome, menus are only limited by your imagination and initiative. For example, if you are in need of a milk substitute for cooking, use baby soy or lamb- based formulas. A ripe banana or coconut in a blender with water or fruit juice can be used in cereal. There are soy, safflower and corn margarines; and even tahini (sesame) can be used in place of butter. Cooked cauliflower or potato in a blender with water makes a milk substitute for creamed soups.

For those who miss the bulk of wheat, they may be able to tolerate related grasses for cereals and flours, such as oats, rice, barley, or corn. Flour substitutes could also include potato, tapioca, ground nut meats, and bean flours. Those who miss bread can substitute rice cakes, rye thins, buckwheat pancakes (for kid's sandwiches), oatmeal cakes, tapioca, potato, popcorn, nuts, water chestnuts, seeds, and squashes, sweet potato, beans of many varieties.

Corn sugar can be replaced by cane, beet, maple, date, or honey. Corn oil can be substituted with olive, almond, safflower, sesame, soy, or peanut. Vinegar (mold) can be replaced by lemon (citrus) or yogurt (milk) or a variety of spices such as lemon verbena. Snacks to have on hand for travel could include small amounts of dried fruits, nuts, seeds, popcorn, carrot sticks, and hard boiled eggs.

With eleven families of vegetables (each with several members), fourteen of fruits, and thirty-nine of protein, there is more food than you could possibly eat in four days. The work is in planning your menu and locating your sources. You will find you eventually spend less time at the grocery; instead you will collect your foods from a variety of individual sources. The pay-off is vastly improved health, and this increased energy will enable you to carry this out.

Rotation Diet Stages

Stage 0

Fasting is necessary. This is only for those who are severely sensitive or badly out of control; these people want to feel better fast. A must for highly chemically sensitive people.

Stage 1

One food a day. For very sensitive patients who have to develop a repertoire of safe, tolerated foods from which to build a diet. Usually used the first two weeks.

Stage 2

Two foods a day. Still there are too many unknown or untested foods, but the total load is being reduced. Patient has to be very careful or he will trigger symptoms.

Stage 3

Three foods a day. You're gaining!

Stage 4

Four foods a day. Many can never get past here without overloading their systems. If you get stuck at any stage and cannot progress further without symptoms, your total load is too high. See the doctor if you can't figure it out. It's partly the chemical load, and most likely you have intestinal hyperpermeability, which must be diagnosed and cured to proceed further.

Stage 5

Five or more foods a day. You've arrived if you can tolerate this rotation, with or without injections. Many people, however, can only tolerate a couple of days a week with this many antigens (usually weekends). They will need to drop back to stage three for the remaining days in order to keep symptoms under control.

By this time you realize that there are two different ways of adding foods back. People with mild allergies (only a few food allergies) should diet to clear symptoms; then they can add back one new food each day. If they have a symptoms that takes a day or two to trigger, they should add the food back for two days to determine if it causes eczema, arthritis, or colitis.

But very sensitive people (people who need to rotate and who need to go through the above stages) should not be in a hurry to add foods back. On the contrary, they are trying to find enough foods that they do not cause symptoms to tide them over until they get better. These people will have to wait months before they test common foods like milk or wheat. They can't afford to be made worse. So they will stay on the safest rarefood rotated diet possible for as many months as it takes to get their total load down.

If you are moderately sensitive, you may not need to fast if you can clear on stage 1 or 2 within two weeks. Remember the goal is to get clear. So do stage 1 or 2 to see just how clear you can get.

If you can't get clear, you may need stage 0 and/or food injections. Only after you clear and identify the problem foods, can you expand your repertoire of foods and move to stage 3. Some people can only eat one to three foods a day for the first month; they need to get their total antigenic load sufficiently simmered down. Only then will they know just how many foods they can tolerate and how far they can spread out the interval between injections if they need those also.

Remember, as you work on reducing the environmental overload of inhalant antigens and chemicals, you will also increase you tolerance to foods. Also, the longer you are off some of your foods the greater the chance of being able to tolerate them after a while.

269

Some people are so chemically sensitive that they can only clear with organic or chemically less-contaminated foods. Remember, the stages are temporary, but necessary. The diet is not a life-sentence, but a diagnostic tool to identify your food allergens; and the stages are designed to match the severity of your sensitivity. Very rarely can a person start at stage 3 and clear. If so, they are probably mildly sensitive. The moderately sensitive need to start at stage 1, and the severely sensitive need to fast at stage 0. These stages correspond with the amount of unloading your immune system needs.

Remember, if you don't feel worse (from withdrawal) sometime between the second and fourth day, you are probably not avoiding some of your worst foods. Between the fifth and twelfth days most people say they feel better than they have in years (and in some cases, ever!)

Masking is an important phenomenon of food allergy to be understood. It is most analogous to a codeine or alcohol addiction. The victim feels temporarily better after having the "fix" (addictive substance), but after a few hours he has to have more because it has worn off and he's now having withdrawal symptoms. Anyone who craves certain foods or must have certain meals at certain times is a good candidate for food addiction.

Once the addictive substance has been avoided for five days, it becomes unmasked; now if it is eaten it will quickly cause the symptoms. It is now easy to appreciate that it was the culprit all along.

An example will illustrate this better. Mike suffered for ten years with severe headaches. They would hit him each night when he got home from his high pressure job. At times he contemplated suicide to get relief. He drank many cups of coffee all day at work and by evening he was withdrawing. He laughed when I suggested coffee could be a cause of his headaches. Anyone could see that logic would have him say, "But coffee can't be the cause because

I have it all day and never have my headaches then. Coffee makes me feel good. It could never be coffee, that's the last thing I would suspect." Now you can see why understanding the masking phenomenon and going on the rare food diet is so crucial to identifying the triggers that make us sick.

Many people who are overweight have a wheat, sugar, Pepsi, milk, or corn (cheapest form of sweetener in processed foods) addiction. They must have that craved food in some form or another to keep them from feeling lousy. As a result unwanted pounds accrue. That's why so many people are able to drop weight effortlessly with a rare food diet. Once they are past the withdrawal, the craving is gone; and how many sweet potatoes can you want on your sweet potato day? It's not unusual to see eighteen to thirty pounds lost in the first two months of the diet.

Four Day Rotation Diet

So you now see that masking is a phenomenon that occurs when you have a food to which you are addicted. It is somewhat like being an alcoholic. You actually crave the food which gives you your allergic symptom. You will actually feel better for a few hours after you have eaten it, but later you will suffer withdrawal symptoms and feel lousy for a day or two. Therefore, by going off this particular food for four whole days, you will go through a day or two of withdrawal and then you will begin to feel better. At this point, your food allergy has been is unmasked. Now when you eat it again, you will experience whatever symptom the food causes, such as severe lethargy, tiredness, headache, wheezing, diarrhea, cough, etc.

In order that you do not develop further food allergies, you should go on a four day rotation diet. This also prevents you from developing masked food allergies that you are not aware of. Basically, you may choose foods from

271

the different groups. If foods are all on the same line, such as lettuce and safflower, you may have lettuce every four days, but two days later you could have safflower oil or sunflower oil.

In other words, you can have a member of the same family within two days if you are not severely allergic to that family. Of course, you could have safflower or sunflower oil on the lettuce, and then rotate the whole combination again in four days. The only exception to this is the wheat family or grasses. Cane sugar, barley, malt, rye, and millet are so antigenically close to wheat, that if a person is very sensitive to wheat, he should not have wheat or any of the other members of the family more than once every four days. However, if you don't have a susceptibility to wheat that you are aware of, you could have wheat one day and rye crackers two days later and wheat again on the fourth day. In this way you are actually having grains every other day. Some foods are in classes by themselves and have no antigenic relationship to other foods, such as sweet potato, sesame (tahini) elderberry, and persimmon.

It is best to make optimum use of your freezer, so that the four day rotation diet becomes easier. At first it seems impossible, but when you really analyze it, you find it is not only possible but also an extremely healthful way to eat. It avoids the refined sugars, over-processed flours, and excessive fats and oils that are so bad in the American diet. Instead, it concentrates on organic, wholesome, nutritious foods and avoids adulterated foods which are contaminated with many additives, colorings, preservatives, and other chemicals. It substitutes more nuts, berries, and fresh fruits. Many people, who have gone on a four day rotation diet because a member of their family had to, have acclaimed the vigor and good health that they felt while on it. This probably means that they had a sub-clinical hypersensitivity to some food antigens or that they were overdosing on the chemicals present in the sugars, over-processed flours, fats, and oils that play such a large part in the daily diet. Granted it is more difficult, but with planning it can be attained. The convenience or fast-foods, which got us into this trouble to begin with, are basically avoided.

The diets that follow are suggestions for living. Most people staying on the rotation diet have severe sensitivities and are also on food injections. The rotation, combined with the injections, help them tolerate the more common foods. Needless to say, we're all very different. You may not tolerate some of these foods (or be scared to death to even try them) for three to forty-eight months. So omit them and you can test their tolerance when you suspect you are ready. Remember, some foods are fixed allergens, and you will lose your sensitivity to them; they should never be tested because they could cause immediate death. When in doubt, see the doctor.

Days 1-4
Examples

If you need the choices made for you and don't want a pre-planned menu, try this. On Day 1, you can eat any food from all Day 1 categories. On Day 2, you can eat any food from all Day 2 categories, etc.

A far superior source is Natalie Golas', If This is Tuesday, It Must Be Chicken. It's silly not to own a copy if you're on food injections. No sense investing all the time or money to be on this and not spend a few dollars to get one of the most thorough sources on rotating.

Animal Protein

Day 1   swordfish
               flounder, halibut, sole, turbot
               duck (eggs)
               chicken (eggs), pheasant, quail

Day 2	clam, oyster, scallop
	squid, bass, perch, trout, grouper, salmon
	rabbit
	bacon, ham, pork

Day 2
clam, oyster, scallop
squid, bass, perch, trout, grouper, salmon
rabbit
bacon, ham, pork

Day 3
tuna, mackerel
whitefish
pike
frog legs
turtle
turkey (eggs)

Day 4
crab, lobster, shrimp
cod, haddock, herring, sardine
beef (butter, cheese, milk, veal, yogurt
lamb

Vegetables

Day 1
asparagus, chives, garlic, leek, onion,
shallot, broccoli, brussel sprouts, okra,
cabbage, cauliflower, Chinese cabbage,
collards, kale, kohlrabi, mustard greens, radish, turnip, watercress
beans, peas, peanut
soybean

Day 2
Chinese water chestnut
carrot, celery, parsley, parsnip, anise
sweet potato
artichoke, dandelion, endive, lettuce

Day 3
yam
beet, chard, spinach
olive

cucumber, pumpkin, squash, zucchini

Day 4	mushroom
	corn, bamboo shoots
	eggplant, sweet pepper, potato, tomato

Fruit

Day 1	fig
	grapefruit, lemon, lime, orange, tangelo,
	tangerine
	mango
	kiwi

Day 2	date, coconut
	pineapple rhubarb
	blackberry
	raspberry
	strawberry

Day 3	banana
	apricot, cherry, peach, plum
	blueberry, cranberry
	cantaloupe, melon, watermelon

Day 4	avocado
	apple, pear
	grape, raisin

Seeds and Nuts

Day 1	peanut, soynut
	cashew, pistachio
	sesame seed

| Day 2 | coconut |

filbert (hazelnut)
sunflower seeds

Day 3   chestnut
almond
pumpkin seed

Day 4   Brazil nut, pecan, walnut

Fats and Oils

Day 1   peanut oil, soy oil
sesame oil

Day 2   safflower oil, sunflower oil

Day 3   apricot oil, almond oil
olive oil

Day 4   corn oil, rice oil

Other

Day 1   breadfruit flour
carob flour, lima bean flour, peanut flour,
soy flour
sesame seed (meal), tahini

Day 2   buckwheat
artichoke flour, sunflower seed meal

Day 3   arrowroot starch, poi, tapioca starch

Day 4   yeast
barley, cornmeal, corn starch, millet, oats, oat
flour, rice, rice flour, rye, wheat, wheat flour.

cream of tartar
potato meal, potato starch

Sweeteners

Day 1   clover honey, sage honey

Day 2   date sugar

Day 3   maple syrup

Day 4   corn syrup, molasses
              raisin

Herbs and Spices

Day 1   garlic, chives
              horseradish, mustard

Day 2   kelp (seaweed)
              nutmeg
              anise, caraway, celery seed, chervil
              dill, fennel
              tarragon

Day 3   ginger
              allspice, clove
              comfrey
              lemon verbena

Day 4   bay leaf, cinnamon
              poppyseed
              basil, mint, lemon balm, marjoram, oregano,
              peppermint, rosemary, sage, spearmint, summer savory, thyme, paprika

The book by Natalie Golos', **If This is Tuesday, It Must Be Chicken** is well worth owning and far surpasses the ideas presented here. It even is color coded for the four days and has menus and recipes. (See Resources) Some cooks even color code the foods in the pantry for real ease.

Or if you prefer to create your own four-day rotation diet, choose any number of items. Just don't repeat any line in four days. All foods on the same horizontal line are in the same family and can be eaten on the same day.

Choices I
(Each line is a family)

Vegetables:

1. Lettuce, safflower oil, tarragon, sunflower, sunflower oil (goldenrod), endive, escarole, artichoke, dande lion
2. beets, spinach, beet sugar, chard
3. mushrooms, yeast
4. squash, cucumber, watermelon, cantaloupe, honey dew, pumpkin
5. cabbage, broccoli, cauliflower, brussel sprouts, mustard, turnip, radish, watercress, horseradish, kraut, Chinese cabbage
6. asparagus, onion, garlic, leeks, chives
7. carrot, parsnip, celery, parsley
8. potato, tomato, peppers (tobacco), eggplant
9. olive
10. sweet potato
11. sesame (tahini) sesame seed butter
12. avocado, cinnamon, bay leaves
13. okra (cottonseed)
14. pea, peanut, navy, kidney, lima, pinto, soy, etc beans, soy oil

Fruits:

1. apple, pear
2. blueberry, cranberry
3. rhubarb, buckwheat
4. orange, lemon, lime, grapefruit, tangerine
5. watermelon, cantaloupe, honeydew, cucumber, pumpkin,
   squash
6. date, coconut
7. cherry, plum, peach, apricot, nectarine, almond, prune
8. strawberry, raspberry, boysenberry
9. banana
10. fig
11. grape, raisin
12. pineapple
13. elderberry
14. persimmon
15. mango (cashew, pistachio)
16. currant, gooseberry

Other:

1. chocolate, cola, coffee, tea, (all ferments)
2. wheat, corn, corn sugar, corn starch, corn oil, corn oil margarine, rice, bamboo, millet, water chestnuts, cane sugar, oats, barley, rye
3. tapioca
4. avocado, cinnamon, bay leaves, sassafras
5. cottonseed, okra
6. mint, sage, thyme, basil, rosemary, peppermint, spearmint
7. honey
8. maple syrup

People often ask "What is there to eat on a rotation?" As you can see on day one you can choose any one of fourteen families of vegetables, any one of sixteen fruits, thirty- five proteins, etc. On day two you can have anyone of the thirteen families of vegetables left, fourteen fruits, thirty-four proteins, etc. Obviously, there is more than enough to eat. All that is lacking is organization and imagination.

Protein:

1. cashew, pistachio (mango)
2. peanuts, peas, peanut butter, beans, soy (soybean oil), lima, string, lentils
3. pecan, walnuts, butternut, hickory nut
4. scallops
5. swordfish, trout, salmon, sardine
6. chicken, duck, goose, eggs
7. turtle
8. frog
9. beef, milk, pork, lamb, rabbit, venison, goat milk, butter, cottage cheese, buffalo
10. Brazil nut
11. unusual meats, lion, etc
12. snail
13. lobster
14. crab
15. squid
16. abalone
17. herring
18. anchovy
19. tarpon
20. quail, pheasant
21. turkey
22. squirrel
23. dolphin

24. bear
25. whitefish
26. catfish, bullhead
27. haddock, cod, pollock, hake
28. sole
29. bass, perch, grouper
30. red snapper
31. pompano
32. mackerel, tuna, bonito
33. flounder, halibut
34. frog legs
35. oyster

Combinations:

1. cheese, yogurt, beef - yeast (ferment)
2. cider vinegar - yeast, apple
3. tofu - soy, yeast
4. wine - grape, yeast, beef
5. wine vinegar - yeast, grape
6. soy sauce - yeast, soy
7. bread - wheat, yeast, cane sugar, (egg, milk, raisin, cinnamon)
8. noodles - wheat, yeast, egg, buckwheat (soba)

Choices II
(Summary for quick shopping reference)

Four Day Rotation

I. Flesh

1. beef, pork, lamb, venison
2. chicken, eggs
3. haddock or cod
4. tuna

5. snapper, sole, etc.

Most fish are in separate families, so you could have fish every day and be rotating.

II. Starch or carbohydrates

1. wheat, rye (Ry-Krisp cracker or flatbreads), oats, barley (make soups), rice, corn, millet
2. peas, beans, lentils
3. nut meats ground
4. tapioca
5. potato
6. buckwheat (not in grass or wheat family)
7. amaranth
8. quinoa, teff

For example, you could have rye crackers one day, potato the second, rice the third, and lentils the fourth;, and you still haven't used up all the legumes, tapioca, nuts, bread, fruit, etc.

III. Snacks:

1. peanuts
2. raisins
3. figs
4. dates
5. cashews, pistachios
6. pecans or walnuts
7. almonds
8. popcorn

IV. Sweeteners:

1. maple syrup
2. honey
3. cane sugar, molasses

4. beet sugar
5. corn syrup
6. date sugar
7. rice syrup

V. Spreads:

1. butter
2. safflower margarine (without whey)
3. honey
4. peanut butter
5. tahini (sesame seed butter)

VI. Vinegars:

1. Since these are mold derived, use only one in four days: wine vinegar, apple cider, soy sauce, rice wine vinegar.
2. lime, lemon, another family and without ferment

VII. Oils:

1. olive
2. corn
3. safflower, sunflower
4. peanut
5. soybean
6. almond oil
7. walnut
8. linseed (flaxseed) --- do not cook or heat it.

VIII. Fruits & Vegetables

Choice of fruits & vegetables as on previous sheets.

Remember, you're just trying to find enough food for four

different days. As you can see, there is more than enough!

Stage III
Sample Diet

Four-Day Rotation Allergy Diet (simplified). Do not eat the same food (or any member of its family) for four days after ingesting it. Use sea salt for taste. Use glass bottled spring water (as much as you want).

	Breakfast	Lunch	Dinner
1.	apple cherries almonds peas	string beans teff lentils with garlic & parsley	beef or lamb potato, white broccoli
2.	eggs (safflower oil or margarine) pumpkin seeds banana rice cakes	carrots dates or raisins sunflower seeds	chicken rice squash sweet potato
3.	buckwheat pear juice sesame seeds honey pecans collared greens	beets cabbage spinach pears sardines navy beans	pork cauliflower turnips brussel sprouts peach or nectarine
4.	cantaloupe cashews	tuna lettuce celery watermelon	snapper, lemon asparagus cucumber millet

Stage IV
Day Rotation Diet Example

Day 1

Breakfast   cottage cheese or potato pancake fried in butter, milk tangerine, blueberries

Lunch   hamburg or deli beef slices, french fries or cottage cheese
avocado

Dinner   steak, potato au jus, parsnips, red or green peppers, strawberries in cream

Snack   cashews

Day 2

Breakfast   poached eggs or oatmeal w/cherries and juice, pear, prune juice

Lunch   rye crackers or rice cakes w/peanut butter or tuna or tahini (no mayo!), cucumber or lentils w/garlic & parsley, celery

Dinner   chicken in peanut oil, rice, broccoli or cauliflower, peas, cantaloupe

Snack   almonds

Day 3

Breakfast   banana, bacon

Lunch   peaches, raisins, pecans
Dinner   pork or lamb, carrots, asparagus, pineapple

Snack   figs

Day 4
Breakfast   apple, bagels, and lox

Lunch   whole wheat bread or toast w/corn marga-
               rine and/or honey, spinach & cold beets w/
               cider vinegar, squash

Dinner   white fish or shrimp, sweet potato w/maple
               syrup or corn margarine, lettuce w/apple
               cider vinegar and olive oil, basil, brussel
               sprouts or cabbage, beans, corn

Snack   dates

Sea salt in moderation allowed daily. Drink as much glass-
bottled water as you wish (Mountain Valley)

Four Day Rotation Schedule

Note: I have found it easier to map out a rotation if I
mimeograph my own blank four day calendar. Then I fill
in the dates and put it on the refrigerator. I just look above
instead of counting back four days.

Day 1	Day 2	Day 3	Day 4
Mon	Tue	Wed	Thurs
Fri	Sat	Sun	Mon
Tue	Wed	Thurs	Fri
Sat	Sun	Mon	Tues

Also, you can make the 4 days red, blue, yellow, green and

buy colored tape. Put red tape on day 1 oils, grain, etc., in your cupboard. Blue tape on day 2 oils, grains, etc. It facilitates deciding what you have to choose from.

Seven Day Rotation Diet Example

Day 1

Breakfast	milk, cinnamon toast, butter
Lunch	cheese and crackers
Dinner	steak, potato w/butter or sour cream, strawberries Romanoff (whipped cream or yogurt)

Day 2

Breakfast	melon, prunes
Lunch	cherries or apricot or nectarine, cashews
Dinner	snapper, Avocado, cauliflower, lettuce, safflower oil, wine vinegar

Day 3

Breakfast	pear, poached eggs
Lunch	rye crackers and honey
Dinner	lamb, mushroom, asparagus, parsnip, beets

Day 4

Breakfast	peaches (preferably organic, dried, home-canned or frozen)
Lunch	pecans, raisins
Dinner	sole, broccoli, sweet potato w/maple syrup

Day 5

Breakfast	apple
Lunch	rice cakes, peanut butter
Dinner	chicken, rice, carrots, red or green peppers or tomato, apples

Day 6

Breakfast	macadamia nuts, figs, grapes, tea
Lunch	tuna, banana, tangerine, rhubarb
Dinner	haddock or shrimp, spinach w/lemon juice, cabbage or brussel sprouts or turnips

Day 7

Breakfast	sausage or bacon, pineapple
Lunch	lentil w/garlic and olive oil or lima beans, oat cakes and tahini or sardines, dates

Dinner   green beans, cucumber w/olive oil and cider
             vinegar, peas, minced onion

Avoid refined sugars, over-processed flour and excessive fats and oils; unfortunately, these are the basis of the American diet.

Concentrate on wholesome nutritious and unadulterated (as much as possible) foods. Subustitute more nuts and berries.

As you get more sophistocated. dp away with margarines completely, for you don't want polyunsaturated hydrogenated oils in your kitchen; only cold-pressed oils and real butter. Try to avoid any processed foods and even canned and frozen unless you prepared them from your organic sources.

With time and practice, you will develop more organic sources and grow your own. This has made a tremendous difference in food tolerance for many.

Groceries for One Week

steak	snapper, etc
lamb	sole
chicken or turkey	haddock or shrimp
pork	sausage or bacon
butter, sour cream	crackers, wheat
milk	cinnamon toast
cheese	safflower
honey	eggs
maple syrup	rice
apples	peanut butter
tuna	tea
olive oil	cider vinegar
lentils	

289

Frozen or Fresh:

cherries, apricot, nectarine
red or green peppers or tomato
cabbage, brussel sprouts or turnip
green beans

cucumber	peas
garlic	lima beans
pilneapple	potato
avocado	cauliflower
lettuce	melon
prunes	pears
peaches	mushrooms
asparagus	parsnip
beets	broccoli
sweet potato	apple
spinach	lemon
tangerine	blueberry
rhubarb	grapes
banana	

Health Food Shop:

cashews	pecans
raisin	macadamia nuts
figs	dates
crackers rye	tahini (sesame butter)

If a seven day diet is too difficult, at least it makes a four day diet seem like duck soup in comparison. A four day diet is all that most people need anyway. A seven day rotation diet is for extremely sensitive people. If you require seven days, most likely you can only tolerate a maximum of three to five foods a day; so menus and combinations are out. You'll end up having one or two whole foods per meal. This leaves many foods for the other days.

Note: Many people feel best if they have only fruits for breakfast, vegetables at lunch (and raw as possible) and a flesh protein or bean, whole grain, and vegetable for dinner. They save nuts and seeds for limited snacks and they only have fruits alone (to decrease intestinal fermentation).

An 8 day rotation would be for someone who becomes intolerant of foods when they use them every 4 days. We show how it is done, but bear in mind one thing. If you are that sensitive, you need to step up your reading program and see the doctor. For you may have abnormal intestinal permeability, nutrient deficiencies, need to heal with the macrobiotic diet, to reduce your chemical overload, etc., etc. There is something very much in need of repair in order for you to bring this to a halt before you get into the downward spiral of disease.

Let's take a peek at an 8 day rotation:

Lunch	hamburg, french fries (safflower oil)
Dinner	steak, Potato au jus (or safflower margarine) asparagus,
Snack	pistachio

Day 2

Breakfast	rice cakes w/peanut butter
Lunch	cauliflower or brussel sprouts
Dinner	chicken in peanut oil, rice, broccoli, strawberries
Snack	sardines

Day 3

Breakfast	bacon, tea
Lunch	bananas, pineapple
Dinner	pork, carrots
Snack	cashews

Day 4

Breakfast	orange juice, melon
Lunch	cucumbers, pecans, figs, squash
Dinner	haddock or sole, sweet potato w/maple syrup

Snack pecans

Day 5

Breakfast	milk & oatmeal w/coconut flakes & sun flower seeds, apricots
Lunch	mushrooms w/wine vinegar & parsley, cot tage cheese & raisins
Dinner	shrimp, macaroni w/cheese and butter
Snack	lobster, French bread, herb butter

Day 6

Breakfast	pears, dates
Lunch	spinach w/lemon juice and olive oil
Dinner	turkey, beets
Snack	oyster

Day 7

Breakfast	apples, rye crackers w/corn margarine, apple juice
Lunch	lettuce w/corn oil and apple vinegar
Dinner	lamb, corn
Snack	walnuts

Day 8

Breakfast	boiled eggs, stewed prunes
Lunch	lentil - garlic, string beans or lima beans cashews
Dinner	tuna, celery, tomatos
Snack	clams

East no factory or fast foods. Eat no foods in a package, bag, box, jar or carton that has to have a list of ingredients and chemicals you can't pronounce, or that fail to tell what they are derived from antigenically. Try to eat as purely as possible for the first month. The first 2 weeks you will get an injection daily if possible. Then you will extend to 1 injection 3 times a week, or every other day. If your symptoms are not as well controlled, go back to a daily injection for a few more weeks or months.

Do not eat anything for the first month that you know you are allergic to.

At first, adhere to the four day rotational diet eating only foods to which you have been tested and which are included in your injections until you are totally clear of symptoms. This occurs within 1 to 4 weeks in most people. Stay on daily food injections until you symptoms are clear. If you cannot clear, let the doctor know because there is something still missing in your treatment plan or you have too much of a chemical overload (as usually is the case).

For example, I needed my food injections every single day for the first two years in order to be the clearest. It wasn't until I made my home and office chemical environments cleaner, detoxified some of my body fat stored chemicals, and corrected my many nutritional deficiencies, that I could go four to six days without needing a food injection.

Once you are clear, then you may try to reduce the injections to 2-3 times a week and still stay clear on the rotated diet. Then you may add-in once every four days a small amount of food to which you were allergic. When you eat a food to which you know you are allergic; give yourself an extra injection above and beyond the twice a week that you normally get. Eventually, you will find how much you can veer from the rotational diet. Often people are clear of symptoms with just two injections a week and an extra one if they eat a large portion of something to which they know they are very allergic.

Some foods are fixed allergens and you cannot now or ever eat them, regardless of injections. Other foods you will find you develop a tolerance to with time and can eat cautiously.

For example, I would wager I would never ever have a tomato or orange again in my life. I'm just too sensitive to them and the forms in which I most prefer them are concentrated so that I would be really overdosing myself (tomato sauce, orange juice).

Before I started injections I would take one bite of a pear and start breaking out. After a year of rotating and injections I could eat 3-4 pears if I had an extra injection and have no symptoms. Three years later I could eat 6 or 7 pears and not even require an extra injection. If that wasn't a scheduled day for a food extract injection, I wouldn't require one. Today I can eat them by the dozen, have no injections and no symptoms.

You will notice the diets that preceded contain many of the common foods that were never allowed in the 4 day rare food rotation diet. That is because that was a brief 2-6 week diagnostic elimination diet. The diet for very sensitive people who require food injections is for life and gradually more and more food tolerances are acquired. Do not be discouraged if you get worse going from a daily food injection to every other day. Just go back to daily as long as you need. I was on a daily injection for the first two years! Even years later, if I was even hours late for an injection I started breaking out. later my interval between injections now was anywhere from every 2-10 days, depending on what I was eating. If I was traveling I would get one every 1-2 days because my (chemical) load is up. At home I can go six to ten days. I know many patients who can go every 1-3 weeks. Just remember if you need to, you can always return to daily until you get simmered down.

As we did with inhalant allergies, we will still attempt to help you make yourself well with controlling the environment first. Only if this fails are injections utilized.

HOW ARE FOODS TESTED?

Foods are tested by the provocation-neutralization technique. It seems at the outset to be a very simple technique, and yet it is the most easily abused and poorly done technique of all in environmental medicine I feel. In fact, doctors set out to disprove it and published their work in the **New England Journal of Medicine** (Aug. 16, 1988). They were so blatantly ignorant of the technique that they used the dose that turns on or causes symptoms for the dose that is supposed to turn off or treat the symptoms. So you can see why they were able to "prove" it did not work: they had the technique backwards!

It takes weeks of practice for the allergist to be able to do it proficiently and still, he continues to learn and improve the longer he does it. Unfortunately, many conventional allergists feel it is beneath them to do any testing and yet it is very crucial for the allergist to become proficient in this so that he can always monitor the proficiency of the people that he has doing the testing for him. They really sink to disgusting depths when they use the

296

multi-test: a plastic board with a dozen needles that they plop on your arm and test all antigens at once. Sort of like branding cattle—and just about as accurate!

The difference between the serial dilution end-point titration technique and provocation-neutralization is that they both start out testing various strengths, but with serial dilution titration several dilutions of one or more antigen or one dilution of several antigens can be put on the skin simultaneously. However, with provocation- neutralization, one antigen and only one dose is tested at a time.

Therefore, it takes about three or four days for a person to be totally tested to say 50 foods. They arrive a 8:30 in the morning and begin testing until late afternoon each day. Beef is the first food tested and a screening dose of a small amount of a weak dilution is first put on. If the person does not have skin reactivity (wheal and flare) or symptoms induced, then a higher starting dose may be used and it will be assumed that the dose can be used for most of the rest of the foods. Exceptions are those that the patient suspects are a problem, those that are known to be a problem in many people and those which he ingests frequently.

So one dilution of a food is injected under the skin forming a bleb or a wheal. This wheal is measured in millimeters and it is palpated for certain characteristics. Dr. Miller has written a book describing this technique, but even the book will not replace hands-on, in the office, one-on-one training and no person should call themselves a specialist if they have not had intensive training in the offices of those who do provocation-neutralization proficiently.

In 7-10 minutes the symptoms that the patient has written down or we observe he is experiencing are noted. Also, the wheal and its characteristics are noted. If the wheal has grown 2 millimeters or more, that is a sign of positivity. If the patient has a symptom induced by the food, that also is a sign of positivity. There are many fine gradations of positivity that lie within this realm and as I say, it is a technique that is done poorly if not learned with extreme conscientiousness. It's also the most fun technique I think in allergy, because it never ceases to amaze us how foods and chemicals and hormones (which are also tested in this fashion) cause and clear such rapid and unexpected symptoms in such tiny amounts. The next weaker solution is then applied and the whole symptom complex is neutralized.

For example, we were testing Jane, a pretty and charming young redhead with asthma and eczema. The asthma had been cleared years ago with inhalant injections and now she was developing eczema and knew that foods were incriminated. When we applied lemon, she burst into tears. This is in contrast to her general personality makeup. When the next neutralizing dose was applied, she felt perfectly fine. She describes the feeling as that of being out of control of her emotions at the time.

Another woman who had severe asthma had potato tested and immediately she started wheezing. She exclaimed, "No wonder I could never get clear when I left the house. I always figured if I left the house at least I would be good for a few days. But wherever I go, potatoes are one of my favorite foods, so I always make sure I have them and I always have just as much asthma wherever I go".

Tomato seems to be one that is particularly bad for inducing arthritis in people who are testing for food-provoked arthritis. Many of the hidden food antigens such as corn, pork (lard), egg and soy are in so many of our foods that we don't even assume that we are ingesting them.

FOOD INJECTION CHECK LIST

1. Test at least 50 foods. Be sure you are not testing only to find out what you react to. That is not the purpose of food

testing. The rare food diet is much clearer and quicker at helping you identify food allergies. The purpose of testing is to find the neutralizing dose of a food to help lower your total load and increase tolerance to foods. I need all 85 foods in my shot.

2. Get nurse instructions for self administration of injections. You'll need a "buddy" at home to give the injections.

3. Get syringes, injectable Benadryl, adrenalin (Anakit), and Epi-Pen (also Lufyllin if asthmatic).

4. Order extracts.

5. Rotate only tested and known to be safe foods. Start with only one food a day. Work up to one food per meal as soon as your symptoms allow. When your symptoms are still clear with one different food per meal on a four day rotation, then go ahead and have two or three different foods per meal. If you get worse always back off to where you had no symptoms and stay there a few days or weeks longer. Then try to move ahead again with different foods. Do not advance ever until your symptoms are clear. Stay with one food a day, rotated, until symptoms are clear.

If not clear after a week, switch to four other foods that you consider to be safe. If a third trial is necessary and not effective, check your chemical environment because that is probably what is making you react. Be sure you're not drinking chlorinated water.

When you are up to five foods a day or more and your symptoms are clear, then you can go to every other day with your foods injection. Anytime you get bad, go back to daily food injections and as few foods a day as necessary to be clear of symptoms.

When injections are every other day and symptoms are clear, you can experiment with adding one new food every other day. Gradually build your repertoire of tolerated foods. When you have a repertoire of a large number of foods, then go ahead and extend the interval to every third or fourth day as your body tolerates.

6. Keep a food diary of what foods were eaten, when the injections were given, what symptoms occurred and what medicines were necessary.

7. See the doctor in 1 month, 6 months and 1 year. If you're doing fine, you can just send a note telling what symptoms are better, what symptoms are only partially controlled, how frequent your injections are, and how much medication you need. If we don't receive something or see you, your orders for new extracts will be rejected and this will hold up your progress.

8. As soon as you receive new vials, write the date when they will be half finished on the calendar so that you may re-order. We need at least 3 weeks for processing.

9. Refrigerate your current vial of foods as much as possible. Take them preferably before the biggest meal of that day. Some people get away with giving them sublingually, but you shouldn't try this until you are without symptoms and able to go at least every other day with an injection. Usually when you start sublingually you need them more frequently than you would by injection route, which is why we don't advocate it except in special circumstances where people are really afraid of injections. The foods should be refrigerated.

10. Freeze the other vials until you are ready to use them. Never defrost and refreeze.

11. Do not be misled by the neutralizing dose of a food. It

has little relevance to your degree of sensitivity and is only useful for me to know what strength to put in your injection. It DOES NOT mean you are or are not sensitive to a particular food. You can only determine that by the 4-day rotation rare food diet. The only two exceptions where we pay attention to food test results other than for determining the dose in your extracts are (1) if obvious symptoms are induced in testing, and (2) if a dose stands out from your other doses in being particularly different from the rest of your doses. Those foods in the last two examples should not be included in your safe foods during the first month as you attempt to bring all your symptoms under control.

12. After a month a strict safe rare-food rotation and daily injections, it's wiser to attempt to decrease your injections to every other day for several weeks. If your body tolerates this, then you are ready to start introducing one new food every few days and build your repertoire. Remember, if your symptomatic, to fast; clear your system and go back on safe foods and daily injections.

13. Be sure you have seen the two VTR's, Food I & II. They answer every question that was asked during the first year we did food testing.

Summary:

So there you have it, everything we can possibly teach you about rotation diets. If you need further information, consult the many references in the Resources, Mandell's, Golas', Randolph's, etc., the audio cassette on diet and the video cassettes on Food diets I and II. If you're still stuck, then you can schedule a consultation with the Allergy Assistant or the doctor.

Unfortunately, we don't know how to give you the one thing you need the most right now, will-power. Every time I ever fasted I was in such bad shape that there wasn't anything I wouldn't do. Still it was difficult until a couple of days passed. Rotating with only one food a day is likewise a struggle. The biggest part is over once your spouse realizes how important and necessary it is. When your friends treat it as natural or accept it because they want to see you better, they have done much for your self-esteem, guilt, embarrassment, laziness or whatever else keeps you from getting better. Remember, without love and encouragement, not only won't you be able to fast or do the diet, but your immune system won't be able to heal as fast.

A final note: As you improve and you get more proficient at locating organic foods, some days will present a tough choice. When in doubt, I opt for organic, fresh, whole, raw, living food over rotation. As your immune system heals, rotation is no longer so crucial to keeping that immune system vital.

Caution: There's a peculiar unmasking that occurs in some very select universal reactors. They get worse on the diet and more chemically sensitive. Some trade horrible symptoms like years of back pain for reactivity to all sorts of chemicals that they never noticed bothered them before. As in many oriental modes of healing, they actually get worse (detoxification, discharge, crisis, further deplete nutrients crucial for keeping them adapted?) before they get better.

Addendum: We have seen universal reactors who were intolerant of all food injections and nearly all foods, heal themselves over a period of 1-2 years with macrobiotics. It is not advised that you do this, however, without excellent macrobiotic counseling, one who has had experience with E.I. victims, and who is comfortable working with you to help you maximize your wellness. We will be glad to help you in this area. You start with **You Are What You Ate**, which introduces you to the principles, then proceed to **The**

Cure Is In The Kitchen, which is the strict healing phase. Then schedule your first "macro-consult" in the office. This diet is so powerfully healing that I myself and thousands others no longer need any injections or medications and have no symptoms. And we no longer have to stay on the diet. This is the same diet many used to reverse end-stage fatal cancers when they had been given only a few weeks to live. Our book **Tired or Toxic?** gives over 33 bio-chemical explanations of why and how it works to heal cancers, E.I. and just about anything you need to heal.

HIGHLIGIITS:

*   You must know food families or have a readily available chart.

*   You must plan your shopping, menus and meals away from home.

*   Eat only 0-3 foods a day until you get symptoms controlled, then start adding foods.

*   Stay on daily food injections until you have enough foods to eat, then reduce to every other day.

*   Never forget to go right back to fasting, then 1-3 very safe foods a day and daily injections if you get into trouble. Hooray for you! You have just learned one of the most difficult therapeutic techniques in environmental medicine. 99% of doctors do not know this very important tool that has enabled countless people to become symptom-free.

*   See the doctor if you keep developing new food sensitivities. You could have correctable intestinal hyperpermeability or leaky gut syndrome,

303

which causes food allergies. More about that in WELLNESS **AGAINST ALL ODDS** and ever more in **THESCIENTIFIC BASIS FOR SELECTED EN VIRONMENTAL MEDICINE TECHNIQUES**, and ever more in the soon to be released **LEAKY GUT SYNDROME**. All from this publisher.

So in essence, if food allergies are a problem, your first priority would be to identify what you react to (via the rare food diet), then avoid it and rotate the rest. If you still have too many intolerances, it is time to test to foods and learn to give yourself injections to them to build tolerance. Or you may need to do the intestinal hyperpermeability test to see if that is part of the cause of your food allergies. If food allergy is still a problem, the strict phase macrobiotic diet (**YOU ARE WHAT YOU ATE** then **THE CURE IS IN THE KITCHEN**) or the juicing, enzymes, enemas, etc. in **WELLNESS AGAINST ALL ODDS** have come to the rescue.

SECTION V
CHEMICALS

The Chemical Connection

My respect for chemical hypersensitivities came most slowly and in unexpected ways. I really was initially quite unimpressed with the potential harm that lurked beneath chemical hypersensitivities. Probably this was good. I had enough to think about with my food hypersensitivities. If I had also realized the extent of the chemical problems I would have been overwhelmed.

Probably my first realization of chemical hypersensitivity came while at Dr. Miller's office where I was testing foods. A nurse there developed laryngitis whenever someone entered the office with perfume. Her throatwarning very swollen and she could barely speak. They gave her neutralizing doses of the petro-chemical ethanol and it helped simmer her down. They also had to repeat this shot whenever the building was sprayed with insecticide.

However, I was too busy with my discoveries about food allergies to find all of this very exciting. What happened to give me such a healthy respect for chemical hypersensitivities was that I gradually developed more and more such sensitivities myself. In addition, I began to meet more and more people who had hypersensitivities to chemicals. Many of them already knew that they were sensitive to chemicals and so they made my work easier. I had only to suggest ways to avoid the chemicals. If this was impossible, I found that some could be neutralized, but this did not work for everyone. There were too many factors at work in some people.

These experiences enabled mformaldehydeingrepertoire and identify people who had chemical sensitivities which they were not even aware of. This has been happening oheadachesast few years all over the country in the offices of many ecologists. If we were suspicious of a certain chemical, we could test. Sometimes the testing would not only give the neutralizing dose to be given, but would provoke the very symptoms that exposure to that chemical could produce. Then we could find the maintenance levelshe reaction and that would be the one to be used by the patient. In other cases, testing did not provoke and injections were not helpful, but directmaintenance levelsthe chemical established that it was the offender and so avoidance was the treatment.

Now we know that a chemical hypersensitivity can mask itself as any disease thinkable. In addition, we know that in some very difficult cases the only way to effectively test is to have the individual in a totally hypoallergenic environment such as Dr. William J. Rea's environmental unit in Dallas. Dr. Theron Randolph of Chicago had the first unit in the world, since he was the first person to discover, in 1951, that people actually react to chemicals. (Forty-four years later the majority of the authoritarian medical establishments choose to deny this discovery.)

If the symptoms clear, then we can be sure that the patient is sensitive to something that he is no longer being exposed to. By putting him in a chemical booth and reintroducing chemicals one at a time, the offending antigens can be found. Often it is a sensitivity to multiple chemicals as well as multiple foods and multiple inhalant antigens that is responsible for the total symptom complex.

With time, hopefully, many more of us will have these very same units. In the meantime, fortunately, many people are not that sensitive and can even testtrichloroethylenethers, we can onlformaldehydee office. There is such a vast spectrum of people and symptoms that there is no one rule of thumb that can hoformaldehydeases. Again, individuality reigns.

Why are we becoming allergic to these chemicals of the 21st century? Obviously, the answer to this is in the fact that there are more chemicals in the environmenantibiotics before. Some sources say a new chemical is synthesized every minformaldehydentinually tighten buildings (to conserve energy), thus trapping the chemicals.

Insecticides are used on food crops before and after harvesting, in storage bins, in transport and even in the store itself. Herbicides, which are used to kill weeds, get absorbed into the food substance and cannot be washed off or peeled away. They penetrate the skin and remain even after boiling.

Many of these chemicals persist a lifetime, others take years beforcbloatingss out of the system. For example, DDT was partially restricted in the 1970's, but I still have an abnormally high level of DDT in my blood. I have found similarly high levels in most of the people that I have checked. DDT persists for years. BHT also persists in fat tissue for years. It is added to hundreds of foods to retard rancidity and prolong shelf life. It is in packaged cereal, gum, oils, shortening, pmineralsips, rice, candy, etc.

Fat substances accumulate insecticide residues aformaldehydeis notorious for its high fat diet.antibioticson, every cell membrane is made of fat. The reason some people feel terrible when they diet is that they have lost so much fat that the insecticide (which was originally bound to the fat) is now free to circulate through the bloodstream. They are actually feeling the toxicity of this free-floating insecticide in the bloodstream.

Chemicals abound in exhaust fumes from factories, trucks, cars and buses. One plane taking off is equivalent to anywhere from six hundred to over a thousand cars in traffic. Among the chemicals are formaldehyde, sulphur dioxide and nitrogen dioxide. The sulphur dioxiinstresstress with water in the air to form acid rain which kills fish in the lakes, destroys forests, etches destruction on the faces of time-worn buildings and depletes the soil of trace minerals.

Formaldehyde, of course, is in insulation, clothes, carpeting, furniture, draperies, bedding, pillows and mattresses. It makes fabrics stain resistant, wrinkle resistant, permanent press and "wash and wear." It's in shampoos, cosmetics and toothpaste. Conventional allergists are now even working on a new allergy injection that has a form of formaldehyde for its base. Of course, cadavers are pickled in it and the hospital is one of the worst places in the world for anyone with a formaldehyde hypersensitivity because the floors are washed with it and the bedding is permeated with it. The formaldehyde spot test has shown us that the drapes that divide semi-private rooms are about 100 parts per million of formaldehyde.

It's even in ice cream; it's in paints. Now the threat of formaldehyde is compounded. Not only do we have morstressstressf formaldehyde, but our technology has enable us to tiinjectionshe houses and offices to prevent outside air from entering. Some offices never exchange air with the outside without first putting it through a system which chemically contaminates it via the duct materials, coatings and adhesives.

Our enformaldehyde loaded with plastics, which not only can emit formaldehyde but phenols, pthalates, xylene, toluene and trichloroethylenes as well. Many of our medicines contain phenol. People who suck on cough drops all day may be ingesting phenol. Of course, it also is in conventional allergy injections. Even the lining of tin cans often contain phenol to prevent the food from losing color.

Chlorine is in laundry bleaches and cleaning solutions. Chlorine, you would think, would not be such a problem. You might even wonder where you come in contact with it until you see someone who is stuffy every morning after shaving, has a headache every morning after a shower or gets flushed, a rash or depressed. Some people have cerebral symptoms from just drinking water and believe me, when you have symptoms from drinking water you really begin to feel paranoid. (More on chlorine and how it can cause hypertension, cancer, and other diseases in **Wellness Against All Odds**.)

It's bad enough to be walking around talking about chemicals when everyone else seems to be functioning with no problems. When you start talking about being sensitive to the water, you really feel like it's time for them to come and carry you away. Every U.S. municipality chlorinates the drinking water with 1 ppm to discourage bacterial growth.

Many of us now cannot even so much as bring a glass of regular tap water up to our noses, much less drink it. The smell of chlorine to a chemically sensitive person is overwhelming. I remember a time when drinking tap water caused no problem for me. Now, if I lift a glass up to my face, I would not for a moment forget what it contained and drink it down absent mindedly. For the odor of chlorine that is emitted from it seems overwhelming to my senses. This is the case with many chemically sensitive people who have a heightened response and now react at levels where normal people never do. Chlorine sensitive people need to filter the drinking water and put sodium thiosulfate crystals in the bath water to neutralize the chlorine. They get so ill from the fumes that someone else has to draw their baths.

Yet, statistics tell us that our water is clean and pure and we have nothing to worry about. Various labs are currently analyzing various waters. It's an expensive task, but they are able to show that there are hundreds of chemicals, mostly coming from our factories, that are polluting our waters. Believe it or not, chloroform is one of the commonest contaminants. There formaldeheinous data on city waters, as most contain over 500 chemicals! When the cover of USA Today tells us that most city waters are highly contaminated with hundreds of chemicals, we know we're in deep trouble. I was afraid to mention this 15 years ago, but now even the average person knows it. How soon before the average Doc does?

People have a variety of symptoms from chemicals; unfortunately, most of them are cerebral - headaches, tremendous tiredness, depression, moodiness, irritability and an inability to concentrate. Not only are these symptoms more dangerous but they are also more nebulous. We feel intimidated and hesitate to mention them even to our loved ones or physicians for fear of being thought of as hypochondriacs. Even when you know which chemicals cause your symptoms, there's a loneliness that stems from trying not to let the rest of the world know. It's like being a leper!

I know a nurse who, after riding in an airplane for an hour, has profound muscle weakness. If she were to fall down, shethalidomidebe able to get herself back up. Yet, after a few hours out in thewarningy, her musculature is markedly improved. She is only 32-years-old.

Other people are such good barometers of chemical contamination they can tell if foods are organic or bogus. If insecticides or herbicides contaminate the food, they will experience a burning mouth, muscle achiness, tiredness, headache or nausea. There are a host of other symptoms, but these are the most common.

One dangerous symptom caused by traffic exhaust is mental disorientation. We have seen many people who have had such a problem. Usually it is a cold, wintery night and they have left work and are caught in a traffic jam trying to get out of a parking ramp. Within half an hour of being exposed to the heavy exhaust in this enclosed garage, they can hardly remember how to get home. When they do get home, it takes them several hours to recuperate. They may feel tremendous nausea and headache along with this cerebral disorientation. It makes you wonder how many auto accidents are caused by someone driving behind a large truck or bus and becoming overwhelmed by the exhaust fumes.

Many times I have had a tremendous headache, nausea, burning eyes and just felt like killing someone when I was sitting in a plane on the runway. The pilot would be formaldehydeuncing, "There are only three more planes ahead of us folks and then we'll be taking off." Everyone seemed to be happy sipping their drinks and chatting; I usually felt like I was going to throw up on my seatmate at any moment. We have testeNorman Cousinsave the same reaction after waiting in the blast of fumes coming from the jets ahead of them. Doesn't this affect their ability to navigate the plane? In fact, shouldn't this be part of the test of all pilots? Shouldn't they be put in a booth filled with diesel exhaust and then given a motor function test to see how they do? Perhaps this is a major cause of pilot error.

Plastic abounds everywhere. You're not even free from it in your auto. In fact, it's even worse there because many of the seats are totally fabricated of plastic compounds and, when heated by the sun, outgas even more than usual. Some people get body achiness, nausea, dizziness, confusion and depression when they get in their cars. In fact, they find they hate to travel or hate to shop, and it's not those activities at all that are actually bothering them. A car air cleaner, foil on the seats and a charcoal mask could work wonders.

Newsprint gives some people symptoms, such as burning eyes, runny nose and headache. It's easy to tell if you have this problem. Just sniff the Sunday paper; it's usually quite fresh and voluminous. People with this problem need to let someone else read it first and air it out in the sunshine. Some put it in the oven for twenty minutes at 180 degrees to accelerate the outgassing of the chemicals.

Natural gas is an expensive culprit to correct and probably the number one chemical causing sensitivities. However, it is one of the last ones thought of and least easily remedied because in order to get rid of it, you must totally remove it from the house. Turning off the gas is not sufficient for many people. The gas oven, the gas stove, the gas dryer and the gas hot water heater must all be totally removed from the house and electric units installed where needed. Even then, pinjectionsn ensue because outgassing from hot motor parts in heating systems of any sort can trigger symptoms in those chemically sensitive.

Many people get arthritis and body aches from natural gas. Some people get sick just eating food cooked in gas ovens or over gas barbecues.

Paint causes a variety of symptoms as does recent renovation, new carpeting, new wall-covering and new furniture. Newness means formaldehyde and not one of us knows how much it will take to increase our sensitivity and unleash a host of chemically-induced symptoms that we never before had.

Even the medicines that we take contain chemicals which can damage the integrity of cells in our body and hasten the advent of chemical hypersensitivity. One of the 14 ingredients in Premarin (the leading estrogen prescription) is shellac, and cough drops contain phenol. And what is worse is many medicines (Zantac, Tagamet, Pepcid, as examples) compete with the body's detox paths thus jeopardizing one's ability to detox other chemicals. More of this in our other books. Conventional allergy injections contain glycerin and phenol; all these chemicals can eventually make someone chemically sensitive, and worsen anyone who is already sensitive.

Of course, alcohol is a chemical that is frequently ingested and it leads to a great deal of chemical hypersensitivity. Many people are seriously and sometimes criminally different with it.

CHEMICAL VICTIMS

So, what do people with chemical hypersensitivities have to do? Everything in life seems to be against them. They require so many changes in their entire life-style, clothes, homes, friends and cooking and food storage utensils (they can even sense the presence of aluminum, plastic (from storage and freezer bags and tubs) and Teflon in their food). Fortunately, very few people have such exquisite hypersensitivities, but they are excellent models from which others can learn a good deal of what they have to do to overcome their chemical hypersensitivities. Each person can then modulate these controls according to his or her needs.

For those with exquisite chemical hypersensitivities, they need homes constructed of terrazzo floors and porcelain steel walls. Sometimes natural woods, other than pine, can be used. Aluminum wallpaper with a water soluble glue over wallboard is another solution which some have found tolerable. There is no universal prescription that can serve the needs of all hypersensitive individuals.

You probably realize that we have to switch gears and pay attention to every symptom, for early symptoms are a lot easier to treat than waiting for a full-blown reaction that may take days to clear. Often a spouse can tell we are reacting. In fact, we may be so far into the reaction that we'll vehemently deny any problem. They need to remove us from the area fast and they'll see they were right.

Heating systems should be electric. Even this is not foolproof. I bought an electric heater and the smell gave me such a headache that I had to run it for a year before the enamel covering stopped outgassing. Now you can order it without the paint on it! There should be fans and vents everywhere, especially in closets which contain typewriters, television sets, computers and other appliances with electric motors.

313

Any appliance that heats up or has a motor can also outgas numerous odors which have the potential to cause symptoms. The wires outgas phenol, formaldehyde and other chemicals. The motors and the motor oils outgas a number of hydrocarbons.

The pillows, beds, carpets, sheets and blankets should be of cotton or natural fibers that are tolerable. Foods need to be organic and should not be wrapped in plastic. Cellophane is tolerated by many and can be used for storage and freezing (Janice Corporation). I froze organic foods in plastic bags one year and threw them all away. All I could taste was plastic. Glass is even better than cellophane. I use my old Corning jars.

People with environmental illness, or E.I., are often prisoners in their very own homes, because there are no other environments quite like theirs that will provide freedom from exposures and subsequent symptoms. In order to heal our immune systems, we all need time out for a few years in chemically clean environments.

How do chemicals damage the cell membrane? By numerous mechanisms, as they can not only damage the cell walls, but also the internal proteins including the genetics. Damaged cell walls have an increased permeability to substances. Can some of this long-standing chemical damage present itself as arteriosclerosis, chronic arthritis, hypertension, heart disease, strokes and cancer? As you will see in subsequent books, yes. Also, new antigens are formed through chemical exposure; this has been proven for TDI, a common chemical in the plastics industry. And this happens with many other chemicals as well. When this happens, any organ can be the attack site, from the thyroid to the leg or coronary vessels, to the brain.

We never bargained for this. We used our chemical technology in good faith that we were creating a better world. We never realized that there would be people who would have to turn back the hands of time and live in a pioneer spirit with homes of wood, metal and natural fibers.

We never dreamed that the chemicals we were using, and are still using, in our foods and drinking water, and the outgassing from plastics, polyester, formaldehyde resin and building supplies would produce such insidiously lethal effects.

Now, however, the assault on modern man from the environment has become awesome. Besides obvious sources of chemicals, there abound thousands of hidden ones. Over the years, we have seen people react to the gas residue from oven cleaners and to food cooked in gas ovens, gas in roasted coffee beans, fumigants in herbs, seeds and grains, waxes in produce, eggs dipped in formaldehyde, clams and shrimp dipped in Clorox, plastic fumes from microwave dishes and wrap, pthalates in water stored in plastic, mercury amalgams in dental fillings, phenols and formaldehyde used to preserve root canal cavities and formaldehyde and phenol in tin can linings.

These are immediate reactions but slower ones occur too. There is evidence that aluminum from cookware, utensils, cans, processed foods and antacids is implicated in causing Alzheimer's presenile dementia. We have seen an alarming number of patients with elevated whole blood and urine levels of aluminum in the office on routine checking.

Of the twenty worst toxic waste sites in the U.S. as of 1983, six were in New Jersey. Not only does it possess more than any other state but also it has one of the smallest total areas. It is no coincidence that it also has the highest incidence of cancer of any of the states. These chemicals, though often ignored, are far from innocuous.

Chemical damage to cell membranes in the vascular areas (Dr. Rea's study in the **Annals of Allergy**, 1981, see Resources chapter) can cause serious phlebitis. Phlebitis, or inflammation of the blood vessel wall, results in dangerous blood clots that can break loose from the wall and flow along, eventually getting stuck. No blood can get by this occlusion and the remaining structure can die for lack of oxygen. The possibility of requiring an amputation is ever-present. And, of course, it can be the cause of a heart attack or stroke.

In his studies, Dr. Rea divided the patients into two groups; those who temporarily used the environmental unit to see if chemicals and foods could be the cause of their phlebitis and those who did not. After five years, all of the people who had identified their triggers were back to work, had spent very little money and had had no hospitalizations for phlebitis. The other group, who had had medical management, had spent thousands of dollars in recurrent hospitalizations. Some had had amputations; none were back to work.

Since that terrific study many of us have found that vessels, the heart, and any part of the body can be the target organ for chemical sensitivity. More on this in the **TIRED OR TOXIC?**

This shows that we are headed in the wrong direction by attacking heart disease with expensive heart transplants, whether artificial or real. We need to really back up and try to find a cause, not just treat the symptom. We need to examine what effect our environment is having on the vessels of the heart, lung and brain. The chemicals in our environment, in our home, in our offices, in the air we breathe, in our drinking water, in our food and on our very person deserve scrutiny.

Right now, if a vessel or heart is bad, they cut it out and replace it with a new one. If a segment of the bowel bleeds beyond control, they cut it out and throw it away. If uterus hemorrhages beyond control, they cut it out and throw it away. Thank God this approach is not used in treating severe headaches or V.D.!

We know there is damage to vessel walls in arteriosclerosis and allergy. If there is a tiny localized area of increased permeability or damage, a small amount of fluid leaks out and puffs up under the skin. We call this a welt, hive or wheal. If a small amount of blood leaks out, we call it easy bruising. If larger amounts of inflammation occur, we call it phlebitis. Clots form, break loose and block off or occlude circulation. Amputation is all that's left for the tissue that died for lack of blood supply. If these clots occur in the brain, we call it a stroke. If they occur in the heart, we call it a heart attack. It is all the same pathology or process.

Long before I was ever aware of any of this, my very own father went to a restaurant one evening and as he sat down, the waitress lit a candle. Within seconds, one side of his face was drooping and he was unable to speak. Because he was in his fifties, everyone immediately thought he was having a stroke and rushed him to the hospital.

Later, he told me that he knew as soon as he sat down that he didn't like the smell of the candle and that the fumes from it were affecting an area in his brain. He felt that the fumes were making it difficult for him to speak and control his facial muscles. He knew that as soon as he got away from these fumes that he would be okay, and he was. He knew this without ever having any knowledge of allergy or ecology himself. In fact he died years before I ever heard of this specialty. In his 50's he died of a heart attack. He had been plagued by angina for fifteen years. Was it possible that he had a vascular system sensitive to chemicals as well as diet? We'll never know.

So, if arteriosclerosis in the United States is the hallmark of old age, why did autopsies of teenage soldiers in Korea show arteriosclerosis? Could it be that it does not totally correlate with age and diet, but that chemical exposures (chemicals in our foods, water and environment) are actually adding to this vascular change? For instance, chemical analyses of the coronary artery plaque in men who died of heart attacks show a presence of plastics,

317

pesticides and benzene. Once these office, home and garage chemicals get into the bloodstream, do they possibly combine with other substances to produce these fatal deposits in blood vessels? Is this the missing factor that is eluding investigators? As you will see in subsequent books (all referenced for physicians) we now know how chemicals can do all of this.

Since the 1940's, the removal of vitamins E and B6 from all grains and oils has contributed to an increased shelf life for these products. It is, however, inversely proportional to our "shelf" lives! You are just not "in" today if you don't know anyone having bypass surgery. The market for cardiac drugs grows so fast I think they will soon run out of product names. The low cholesterol diet is a joke and one reason it isn't as efficacious as initially hoped is that they forgot to put back in the food what's missing. So most victims of high cholesterol are missing the nutrients with which to properly metabolize their cholesterol.

The hoax is, once you are told you have high cholesterol, you eat increasingly more plastic food. Since you shouldn't have cream (real cream from a cow before it has been homogenized has lipid-lowering substances in it, but by the time it passes through the factory, they have been removed), you use some form of plastic milk. This is usually a hydrogenated coconut oil derivative which is dangerously saturated. Or, you are told to use corn oil margarine; this product has been subjected to exorbitantly high temperatures and molecular change which is destructive to the body and potentiates arteriosclerosis. You are happy because your level of cholesterol is down and you will never know what insidiously killed you. How ridiculous can we get —instructing people to go out of their way to make themselves unhealthier! Plastic eggs, plastic sausages, plastic cheeses and hydrogenated corn oil margarines that are known to cause arteriosclerosis are recommended by cardiologists world-wide. However, it sup-

318

ports the food industry.

So we see that chemicals can cause a variety of symptoms and that they are the sneakiest little buggers to figure out. By no means do we intend to displace the conventional medical physician. Certainly, you should have a complete medical workup to rule out any known causes for your symptoms. Then and only then should you entertain trying to find a biochemical (nutritional) and environmental cause for your symptomatology. '

The primary treatment for chemical sensitivities is always to avoid those chemicals. Empty your immunologic rainbarrel by reducing the load of exposures to your system. Some people harbor large amounts of chemicals that persistently overload the immune system. They never begin to recover until they have been through a detoxification program. Years of residues from drugs, pesticides and other xenobiotics (foreign chemicals) must be flushed from their systems before they are able to initiate healing.

The pesticides are potentially the most dangerous of chemicals because they are specifically designed to be poisons and are stored in the body for years. There is much evidence in the scientific literature that they damage various parts of the immune system as well. Dr. Rea, himself, and many others traced the onset of their E.I. to pesticide exposures.

Medicine will soon catch on, and probably in ten or twenty years it will become routine to measure your serum insecticide levels. Right now there are very few places that do it. My serum DDT levels are abnormally elevated and so are my hexachlorobenzene levels. DDT, of course, is an insecticide that has been partially banned (a special permit is now needed to use it); unfortunately, it persists in the body for many years. Hexachlorobenzene is a fungicide that is still used as a fumigant for grains, seeds and nuts. Bread was one of my addictions and I ate horrendous amounts of it. As I move more and more to a truly organic diet and lose some of my fat (fat is where extra levels of insecticide are stored), hopefully I will be able to lower my levels to zero. At this point in time, the only person in the world who is known to have a negative levels is Dr. William Rea. It would be a good start for you to know your pesticide levels and then work at trying to reduce them to zero. No one knows the long term effects of having these potent chemicals stored in the body at all times.

So we have people sensitive to natural gas. We have people swaddled at night in formaldehyde. Do you remember the poor lady with the formaldehyde induced laryngitis? What would have happened if her target organ had been her brain instead of the larynx and she had become comatose or overtly schizophrenic? I wonder if anyone would have ever thought of taking her to her mother's for a week and thereby getting her out of the high formaldehyde level in her home? If they had taken her to a hospital, she would have remained just as bad (in fact, this did happen). What if she had been a baby instead of an adult and couldn't speak? Would anyone have thought of chemicals since no one else in the house was affected?

How do we avoid these chemicals? First, we must have a great deal of knowledge and second, we must slowly eliminate them one by one from our environment. At first it seems overwhelming. How can I live in a world without chemicals? You must remember that a journey of a thousand miles begins with one step. When you start feeling good, you will become hooked on feeling good and you will do anything to keep it that way.

I needed many tests and trials to be sure that chemical exposures could exacerbate an area of previous injury and weakness in my back. Now, it is no longer a problem for me to do what I have to do to keep from having this pain. Compliance improves with practice. Still, it is hard to believe that chemical hypersensitivities can single out an area of previous weakness (an old injury or infection like polio years earlier) as the target organ.

For the uninitiated, I know this sounds absolutely totally bizarre and ludicrous; it did to me and I was one who was in need of it. However, once I saw for myself that I could provoke and then relieve my back pain by controlling the chemicals I was exposed to, I became a believer. When I realized that now I could have pain-free days without the nausea caused by medication, I became more serious about pinning down the exact cause. Now I know what chemicals to avoid. By watching my foods, I can enjoy an increased state of well-being and a decreased need for injections for foods and inhalants. My skin has cleared and I no longer suffer with headaches, sinus infections, asthma and a constant clearing of my throat. Now I am addicted to feeling good. I am hooked on feeling well and it would take a tremendous force to make me return to my old ways.

I used to go to bed in tears many nights feeling sorry for myself for having such an ugly eczematous face. I also felt sorry for my husband for being saddled with this self-pitying mess. Then when I hurt my back it seemed that life was totally stripped of pleasures. I either couldn't do something because it hurt my back or it caused an allergic reaction. Just about the only thing I could do, which is ironic considering the severity of my symptoms during those 16 years, was practice medicine. I see that God had a plan. For I would never have become involved in all this and would never have been able to reach so many people had this not occurred.

Unfortunately, there are many other people who have these very same sensitivities and most likely the number will increase. In the early 1980's, the **New York Times** (December 26) contained an article that was indeed a sign of our times. The article described how toxic chemicals were discarded by several factories in Minnesota, causing the drinking water to be unfit for two large cities. The ground water was seriously contaminated with trichloroethylene and other carcinogenic chemicals. Industrial wastes had been seeping into the water supply for an indeterminate amount of time. Trichloroethylene is a solvent and degreaser and it is used in dry cleaning clothes, making plastics, manufacturing lacquer and in decaffeinating coffee. It has caused leukemia.

Testing of the water showed that these chemicals were in the hundreds of parts per billion; drinking water should have no measurable amounts of such chemicals. Predictably, there were many people who had bizarre symptoms for which medicine had not been able to find the cause. These people obviously could no longer even trust their government to look after their welfare, for it had failed them miserably. It had allowed industry to poison their water supply.

One person had stomach symptoms and diagnostic tests could show no cause. It made me wonder how long it would take for this person to develop leukemia or just how much water a small child could drink before becoming seriously poisoned.

The problem is these chemical compounds are tasteless and odorless. Their presence is only detectable with very sensitive and expensive chemical tests. What guarantee do we have that the appropriate tests are even done, much less done correctly? One of the offenders was an ammunition plant, another was a cartridge company and another was a creosote treating plant.

Since that time, there have been dozens of cities across the U.S. that have discovered the same problem in their water. The only difference is it no longer makes the **New York Times**. In fact, it's lucky to go beyond the local rag. We have accepted gross chemical contamination as a part of life.

In a second article in the very same paper, we see that modern man has contaminated the ground in another town in Missouri. There had been floods in the wintertime and people were saddled with the depressive task of going back home to clean up the mud from their homes. To make matters worse, it was the discovered that dioxin (the culprit in Agent Orange), which was sprayed ten years earlier on children's tarvia playground, now contaminated the ground and water of the entire area, making it unsafe all along. These people feel betrayed by their government. For years, many of them had even been growing their own food in their gardens and were under the illusion that these foods were safe and healthful. They probably had absorbed a great deal of the dioxin. They laughed when the government told them to move. They asked how the government knew that wherever they would go would be any safer. Of course, their biggest worry was the medical future of their children.

I recently went to an allergy meeting to show my mycologic (mold) research and realized that I spent the day in a man-made environment. I started out in the morning encased in the gaseous cocoon of an airport, then in a limousine, then in a large convention hall, then in an underground shopping mall, then in a smoke-filled restaurant and finally in a hotel with windows that did not open.

Most of us are constantly indoors in enclosed malls, offices and houses with the hatches battened down. We have neglected to consider along the way whether or not man has the ability to adapt to these fake environments; these environments where we have added a host of chemicals that many have never before been exposed to; an environment where we are not permitting clean air to dilute these chemicals, but instead are concentrating them by keeping it airtight. Add to this the problem of individuality and the fact that diseases are caused by these chemicals in a vast portion of the population, and we have a very difficult problem indeed.

Where will it all end? Don't kid yourself. I think it is just beginning.

Scientists keep saying cancer is caused by a virus, but they have yet to find it. The American Cancer Society is no longer blind to the evidence of the thousands of environmental chemicals that have caused cancer. People have tremendously individual biochemical make-ups. Susceptibility to chemically-induced cancer is highly individual. Laboratory tests are performed on highly inbred strains of animals; they are all genetically very similar. No wonder it's hard to prove cause and effect. That's why 1/100th of the dose of thalidomide found safe in rats caused deformity in humans.

Anything you can breathe can get into the bloodstream. That's how people die of odorless carbon monoxide poisoning! To save a few hundred dollars a year in fuel bills, people have tightened up their houses to decrease air turnover. As a result, they are spending thousands of dollars on diagnostic tests to figure out the cause of symptoms induced by chemical inhalations.

By the time they are diagnosed, their sensitivities have multiplied. It often takes two to seven years after returning from a unit to heal and increase tolerance to normal exposures. During this time, they are prone to frequent backslides in their progress with the slightest exposure. Depression is hard to fight and they are wise to form support groups with other sensitive people that they meet in their doctor's office.

The commonest symptoms are cerebral and neuromuscular; they are bizarre and defy medical diagnosis. Any symptom is possible. The situation is urgent for the many affected. Remember, if you have stomach problems, you get x-rayed, medicated or surgerized. Then if you're lucky, someone will think of allergy before hypochondria. If your symptoms are cerebral, we don't have many tests, so the diagnosis of a "nut" is arrived at sooner.

Out-of-doors used to be a safe place to go, but in cities we have sulphur and nitrogen dioxides, formalde-

hydes and other chemicals that are spewed out from vehicles and the chimneys of factories. Many people cannot
even walk in their neighborhoods because of wood burning
stoves and clothes dryer fabric softener sheets that are
exhausted to the outside.

Many patients become overtly ill from city traffic
fumes. In fact, cerebral dysfunction is one of the most
prevalent and dangerous symptoms in a situation that calls
for split second decisions and coordination.

These exposures leave unmentioned another chemical source, medicines. We are a drug culture. No one
knows the long-term effect of so many drugs in one body.
We do know they deplete a host of vitamins, but we were
never trained to replace them or even check for their
deficiencies. We're just starting to realize that in some
people. Lasix can cause irreversible auditory nerve damage, or deafness, and arthritis medicines can cause permanent damage to the eye after years of use, or the development of food allergies after just a month of use. We already
know many of our cytotoxic drugs or cancer drugs may
clear cancer in one organ, only to cause it in another later.
Not only has our environment changed in the last few
decades, but mankind has changed. We now have generations of people who would not have survived were it not for
antibiotics and insulin. In other words, we have genetically
weaker or maladapted people.

So, here we have a perfect set up: a genetically
weaker race exposed to a sudden burst of thousands of
chemicals. Is it any wonder that at least 20% of the population is affected by ecologic or environmentally-induced
illness? Is it any wonder that at least 20% are unable to
adapt to their environmental overload? These chemicals
then injure the immune system and damage some of the
suppressor cells that regulate the way in which a person
either over- or under- responds to foreignness. We already
have direct evidence how chemicals involved in making

plastics induce changes in body proteins, causing the body to make antibodies against its own tissues; the result is asthma or a myriad of other diseases.

Most people do not know that they have chemical or food sensitivities. They just go through life at half-mast assuming they have to "learn to live with it." They learn to live with chronic tiredness and depression that come and go for no reason and a host of other symptoms. They have exhausted all that medicine has to offer and when all the tests are done, they're either told one of two things: "You have to learn to live with it," or, "Why don't you see a psychiatrist?"

Yet, their intuition tells them that it's not normal and they are correct. Indeed, they are victims of a maladaptation to the new 20th century environment. Addendum: In November 1993, I went to the American College of Allergy and Immunology meeting. They spent a day teaching doctors that chemical sensitivity is a psychiatric illness! And they did not present one shred of evidence, nor did they discuss the biochemistry of chemical sensitivity at all. These are the people whose commercial exhibits at their meetings are 99% drugs, as opposed to our meetings where they are 99% air cleaners, cotton products, nutrients, hypoallergenic foods, books for patients and doctors, environmental units, special laboratory tests to diagnose chemical sensitivity and toxic levels of pesticides and other chemicals, special mold plates, formaldehyde spot tests, and all sorts of special patient resources.

This was initially written in 1984, and lightly edited in 1994. For more information, complete with references from the scientific literature, see **TIRED OR TOXIC?, WELLNESS AGAINST ALL ODDS,** and **THE SCIEN-TIFIC BASIS FOR SELECTED ENVIRONMENTAL MEDICINE TECHNIQUES.**

General: Chemical incitants are found in our air, water, foods, drugs, cosmetics, furnishings, appliances, construction materials, office supplies, heating systems, cleansers, fumigants, and textiles. They are hard to pinpoint because they are taken for granted; they are not suspected. Even when they are recognized, it is hard to avoid them because they are so commonplace. Few people are able to adapt to the new chemicals and live with them. There are many people whose adaptation decreases with constant exposure and/or with stress. They become increasingly susceptible to certain materials and their symptoms become chronic, that is, always present. People suffering with chronic sensitivities may have many mild, vague symptoms that together are not severe enough to impel them to see a doctor. They may be tired, drowsy, droopy and irritable and they do not realize that these symptoms are a result of something in the air or something they ate, drank or touched.

For example, Charles had arthritis for a year-and-a-half. He was a 39-year-old consulting engineer and he developed his pain shortly after moving here. He consulted many rheumatologists. He noticed that when he was out of town on a job for several days, he didn't hurt. We tested him to formaldehyde and caused his pain to reappear, then we neutralized it within minutes. Measurements of his blood level of formaldehyde were twice as high after a weekend at home than after a day at work. The source? His 2-year-old home had particleboard subflooring (formaldehyde), new carpets (formaldehyde), new furniture (formaldehyde) and gas heat (formaldehyde as a byproduct of incomplete combustion).

Moving to a 20-year-old house with electric heat and hardwood floors and going to house sales for older furniture brought relief. Some people test chemicals beautifully, as he did. One dose turns him on and another dose turns

327

him off. This only happens if the person is not too over-loaded.

For years I had severe symptoms from formalde-hyde and natural gas, but testing produced no reaction. I was chronically overloaded. This is an important point, for some people assume a negative test means they are not chemically sensitive, when in reality nothing could be further from the truth. Much caution should be exercised in deciding the interpretation of chemical testing and a consultation with the doctor is recommended.

In cases where legal proof is needed, the chemicals are tested single-blind on two different days in different order. Also, a random sprinkling of normal saline placebo controls is used. In this way, no one can accuse the patient of malingering. If the person reacts to the control as well, he is most likely overloaded and needs to return after a few days in an oasis. Then his reactions are dramatic.

For example, a dentist tested chemicals and reacted to every test, even the control or salt water. He then spent a night in a farmhouse in the country. The next morning he was beaming. He had had his best sleep in years. This told us that the air in his own city was too contaminated for him to ever get better because even sleeping in a cabin in the outskirts of that city for one week didn't make him as clear as a night in that farmhouse did. When we tested him the day after having slept in the farmhouse, his reactions turned on and off like a switch, providing the proof he needed.

Basically, we do not like to give injections for chemi-cals. There are some exceptions, but, in general, it is best to avoid them to reduce the total load and allow the body to heal and overcome chemical hypersensitivities by healing the detox pathways as many of us have. As well, once someone reduces his chemical overload, he finds his food, inhalant and Candida sensitivities improve.

Again, natural gas is one of the most common causes

of symptoms. It is used in hot water heaters, clothes dryers, ovens, ranges and heating systems. Many peoples' symptoms become worse in October when the heating system is turned on. In between heating cycles, the exhaust flue for the furnace becomes cold. The cold flue does not conduct heat upward, so when the thermostat sends the message that more heat is required, the gas ignites again. Until the flue is warm and a draft is created, there is a backflow of the products of combustion backup into the cellar and eventually into the whole house. Formaldehyde is one of these products.

A government EPA official, James Repace, wore a pollution monitor for 24-hours. He wore it as he traveled through the Washington rush hour traffic; he wore it in his office; he wore it in meetings where he was surrounded with cigar smoke and aftershave; he wore it in the smoke filled EPA cafeteria, etc. The peak of pollution measured was surprising: it was in his own home while having dinner in the kitchen near the gas oven and stove.

Some people cannot go outdoors in the winter because their neighborhood has many wood burning stoves. The burning wood triggers their asthma or headaches. In fact, they must devise an air filtration system of activated carbon and purafil so that when they open the window they can filter the outdoor air coming in. Since most of the chemicals we react to are below the threshold of perceptible odor, this is the spookiest allergy of all.

We once waterproofed our basement walls. I couldn't smell the petrochemical but knew I was reacting badly because throughout the afternoon I developed the most severe headache I had ever known. By evening, I was trying to finish up seeing patients when I suddenly couldn't read, think or speak. It was literally a blinding headache. I could not see. As soon as I got away from these premises, all my symptoms disappeared within three hours.

After an hour-and-a-half in a shopping mall, it used

to be I wouldn't know if I was going to throw up or pass out because of such severe back pain from an old horseback riding injury. After getting back outside awhile, I was back to normal. Another time I arrived at my hotel in St. Louis. I was going to give two lectures at the Advanced Course for Physicians Learning Clinical Ecology Techniques. The first night I woke at 2 a.m. feeling so agitated I thought I would jump out of my skin. After an hour of pacing in the room, I realized I was reacting to something in there. I dragged my mattress to the floor and slept with my nose out the patio door. Some of the worst problems of chemical reactions are:

(1) Often no one can smell the chemical; however, if someone can, it's usually only the person reacting to it who does.

(2) The person reacting gets either a physical symptom which he would never dream of blaming on a chemical or a cerebral symptom which causes sudden mood changes.

(3) Once the person starts reacting he is usually helpless in terms of being able to diagnose the problem or even get out of the area. Often he is hostile to well-meaning friends who try to help him or suggest he get out of the area.

I arrived at a beautiful hotel in Rome with my husband. We were having the best vacation we had ever had. We walked into our room and within five minutes I was in tears, denigrating the room and being about as negative as possible about anything that popped into my head. We went for a walk and I cleared. When we came back, we were on the lookout and recognized the cause; there was a noticeable odor of a glue that had been used with the new wallpaper. We got another room that had not yet been refurbished and I was fine.

Chemical reactions can be very stressful to personal

relationships and draining on the uneffected spouses. Not only do the spouses have these bizarre episodes to contend with, but they also have the added burden of executing the responsibilities of the one who is sick. A dangerous reaction is the mental fogginess that occurs when some people are exposed to traffic fumes. This can be very heavy in a parking garage or in a tunnel or behind a diesel vehicle. Your reaction time and judgement can be dangerously altered. One young secretary was having enough problems with the cigarette smoke and perfumes at work, and by the time she sat in the parking garage lineup, she became so drugged she could hardly see her way home. Once home, she was finished for the evening and only able to go to bed. Another young engineer was so drugged by the time he got to work in his car (because of new vinyl interior) he couldn't function. The pre-fab cubical walls (formaldehyde), felt pens, inks, and oils from a nearby copy machine finished him off.

If the office is the source of chemicals causing symptoms, it's easy to diagnose since the person will usually clear out on weekends and vacations. The commonest source of pollution is the home and, therefore, the most commonly affected victim is the wife. She rarely gets out into a cleaner environment (shopping malls are worse than the home usually) long enough to get clear (it could take days).

One teacher had been bedridden with rheumatoid arthritis for several months. She was very lucky because her proof came easily. In four minutes we were able to neutralize her out of pain and stiffness with an injection of phenol. Even though she lived over one hundred miles away, she came to Syracuse several times to allow us to test her double-blind and film her so that other doctors could learn about environmental medicine. Within minutes she was laughing, touching her toes, skipping down the hall and waving her arms as if about to fly. She was rightfully excited for good reason - for months she had been unable to touch her toes, comb her hair or even peel a banana. She needed the assistance of her husband, a college English professor, for just getting up the single step to our office door.

Even though she was lucky in having dramatic proof that 20th century chemicals were the cause of her misery, it didn't make environmental controls come any easier or quicker. We know she will never get completely better until she gets rid of the natural gas, new carpets, newly upholstered furniture and the many objects that outgas formaldehydes and phenols. The house is old enough, but they also built a couple of new rooms prior to the onset of her arthritis. Whether she will be able to tolerate the building materials in those additions will only be determined after all those other items have been first removed. However, another culprit is the presence of the nearby super-highway. Moving would be best, but they've spent years adapting this home to their needs.

So you see, the chemically sensitive patient indeed has the toughest sacrifices of all in order to be disease-free. He really needs a house devoid of all modern day chemicals which got him in this predicament to begin with. You can easily appreciate that we've created a monster by introducing these thousands of untested chemicals into our modern world. We neglected one basic biological principle, and that is to be sure that the organism (man) can adapt to these. Many of us can't.

For instance, there is the child who fails his math test because strong phenol solutions were used the night before to clean the classroom floor; there is the secretary with migraines due to NCR paper or the copy machine; there is the engineer who can't concentrate by afternoon because the air intake is on the tarred room which is heated by the midday sun; there is the wife with chronic depression from natural gas or chronic cough from plastics.

When my secretary used to book me into a hotel to give a lecture, she had to request an older, non-renovated room with a window that opens. It must not be on the traffic side of the building. There should have been no cleaning solutions used that day, and preferably should not have been previously occupied by a smoker. Even with all this, there still were many items that I used to bring with me to increase my tolerance in such a highly chemical environment. Some hotels have been so badly contaminated with natural gas from their many restaurants that I've had to rent oxygen for my entire stay in order to survive and deliver my lecture.

I appreciate permission to borrow some of the following technical information from Dr. William J. Rea's **Office Manual:**

Indoor Pollutants: You may have noticed an increase in symptoms (particularly in the eyes, nose, sinuses or bronchial tubes) when you have been exposed to smoke from a poorly vented fireplace, fumes from drying paint or exhausts from cars in a tunnel.

Did you know that you may be sensitive to odors? Some people are sensitive to odors from hydrocarbons, such as oil, gas and coal. They react to the leaks of natural gas from the gas range, refrigerator, dryer or water heater. Also, they may be sensitive to the odor of oil from the garage, furnace, appliances (with lubricated electric motors or fans) or oil-soaked filters used in air conditioners.

Even odors from a warm-air heating system may cause symptoms. Steam heating systems may affect people susceptible to the odor of chlorine in the water. Leaking refrigerant gas from electric refrigerators and air conditioners may be an unsuspected incitant. Other sources of possible incitants include soft plastics, vinyl, rubber, polyester, rayon, nylon, carpeting, pads, upholstery, drapery, clothing, bedding, city tap water, solvents, dyes, scented cosmetics, household cleaners, polishes, waxes, ammonia, detergents and cleansers.

The person whose symptoms are usually worse at night may be reacting to odors from rubber pillows, foam mattresses, rug pads, plastic pillow or mattress cases.

In public places you may be exposed to disinfectants, pine-scented sweeping compounds, deodorants, insecticides, or oil or gas space heaters in small shops.

School children may become overactive, irritable or tired as a result of air pollution, particularly if the classroom is over the kitchen, furnace room or near the swimming pool, restroom, supply room or incinerator.

In an office, you may react to inks, carbon paper, duplicating machines, rubber cement, typewriter ribbons or pads, perfumes, fabric softeners, deodorants worn by fellow workers or smoke from cigars and cigarettes. NCR "carbonless paper" causes burning eyes and severe headaches in susceptible people while others are seemingly unaffected. Green and pressure treated lumber contains pesticides and fungicides that affect susceptible people. Use only kiln-dried lumber.

Outdoor Pollutants: When outdoors, the susceptible person is likewise exposed to many potential incitants.

Probably the worst offenders are gasoline and diesel motors. People living near certain manufacturing or processing plants, refineries, storage tanks or coal-fired factories are assailed by smokes and gaseous discharges that can call forth sensitivities, especially, but not exclusively, in body organs concerned with breathing. You may be afflicted by odors from tires, car rust-proofing, upholstery, gasoline pumps or leaking automotive fluids. Other troublesome odors include fogging for insect control, spraying for weed control, tarring of roofs and roads, burning rubber from incinerators, creosote from railroad ties, waxed cartons and oil-soaked rags. Wood burning stoves are now creating more of a problem than industrial effusions.

Additional common offenders include coal, oil, petroleum by-products, natural hydrocarbons such as terpenes, marsh gas, alcohols, glycols, formaldehydes, insecticides, herbicides, pesticides and chemical fertilizers.

It is important, therefore, that the sensitive individual be aware of his reactions when exposed to chemical toxicants; only then will he be able to identify troublesome substances. The most common reactions include headache, fatigue, depression, forgetfulness, nervousness, diarrhea, dizziness, irritability, impaired reading comprehension, difficulty in coping with figures and other abstractions, mental confusion, learning disabilities, respirator problems, hives and dermatitis. However, the symptoms may be highly individualized and unique to a given person.

Minimizing Chemical Exposure: A few precautions and recommendations are described here which will aid in minimizing chemical exposure. All products mentioned have been successfully used by chemically sensitive patients, but should not be regarded as safe for everyone. Before using any product, be sure to test it in small quantities to determine your individual reaction to it. We are all different.

The Home: Oil, coal, gas ranges and gas utilities rank highest among primary offenders in the home. Electric utilities are recommended. All odorous products, including cleaning supplies, insecticides, paints, solvents and laundry products should be kept in a separate building away from the house. Felt tip pens, cosmetics, perfumes, shoe polish, lighter fluid, glue and the like should be kept in tightly sealed containers. Large coffee cans with plastic lids are ideal for this purpose.

In cleaning, utilize less toxic products and **avoid all types of aerosol sprays**. Vinegar (one tablespoon per quart of water) is excellent for cleaning mirrors, glass, tile, chrome and stainless steel. It may be used in rinse water when shampooing or laundering to remove detergent residue. **A dish of vinegar and water left uncovered makes an excellent air freshener.** Cake Bon Ami and unsoaped steel wool pads are recommended for tough cleaning problems such as ovens, stove burners and cookware. For wax build-up, furniture refinishing and pipe and drain maintenance, use Sal Soda concentrate. For **dusting** and polishing, a lightly dampened cotton cloth works well. Zephiran mixed with water makes an anti-bacterial and anti-fungal agent and may be used in skin care as well as in household cleaning. For **dishwashing**, 1/4 cup of borax may be substituted for dishwashing detergents, such as Amway, Shaklee or Neo-Life biodegradable non-scented products.

Use heat, dryness and fresh air to prevent mildew. Do **not** use paraformaldehyde crystals (formaldehyde), Lysol (phenol), or such other smelly cleaning and air freshening products since the fumes are too toxic for a sensitive individual.

Clothes moths cannot stand much activity, sun, light or even air movement. Therefore, remove your clothes periodically from dark closets and brush and air them in a well ventilated area. Use your vacuum cleaner frequently to keep dust removed since dust is an excellent breeding place for moths.

For insect control, do not use sprays or aerosols. Boric acid powder can control roaches. Use diatomaceous earth for fleas. A mixture of honey and boric acid is usually effective against ants. It is also said that ants can be kept out of your house by putting coffee grounds or red pepper around the outside of doors and windows. (Check other books at N.E.E.D.S. on non-toxic pest control).

Wash clothes, all bed linens and towels with washing powder distributed by Shaklee, Neo-Life or Amway. Or, use 20 Mule Team borax on a one-to-one basis with baking soda. Do not use bleach, fabric softeners, starch, etc.

Rinse twice. Vinegar may be added to rinse water.

Remove all feather pillows. Make your own by stuffing a pillow case with cotton batting or cotton blankets or a pad of twenty Curity diapers. Or, buy a cotton pillow or send for one yard of muslin and one pound of cotton and make your own for one-third the price. Put several layers of cotton sheets and blankets over conventional mattresses. The very sensitive should place five layers of heavy duty aluminum foil (shiny side up) under the cotton sheets and two cotton mattress pads.

Make an ironing board cover with old sheets washed with Borax and one of the above mentioned powders.

Personal Hygiene: Tobacco smoke is particularly dangerous for the chemically sensitive patient and must be avoided. When possible, wear garments made of natural fibers, such as cotton, silk or linen which have not been chemically treated and which may be home laundered. For items which must be drycleaned, utilize cleaning services which do not use insecticides in their cleaning solution. dispose of plastic bags and air all drycleaning before hanging it in the closet.

Use nothing in or on your body except the following:

Shampoo: Almay or Ar-ex, Castille soap, Johnson baby shampoo. Do not use rinses, dyes or conditioners unless totally unscented.

Bathing soap: Ivory, Basis or Nivea Basis soap or Oilatum or Rose Petal Liquid.

Deodorants: Baking soda, Almay, Cheq. (Once your body is cleaned out, you no longer will need deodorants of any type).

Teeth Cleaning: Baking soda wet with hydrogen peroxide is a great whitener, but too abrasive for every day. Polish teeth with towel and rubber tipped pick often. Do not use mouth washes or breath fresheners. Tom's toothpaste is okay for many.

Shaving: Colgate shaving bar soap. No creams, lotions, etc.

Do not use perfumes, cologne, scented cosmetics, hair spray, bath powder, body lotion, hand lotion, face cream, etc. If a cosmetic is used, it should be with no scent. Sometimes Almay, Marcelle or Ar-ex can be tolerated.

Travel: Automobiles should be equipped with air conditioning, manual control of outside air intake and non-odorous fabric upholstery. Manual air control should be set to recirculate air. When driving, keep enough distance between you and the car ahead so that exhaust fumes will dissipate before reaching you. Keep windows closed in traffic. Car ionizers and air purifiers are available. Use no air freshener "stick-ups."

Food Preparation: Drink artesian water or glass-bottled spring water.

If unable to obtain organic fruits and vegetables, wash "grocery store foods" in Neo-Life Green or Shaklee's Basic H and warm water and rinse thoroughly. Or, use a dilute Clorox pre-soak and rinse copiously for fifteen minutes. Use heat resistant glass or stainless steel cookware. Avoid aluminum, copper or teflon coated cookware.

The Rest of the Home: The majority of people with moderately severe chemical sensitivities will clear when the following can be accomplished in the home. (It must be remembered the most reactive triggers are ingested and inhaled. No two people react to the same things nor with the same symptoms.) If one is not able to clear with these measures, a "housecall" made by a chemically-sensitive person will often reveal the culprit.

(1) No carpets. If this is difficult to attain, at least have none in the bedroom and be sure the remaining ones are at least ten years old.

(2) Layer mattress (formaldehyde) with heavy duty alumi-

num foil, shiny side up and two to six layers of old cotton blankets or mattress pads washed in Borax. Cotton mattresses, pillows and zippered covers can be purchased from JANICES (1-800-JANICES for catalog). Use all cotton sheets, blankets and pillows.

(3) Seal off heating vents with aluminum foil and tape and use an electric hot water portable unit.

(4) Remove as much from the room as possible, especially all plastics, vinyls, foam cushions, shoes, cosmetics, new furniture and dry cleaned clothes.

(5) Select an air cleaner with a filter you tolerate and that removes chemicals as well as dusts and pollens. If this does not give you a chemically-less-contaminated oasis to which you can escape, you'd better seriously consider the heating system. Gas forced air can be converted to electric. Gas hot water can be made tolerable if the furnace and pipes actually containing the gas are physically removed from the house. A small shed can be made to house them in the yard.

The same basic measures apply to fuel oil tanks and oil furnace. Some have built a small room around the furnace and vented this room to the outside. While we're in the basement, all paints, oils and other suspicious items should be stored in metal trash cans, or better yet, stored outside the house. Obviously, other gas utilities (stove, oven, dryer, water heater) will not be tolerated by anyone with moderate chemical sensitivity.

It seems that what we have saved in heating bills we will pay with interest in medical costs. If the chemically sensitive person becomes too badly overloaded and cannot clear in a clean environment, there are only four options left: clean the environment further, find another environment, go outdoors (to the ocean or mountains) for one to two weeks or go to the environmental unit in Dallas. There is one other trick that works and that involves fasting, staying on oxygen and having vigorous daily exercise. Fasting helps reduce the chemical overload and is done with nearly every patient who enters the unit. Many of us get too chemically overloaded in airports; however, our tolerance can be greatly increased by taking one tablespoon of buffered sago palm vitamin C and fasting that day. Alka-aid tablets can also help and a hand held charcoal mask is a must, and a battery-operated ionizer (N.E.E.D.S.).

A problem of special note occurs frequently. This is the person who becomes sensitized to only one chemical such as an insecticide, DEAE (a rust retardant in steam heat) or formaldehyde. Often this person is a chemist or laboratory worker and is aware of the source. The problem arises when the victim fails to recognize the spreading phenomenon that may follow. Once sensitized, they start developing a sensitivity to many other substances like foods, molds and other chemicals. Many of us are like time bombs waiting to go off. Regardless of the sensitivity level that we possess today, it is miniscule compared with what it could be tomorrow.

For this reason it is important that home and diet are as uncontaminated as possible. Since the work environment is the least controllable, we must do all we possibly can to reduce the total load to arrest the spreading phenomenon. Environmental controls are difficult enough when one has a devastating disease and the cause is known, but they are doubly difficult for the person who is trying to simply prevent the onset of this disease. Prevention requires higher intelligence.

Marjorie started with classic chemical symptoms of headache, dizziness, brain fog or inability to concentrate, muscle spasms, flu-like achiness and exhaustion, burning eyes, sore throat and depression. She dated the onset to when they started renovating at work. By the time I saw

340

her, she had already spread. She was now sensitive to other chemicals, dust, molds, some foods and Candida. By treating her total load, she was healthy enough to continue at the job she was so good at and yet we did nothing with the actual work environment.

It's important to remember that those of us who do not adapt to 20th century chemicals may be similar to the canaries used by miners to check for gas leaks. Our acute symptoms should be a warning to others of the unforeseen, latent and potentially lethal threats to health. We have indeed created a monster.

Just take one class of chemicals, the insecticides. Forget for a moment the thousands of other chemicals in your indoor daily environment that have come on the market in this century. The insecticides will serve as a prototype of the problems involved. British scientists purposely exposed themselves to an insecticide to see the effects (effects one could not appreciate if testing were done on laboratory animals) They suffered extreme tiredness, lost interest in everything, became weak and frequently ached all over. Each subsequent minute of exposure caused a more rapid, violent and longer-lasting recurrence of symptoms. It took months for them to recover. When they reported their symptoms, they were accused of being psychosomatic by those with financial and political power. No medical journal would publish their findings!

Aside from the fact that there is tremendous biochemical variability and susceptibility among victims, there is also the problem that there have been very few studies of the synergistic effect of these chemicals on an organism. What happens when you are exposed to a half-dozen insecticides daily in the building you enter, in the products you use and in the foods you ingest? What is the combined cumulative effect of these in your body? It does not require large amounts of a chemical to produce permanent change. One molecule of a substance is enough to alter the function of DNA, which then directs the future functions of every cell in the body.

Many of us have had our levels of pesticides measured and I'm astounded at the levels and numbers I harbored. We now have methods to detoxify the body of these since many cannot recover until these levels are purged.

*****

E.I.
Environmental Illness
Environmentally-induced Illness
Environmentally-induced Injury

FORMALDEHYDE IS EVERYWHERE

Part of the following technical information has been kindly supplied by Dr. Doris J. Rapp. Formaldehyde is the first member of the aldehyde group R-C-H. Another common name is Formalin. It exists in gaseous or liquid form.

Uses of Formaldehyde

1) Intermediates in the synthesis of alcohols, acids and other chemicals, especially plastics.

2) Tanning agent (furs, leathers).

3) Used in the formulation of slow-release nitrogen fertilizers and in the destruction of microorganisms responsible for plant diseases.

4) Used as additional agent to make concrete, plaster and related products impermeable to liquids.

5) Used as an antiperspirant and as an antiseptic in dentifrices, mouthwashes and germicidal and detergent soaps. Also used in hair setting lotions, sprays and shampoos.

6) Air deodorant and air freshener in public places, in industrial environments and homes.

7) Destroys bacteria, fungi, molds and yeasts. Disinfects equipment in the fermentation and antibiotic industries. Disinfects floors, sickrooms and surgical instruments. Hospitals have a high level of formaldehyde.

8) Synthesis of dyes, stripping agents and various specialty

chemicals in the dye industry. It also improves the color stability of dyed fabrics. It's part of that "new smell" of clothes and contributes to the burning feeling on the skin.

9) Used in combination with alcohol, glycerol and phenol in embalming fluids. It is also used to preserve products such as waxes, polishes, adhesives, fats, oils and anatomical specimens.

10) Synthesis of explosives.

11) Used in conjunction with other chemicals in preparing fireproofing compositions to apply to fabrics (especially children's night clothes).

12) Used in insecticidal solutions for killing flies, mosquitoes and moths. Also used as a rodent poison. Dry cleaners and rug cleaners frequently use it. Some people have developed severe chemical sensitivities after having their carpets commercially cleaned and "mildew- proofed".

13) Used in the synthesis of vitamin A and in improving the activity of vitamin E preparations.

14) Improves the wet strength and water resistance of paper products. Used in nearly all papers and copy machines (office and home).

15) Preservative and accelerator for photographic developing solutions.

16) Used to make natural and synthetic fibers crease-resistant, wrinkle-resistant, crush-proof, water repellant, dye-fast, flame-resistant, water-resistant, shrink-proof, moth-proof (wool). Used in nearly all clothes, sheets, bedding and mattresses. Formaldehyde is found in many

things, but here are some of the more common sources: Adhesives, carpeting - spot resistant (the newer it is, the worse it is), chalk, chewing gums, cigarettes, cosmetics, deodorants, shampoos, toothpaste, some soaps, nail polish. Construction - particleboard, paneling, plastics, polyurethane and urea foam insulation, pre-fab buildings, renovations, trailers, concrete, plastics, plywood, fiberboard, cabinets and drawers.

Retards mildew. Disinfectants, deodorizers, detergents, dyes for clothing, embalming fluid, explosives and fertilizers.

Stores - especially "5 & 10" discount stores, building supply stores, carpet and fabric stores.

Filters, food (ice cream for example), some maple syrup, injected into some eggs, milk, fuel, fungicide, many fumes, exhausts, smokes.

Laminates - furniture glue, upholstery and foam stuffing.

Laboratories - especially medical and dental.

Leathers - fur, synthetic lubricants, mattress, paints, latex.

Paper - butcher, office, money and mimeograph. Pharmaceuticals - many prescription creams, lotions and oral medicines.

Plastics - auto, appliances, sports equipment, dishes, toys, office supplies and machines, Baggies, tupperware. Rubber. Spray starch. Surface coatings.

Textiles - nearly all clothes, sheets, pillows, blankets, permanent press. Urethane resins. Water softening chemicals. The present of formaldehyde can be determined by applying a drop of the Formaldehyde spot Test to the object. The spot will turn purple if the object outgasses more than 10ppm formaldehyde. (Available at office.)

How to Control Formaldehyde

"So, it looks like formaldehyde is in everything," you say, and you are right. It's one of the primary causes of indoor chemical sensitivity reactions. The reactions can leave you feeling like one of the world's biggest hypochondriacs because there are no x-rays to diagnose its presence. A blood test called a formic acid can detect its presence, but it can be normal in spite of severe formaldehyde intolerance. however. Many physicians untrained in the new specialty of environmental medicine won't believe you even if you tell them the diagnosis.

So, how do you begin to reduce your exposure to it? First, begin with your body. Get rid of toothpastes, shampoos, conditioners and polyester clothes. Get rid of polyester sheets; cover the formaldehyde containing mattress with aluminum foil; remove the bedroom carpet, furnishings, foam cushions, pillows and polyester drapes. Now you have one-third of your life with reduced formaldehyde exposure; now you should be able to awaken without its symptoms.

You can carry these measures into the rest of the house and get rid of other plastics, particle board cabinetry and foam-stuffed sofas. Opt for wood (not glued and no particle board) or metal furnishings and make your own cotton covers and stuffings. Use no unsafe cleansers and ventilate frequently.

Dunk and Bright furniture on Brighton Avenue will stuff a couch or chair in Janice's cotton. (Prewash your cotton and selected cotton fabric in baking soda and rinse with vinegar.) Avoid glues and adhesives and favor doweling in the furniture. Keep the living room in cotton, silks, wools and linens; avoid Scotchguard finishes. A Foust or Allermed air purifier would help at work.

You should allow no smoking in your area and try to discourage aftershave and perfumes by letting people know you are allergic to them. If worse comes to worse, there are a few labs in the country where your blood can be checked for benzene, xylene, toluene and other potentially carcinogenic chemicals. An elevated level after work and a normal level before work is enough evidence to keep you from work until they ventilate the area sufficiently to lower your blood levels. Blood tests can be mailed.

Testing to chemicals in the office, single-blinded, can often document your chemical sensitivity. Some people come for testing so overloaded (from home, car and traffic exhaust) that they react to the normal saline as well. This negates the validity of the test in a doubter's eyes. Others may not react to a test dose, but they react in real life to some unknown chemical that is not yet recognized. If a person tests negative to natural gas but suspects chemical problems, it would be foolish for him to live in a house with gas since his sensitivity can spread at any time.

Mary began to have severe exhaustion, depression, tight throat, leg aches and dizziness from renovations at work. Single-blind testing to the involved chemicals duplicated her symptoms. The evidence became conclusive when blood tests after a day at work confirmed much higher levels of chemicals than blood tests after a day at home. Since these highly specialized blood tests are available in only a few laboratories in the world, very few doctors are aware of their existence.

Quick Chemical Checklist

(the following lists merely skim the surface and are not complete)

FORMALDEHYDE IS FOUND IN:

Apple gum
Grape gum
Particleboard
Carpeting
"Permanent press" clothes, polyester
Facial tissues (some)
Butcher paper, paper towels
Polyurethane plastics
Eggs - some grocery store eggs are sometimes contaminated purposely by injecting formaldehyde into the egg so that shelf life is increased.
Wall insulation (urea foam formaldehyde)
Spray starch
Mimeographed paper
Dyes
Cigarettes
Cosmetic preservatives
Milk
Concrete or plaster
Some soaps, toothpastes, shampoo, deodorants, air fresheners
Foam cushions, padding, mattresses
Cleaning supplies
Chalk
Trailers
Fabric stores
Laboratories

ETHANOLS, PHENOLS AND ALCOHOLS
ETHANOL and other **HYDROCARBONS** are found in:

Anesthetics
Rubber
Hand lotion, perfumes

Flavoring agents
Perfume
Printer's ink - newsprint
Glycerol
Metal polish
Gasline, garage fumes, kerosene
Pine odors
Dried fruits
Much fat of meat (animals and feed are chemically sprayed, hydrocarbons are vehicles for pesticides)
Oil and gas heat, stoves, furnaces
Coal tar derived dyes
Coal and wood burning heat
Sprayed fruits - even if scrubbed and peeled
Sprayed vegetables - especially cabbage family
Lighter fluids
Nail polish and polish remover
Cleaning supplies

GLYCERINE IS FOUND IN:

Cosmetics
Moistening agents
Lubricants
Anti-freeze
Allergy extracts
Marshmallows, candy, fudge, baked goods

PHENOL IS COMMONLY FOUND
IN THE FOLLOWING:

Nasal sprays - Afrin, Neo-Synephrine, etc.
Bronchial mists - always check with your doctor or pharmacy. "Over-the-counter" drugs - cough syrups, eye drops,

anti- histamines, cold capsules, decongestants
Ointments - first aid creams, etc.
Hair products - setting lotions, hair sprays, dyes, shampoo, perfumes
Aftershave lotion, scented deodorants
Aspirin
Scotch tape
Newsprint, wallpaper
Herbicides and pesticides
Canned foods
Epoxy
Cleaning supplies, Lysol

TRICHLOROETHYLENE

Paints, degreasers, printing, drycleaning fluid, plastics, decaffeinated coffee, white corrective ink, carbonless paper, cleansers.

I was in Dallas in 1986 to give a case presentation at the international symposium. That day I felt particularly trashed—just awful. It's hard to explain, but I felt drugged, achey and drained. Knowing I never do well in hotels (miles of carpet, perfumes, gas restaurants, strong cleansers, no windows that open, plenty of glue, smoke, plastic-finished wallpapers, etc.), I tried to ignore it.

That is, until Dr. Joe Miller said, "Sherry, I don't want to hurt your feelings, but your jacket is making me sick."

"Heavens, you could never hurt my feelings, especially when you've taught me so much!" I said, "I've felt awful all day — ever since I put on this jacket." I recalled then that I had had it drycleaned the year before; even then it had made me sick, so I had put it in the back of my closet and had not worn it until now.

I immediately went over to Dr. Rea's office and had

my blood checked for the presence of trichloroethylene (dry cleaning fluid); it was sky high. In fact, I was in the top 98% of people that had ever been measured! Needless to say, I took off my jacket and gave my lecture without it. We never stop learning.

Ethanol (alcohol) and related Hydrocarbons

This is the class name for a group of chemicals recognized as having a certain definite chemical make-up; it contains one or more carbinol groups. This is written C-O-H. H is a hydrogen atom attached to an oxygen atom which is also attached to a carbon atom. This carbon atom has at least three other attachments. These formulas then result in methyl alcohol (also called methanol or wood alcohol), amyl alcohol, isopropyl alcohol, butyl alcohol, ethylene glycol (which is used as permanent antifreeze), glycerine or glycerol and menthol.

1) ethyl alcohol - formed as wine or hard cider by the fermentation of any sweet fruit juice; industrial ethyl alcohol may be made from molasses, potatoes or grain (particularly corn), or synthesized. It

- will dissolve many organic substances such as shellac and oil. It is

- an ingredient in tinctures and many toilet and drug preparations.

- used as body rubbing alcohol.

- used in making ether and sterilizing surgical instruments.

- used in making rubber.

2) amyl alcohol - made from ethyl alcohol.

- used as solvent.

3) isopropyl alcohol

- used in manufacture of antifreeze, rubbing alcohol and solvents, used in most medical offices and hospitals before drawing blood or giving an injection.

351

4) glycerol - used for sweetening, preserving food (coconut, candies) and allergy extracts.

- used in the manufacture of cosmetics, perfumes, inks and certain glues, cements and hand lotions.

- used in medicine in suppositories and skin emollients and injections. In most allergy injections across the world as a stabilizer. There are about 1/2 dozen of us who have glycerine-free injections for highly sensitive people.

- anti-freeze and lubricants.

5) menthol - used in perfumes, confections, liqueurs.

- used in medicine for colds and nasal disorders because of its cooling effect on mucous membranes. Used in liniments and salves for achey muscles and joints.

Products of alcohol:
1) anesthetic
2) cleaning fluid, pine odors, naphtha, lighter fluid,nail polish and remover, pain thinner
3) flavoring extract (vanilla)
4) preservative, sprayed fruits and vegetables to retard mold and insects
5) acetic acid, synthetic chemicals
6) explosives
7) formaldehyde plastics
8) rubber tires (buna), rug pads, overshoes

Alcohol is used in the preparation of:
1) hand lotions, perfumes
2) celluloid - toothbrushes, bakelite products
3) dyes, coal tar derived in foods, medicines, clothes,   rayon textiles
4) drugs
5) photographic film
6) paint and varnish
7) soaps
8) printer's ink, newsprint

Direct uses of alcohol:

    1) Source of light and heat, gas heat, stove, water heater, furnace, coal heat, wood-stove, garage fumes, kerosene.

    2) Motor fuel, gasoline, garage fumes.

    3) Disinfectant, dried fruits, vehicle for insecticides (concentrated in the fats of animals and humans.) Dry-cleaning fluid (also has trichloroethylene which is used to make plastics and decaffeinated coffee) and mattress insecticide.

    4) Sedatives.

    The above sources have been generously supplied by Dr. William J. Rea (Environmental Health Center Manual.)

PHENOL

    Phenol is any of a family of organic compounds characterized by attachment of at least one hydroxyl group to a carbon atom forming part of the benzene ring.

    Phenol is also called carbolic acid or hydroxybenzene. In 1834, a German named Runge isolated carbolic acid from coal tar. In 1843, another German, Gerhardt, prepared the same substance by a different method and called it "phenol."

    In 1845, an English surgeon, Joseph **Lister,** (hence Listerine!), used a dilute solution of phenol to treat wounds, thus established its usage as an antiseptic.

    Other uses of phenol are listed below:

    1) Serves as a starting point for
        production of epoxy and phenolic resins,
        aspirin and other drugs.

    2) Used in the manufacture of picric acid explosives.

    3) Constituent of herbicides and pesticides.

      4) Phenolic resin (bakelite) <formed by reaction

of phenol (C6H5OH) with formaldehyde (CH20)> is used in molded articles, such as telephone parts, thermal insulation panels, laminated boards, children's toys, refrigerator storage dishes, etc.

5) Used in manufacture of nylon, synthetic detergents, polyurethane, perfume, gasoline additives, dyes and photographic solutions.

6) Preservative in medications; preservative for immunotherapy injections. Used in cough drops and throat sprays (Chloraseptic), and mouth washes (Listerine) and face creams (Noxema).

7) Cleaning solutions such as Lysol.

There are naturally occurring phenols such as the toxic agent in poison ivy and poison oak.

With kind permission of Dr. William J. Rea, the following has been taken from his **Environmental Health Center Manual:**

Be sure to read all labels. If you are not sure, ask your pharmacist or doctor. You may also write the manufacturer. Phenol is in all routine allergy extracts unless otherwise specified. Phenol is emitted or outgases from televisions and electrical cords, or anything that has any kind of plastic on it. Our office has phenol-free extracts.

Phenol is in many medications, many over the counter products, and in all allergists' injections the world over. Some people can only get better after the phenol is removed from their injections. There are now over a dozen of us in the U.S. who have phenol-free extracts for the chemically sensitive.

It is difficult and expensive to maintain this. Phenolated extracts are made up into the nine dilutions and then used throughout the entire year. Without this preservative, we need to remake everything every six weeks and throw away all that was unused. So there is eight times more work and some unavoidable waste of money.

A good test of whether a doctor is a serious specialist in environmental medicine is whether he has phenol-free extracts. You should be able to determine this over the phone. If he does not have phenol-free extracts, he can't help highly chemically sensitive people. Also, you can assume that he does not have much experience with such patients and that he isn't sensitive enough to their needs.

Glycerine is a stabilizer in all extracts in the world, and phenol-free, glycerine-free extracts are even more difficult to prepare than phenol-free. However, they are the only ones tolerated by exquisitely chemically sensitive people.

There are even fewer offices in the world who make them. Dr. William J. Rea is the first person to make them that I am aware of. Our office also has them.

One astute mother brought in her seven-year-old son who was starting to do poorly in school. She noticed that on Saturday mornings, after a few hours of TV cartoons, he was unbearably wild and mean. His teacher reported he was like this in school at times also.

When we tested him to xylene, phenol and toluene, we could turn this same behavior on and off like a switch. He even wrote on his test sheet, "I feel mean." Obviously, when the TV was on, the wires heated and accelerated the off- gassing of phenols and toluene. At school his teacher's perfume and the Lysol spray she kept insisting on wiping the desks with throughout the day were the other culprits. Again, I am aghast to think of this young man's future if it weren't for the exceptional analytical intelligence and perseverance of his mother. How many children have these problems and are mainlined into special education classes because their parents and teachers are unaware of the powerful effects of every day chemicals on the brain?

355

THE FORMALDEHYDE NIGHTMARE

Since the mid 70's, formaldehyde has received a great deal of press. We have learned that exposure to it can produce a variety of symptoms. It doesn't matter if the person had allergies before or not. Once he is exposed to formaldehyde and develops the ability to produce symptoms, his threshold for formaldehyde exposure is often lowered. Now, when he is exposed to levels which would not normally cause symptoms, he is acutely aware of its presence and experiences a repetition of his symptoms.

Formaldehyde hypersensitivity can cause just about any symptom you can think of. It has been proven beyond a doubt in carefully controlled environmental units, such as Dr. William Rea's in Dallas, Texas and in Dr. Theron Randolph's in Chicago, Illinois, that formaldehyde is responsible for producing symptoms in a variety of patients. It has been shown to cause headache, itchy eyes and nose, asthma, joint pains, rashes, mental confusion, disorientation, fatigue, phlebitis, laryngitis, depression, nausea and vomiting just to name a few.

CASE HISTORIES

F.N. was a middle-aged female who found that she could not tolerate wearing clothes with formaldehyde in them. (Wrinkle-resistant or permanent-press clothes have formaldehyde in them to create this characteristic.) When she wore them, she would get a headache and her eyes would be irritated, itch and burn, and her voice would become hoarse. She had a hyper-acute sense of smell and could actually smell the formaldehyde in these clothes. She now wears 100% cotton and feels much improved.

G.D. was a young officer who had his house foam-insulated in 1976. A year later he began having headaches, dizziness, extreme fatigue and nausea nearly constantly. It continued to get increasingly worse over the years. It was especially bad when he rode in his trooper car or stayed in the trooper barracks which were located over a firehouse where the firemen frequently warmed the fire truck engines. He got such dizziness and disorientation that he felt as though he would pass out. He was unable to work, his face was flushed and brilliant red, and he got severe headaches. He was exhausted and could not function well mentally. He had been to a neurosurgeon, three famous medical clinics and through three CAT scans. No one could diagnose his problem. We found that his symptoms could be turned on and off with appropriate dilutions of formaldehyde. Formaldehyde is, of course, one of the products in automobile exhaust.

S.N. was an elderly female who, for eight years, had very itchy eczema over her whole body. Her skin was red, flakey, scaley, very sensitive to the touch; it cracked and sometimes bled. She had been to a variety of dermatologists and had tried steroid creams which made her worse. A patch test showed that the chemical she was wildly sensitive to was formaldehyde. formaldehyde is a common ingredient in many creams. It is used to inhibit mold growth so that when you open up the tube it doesn't have mold growing in it. By having her use only creams which did not contain formaldehyde, (she had to use Crisco as a skin lubricant without formaldehyde) and by having her wear only 100% cotton garments, multiply washed, we were able to clear her skin.

F.H. was a young female who, in 1980, had her house insulated with urea foam formaldehyde (U.F.F.I.). She began having symptoms, such as headaches, burning eyes, choking and chest pain. Six weeks later she moved out. A few months later she tried to retrieve her clothes and furniture but could not use them because they smelled strongly of formaldehyde. She lived in an apartment for two years while she had the formaldehyde removed. The outer shell of the house had to be removed to do this and it cost over $10,000. When she moved back in she still couldn't tolerate it since her sensitivity was now even more heightened. She found she could live in the attic (which had not been previously foamed). One of her children now sleeps on the porch all winter because she, too, has become sensitized.

S.S. began having headaches, irritability and extreme lethargy after the house was foamed. The whole family also suffered from sore throats, burning eyes, runny noses, headaches, coughs and extreme tiredness. They spent a great deal of money going to doctors and having the "foam" (U.F.F.I.) removed. Subsequently she has developed a larger number of symptoms and allergies to many inhalant antigens.

M.M. was a middle-aged female. In 1979 she had her suburban house foam insulated. She began having headaches, lightheadedness, spontaneous nose bleeds and laryngitis. She had to sleep in a tent in the yard for a year while her case went to court.

L.M. was a young female. In July of 1976, she had her house foam insulated. She hated to tell me of her symptoms because she felt like a hypochondriac. She had had asthmatic bronchitis, sinusitis, chills, perspiration, headaches, nausea, a tickling sensation in her nose and throat, sore throats, dry cough, tight chest, burning and watering eyes, nasal congestion, skin rashes, copious amounts of phlegm in her throat and tiredness and depression all the time. When she left the house her symptoms disappeared.

One laboratory technician developed attacks of dizziness, glassy eyes and severe headaches. She felt as though she would pass out. After the attacks, she was left feeling intensely drained. A number of other cytologists working there had torticollis, anxiety attacks, bizarre neuromuscular complaints and symptoms that defied medical diagnosis. Many were incapacitated to the point of being unable to work.

A 38-year-old engineer ached all over his body whenever he was in his 2-year-old home. Out of the home he was fine. Measurement showed his particle board sub-flooring outgassed more formaldehyde than a recently foam-insulated house.

One lady suffered dizziness, numbness and nausea from formaldehyde fumes released when she ironed permanent press clothing.

What are the commonest symptoms we've seen in people with formaldehyde hypersensitivity? My very first patient was a lovely woman to whom we all owe a great deal of gratitude. She taught us a tremendous amount about formaldehyde and she showed us how to overcome a great many of the handicaps that it throws in our way.

She was an operating room nurse in 1977 and she bought herself a trailer. When she moved into it, she did not like the new smell and complained. People came out and checked it, but there wasn't much they could do. Financially, she was strapped and had to live in it for two years during which time she became extremely formaldehyde sensitive. She suffered from dizziness, nausea, lethargy, depression, crying, rashes and watering and burning eyes. Her dog even had some of the very same symptoms. Other people, when they visited, would exclaim that they did not like the odor of it.

Of course, the trailer was all new construction and new construction means much formaldehyde because it's less expensive. It's in the particle board that abounds everywhere. It's in the glue that holds these little particles of material together. She has, over time, become so extremely sensitive to formaldehyde that she needs to live now in a very specially constructed environment. We have films of her becoming semi-comatose within two hours of just being in an office such s ours, which has 0.03 ppm formaldehyde. This is the same amount that many older homes have.

After one such filming session, I was escorting her out the back door of the office to her oxygen and truck when she said, "Oh my God, there's gasoline in that room!" She pointed to the closed door of a testing room. When I opened it, I found a man being tested who was wearing coveralls from a garage. She can't tolerate one minute in a room where I have sneaked an open bottle of 1/2 ounce of formaldehyde (even if it's hidden inside a closed metal cabinet).

When she travels to town, because of the formaldehyde emissions from motor exhaust, she must bring oxygen and a ceramic mask. She is unable to go into stores or offices. When we see her medically, we see her in her truck in the parking lot of the office. For her, an allergy to the 21st century is no laughing matter. She needs a home in the country that is quite primitive with no new particle board or plastics in its construction. She has been an indomitable inspiration to many who have experienced the formaldehyde nightmare. She has the intelligence and fortitude to see beyond the physicians who label her psychotic.

Unfortunately, most of the people with chemical hypersensitivities are advised to consult a psychiatrist (that is, if they have nay money left!). I guess we all sound paranoid to the person who is totally unknowledgeable about the effects of formaldehyde.

One lady was the wife of a milk tester and had five children. They had their farmhouse foam insulated and within half-a-year she lost her voice. By the time I saw her two years later, she had only a whisper of a voice, like a severe case of laryngitis. She had been to numerous physicians, including five ear, nose and throat specialists at our medical center. None of them could tell her why she didn't have a voice. Fortunately, she was highly astute. Most of the people with chemical hypersensitivities have to be just to survive. She discovered that if she lived at her mother's for a week her voice would come back.

We tested her with formaldehyde. We had her come to our office when she had her normal voice after having lived at her mother's for two weeks. Within three minutes of one dose of formaldehyde, we were able to turn her voice off. Later we were able to find another dose of formaldehyde that, within seven minutes, would turn her voice on again. So for years she has lived at home giving herself injections every three to four days so that she could have a normal voice. Of course, the best thing would be to get out of the house, but that wasn't possible for her at that time.

In February before treatment, her serum formic acid (a metabolite of formaldehyde) was 9. In April, after two months of symptoms controlled with injections, it was 4. In February her Raji cell (immune complex indicator) was 288; in April it was 33.

We made video tapes of this turning on and off of her voice. Injections were given double-blind, which means I didn't know what was in each injection and she didn't either. This insured that there was no way she could possible have faked her reactions. We showed these tapes on Buffalo television and in lectures around the country so that physicians could see that there are indeed individuals who have extreme chemical hypersensitivities and that some of us may react to one particular dose of an antigen in a good way and react to another dose of the same antigen in a harmful way.

The body does this over and over again with many of its own hormones. We function normally with one amount of thyroid; we function very abnormally with other levels of thyroid. Too low a dose makes us hypothryroid; we become dull, sluggish, tired, cold intolerant, puffy and fat. Too high a dose does the opposite and makes us hyperthyroid; we become irritable, thin, diaphoretic and heat intolerant. The body recognizes different doses of prostaglandins, histamines and serotonins (which are chemical mediators of allergic reactions) with divergent results. It recognizes that some doses are pro-inflammatory and others are anti-inflammatory.

FINDING THE CULPRIT

There are many people who have a variety of symptoms from formaldehyde off-gassing. The problem is that many of them do not know that their symptoms are from formaldehyde. If they do, they cannot find a physician who recognizes it as a problem or who can tell them how to decrease the load of formaldehyde in their environment. If the person is merely sensitive to formaldehyde and can experience relief when outside his house, they he is told to move. If, however, the person's system has changed to such an extent that he has a heightened sensitivity to formaldehyde and is not able to tolerate it in areas where he normally could, then this presents a much more difficult problem.

Many do not have as easily diagnosed stories because they develop symptoms to formaldehyde without ever having had their home foam-insulated. They became sensitized by "normal" exposure levels of formaldehyde. Common examples could be a new carpet, a remodeled kitchen, a new office, a new car or home, a renovated office, a trailer, or undergoing anesthesia either at the dentist's or a hospital. A new house with particle board flooring can have higher levels of formaldehyde than a foam-insulated house.

For this reason, we have developed a formaldehyde spot test. Remove a drop of solution from the vial with a syringe and place it on any material to be tested. For example, you may want to know if there is formaldehyde in a fabric that you are going to make sheets or clothes from. You may want to know if there is formaldehyde in particleboard or ceiling tile that you are going to use. You may want to know if formaldehyde is off-gassing from plastic appliances or toys that your children have. The more you can lower the background formaldehyde level in a home, the less the total load of formaldehyde will be. Consequently, the less the symptomatology will be. Also, in the long run, the less you will be further triggered into a heightened formaldehyde hypersensitivity.

If a drop of solution is placed on material to be tested and it turns into a very faint purple within two minutes, the material is off-gassing ten parts per million of formaldehyde or more. This is way too much formaldehyde and this material should not be used. If it is off-gassing a dangerously high level, it will burn a moderate shade of purple and is exquisitely heavily contaminated with formaldehyde.

So, one way you can help yourself is to drastically lower your ambient formaldehyde level. Discontinue nail polish, smoking (smoking can give off as much as 30 ppm formaldehyde), riding in cars with poor exhaust systems and shopping in department stores where a strong odor of formaldehyde is off-gassing from clothing, fabric, carpet or plastic.

In some people, chemical symptoms may not occur for two to five years after the new materials have been introduced into the house. Because the symptoms occur slowly, the two events are never linked.

There is evidence that high exposure over prolonged periods may be carcinogenic. No one has all the answers, but one thing is for sure - formaldehyde has become a real nightmare for many people who, before 1975, had never even heard the word. Two major clues that seem to point to many chemically-induced problems are awakening tired and achey and experiencing cerebral symptoms that just don't make sense and that you can't control. The gamut of symptoms, however, is endless; they masquerade as many other diseases.

By now, you have knowledge of it and the tools for

proving it. Dr. Rea's unit clears one quickly. Then you go home and gradually sneak back conveniences until you reach your tolerable limit. In the office we do the opposite. We suggest that you make changes and eliminate exposures little by little until you are better. This enables you to find your level of wellness along the way. If you're lucky, you won't have to go to extremes that others do. However, the office method is best for highly motivated and resourceful people for a number of reasons:

1) You may become discouraged and want to abandon the whole process since you're not better yet.

2) The longer you procrastinate, the longer you are exposed, the greater your sensitivity can become and you can develop new problems.

3) It fosters the development of denial. As you eliminate more from your environment and are still not better (because your total load hasn't been reduced enough), you find it easy to say, "I knew this wouldn't work!" We all have that eternal hope that we have only a few allergies or none at all.

4) The longer you procrastinate the longer it will take to clear. The sooner you clean your environmental overload the more chance you have of gaining some of your lost tolerance in the months or years to come.

Camping or going to the ocean is the poor man's unit. All you need is to get clear. One dentist was terribly sick and I saw him just as I was leaving for a speaking tour in China. I gave him a crash course in environmental medicine and Randolph's book and I crossed my fingers he would be able to work through the psychological barriers. He was, to put it mildly, superb. When I returned, he felt better than he had in years and was radiant. He had cleaned out the garage and moved his foiled bed into it. He only entered the house to use the bathroom.

A major problem is the mental attitude of the patient. We want to take a pill and feel better yesterday, not tear up the house and remove our favorite things. Plus, this illness isn't in vogue; it's not socially acceptable. For many, the social isolation they feel is worse than the suffering.

The same stress that Dr. Elizabeth Kubler-Ross speaks of in her book **On Death and Dying** can be explained here. At first there is denial and isolation, then anger followed by bargaining ("Well, can't I just have coffee each day? How do you expect me to go to work without my coffee?"). Then there's depression and finally acceptance. People vacillate in and out of these stages. As Dr. Iris Bell states in her book **Clinical Ecology** there is another stage we have that the dying don't have, and that's the crusader's stage. It can be put to good use or it can turn people off and alienate them.

So, when people offer up a host of excuses why they can't do any of these environmental controls or diagnostic trials, I just recount that I, too, faced choices. I could eat all that I desired and have my face a mess or I could rotate and be clear. It was totally my choice. I could deny that chemicals played a role and be incapacitated with unwarranted depression and back pain or I could eat organic food and use the foil and cotton and feel better. It simply depended on how good I chose to feel. The same goes for you. When you're bad enough, you'll do anything to make yourself better.

If you "just can't do it," then you're simply not that bad. I'm happy you're not, but watch out — you may get worse.

The Car

The car is often an overlooked source of severe chemical exposure. You can lessen the load by installing a Foust or Allermed air cleaner, installing an ionizer and putting a homemade framed layering of filter-charcoal-purafil-filter over the air vents. If possible, choose an older car that has a cloth interior (not vinyl) and that has metal rather than plastic surfaces. Be sure to check for muffler leaks and keep windows closed in traffic and avoid newly tarred roads. Some people travel with oxygen and a ceramic mask. If the engine could be in the rear and the car tightly sealed against entering fumes, this would be a plus.

If you are exposed long enough to produce symptoms, take six alka-aid tablets, quickly put your charcoal mask over your mouth and nose, go home, take your buffered sago palm vitamin C, shower, retire to your oasis, use oxygen if needed and fast until the symptoms are gone. There are other measures but you would need to see the doctor for these.

Dr. Rea, myself and many others also have to carry a "seat" with us everywhere we go or we get symptoms from sitting on plastic chairs or foam-filled cushions. Dr. Rea gets weakness; I get severe back pain where I have no disc. I know it sounds insane, but try it to see if you are that chemically sensitive. Your body won't lie to you.

The aluminum foil on the seat sounded particularly crazy to me when Dr. Rea first recommended it. "What?!?" I squawked. "You want me to sit on a foil pad and that will stop formaldehyde from the foam seat cushions from getting into my body and setlling in my back? Are you nuts?"

But he was right as usual. In fact as you will discover later, a six-layer spread of restaurant grade aluminum foil over a mattress can make a world's difference. And being a real doubting Thomas I stupidly had to suffer many times when I thought I could forego this insanity.

Once when my husband and I had arrived in London (I was giving lectures there), we settled in for a much needed night's sleep. We must have had new mattresses, because at midnight I was awakened by excruciating back pain and felt so edgy I thought I would jump out of my skin. So here was Luscious, combing the streets of London for a cotton blanket and heavy duty aluminum foil. Being a highly resourceful person, he was back with them within an

366

hour and I slept like a baby. And I did not travel without my foil blanket roll again until I was well.

*   Many "undiagnosed, chronic or incurable" symptoms can be proven to be caused by chemical sensitivity.

*   Only intelligent, motivated and resourceful individuals will be successful in identifying and eliminating the causes.

*   Uncovering the total load for each individuals can be a very complex task, requiring constant education and vigilance.

*   Only phenol-free extracts will be tolerated by very chemically sensitive people. Glycerine-free, phenol-free extracts are the ultimate in purity.

*   Candida hypersensitivity, food hypersensitivity, severe mineral deficiencies, pesticide and hydrocarbon toxicities, fatty acid deficiencies and other aspects of the total load are frequently the missing factors necessary in the healing of the immune system.

*   Many struggle along in misery for months and years hoping to find some "cure" that negates having to do environmental controls. Others, like the dentist who went home and moved his bed into the garage, improve dramatically.

*   Testing to chemicals only works for diagnosis if the testing environment is clean enough to not provoke symptoms. Likewise, the individual being tested must be sufficiently "cleared out" or unloaded to respond. It is usually preferable to avoid the chemicals once they are identified as opposed to getting injections for them.

*   Some victims are too overloaded and require a detoxification program in order to unload the body of xenobiotics (foreign chemicals).

*   Drastic temporary measures are often necessary; new carpeting, new furniture, gas heat, and gas appliances must be removed from the house.

*   H.E.A.L. groups, a supportive family, friend or

spouse are essential to faster recovery. A person trapped in a house with a spouse who prefers to know nothing about E.I. will not recover fully, if at all.

*   One manual cannot encompass all that a person with E.I. needs to know. Frequent consultations with the doctor and other E.I. victims, reading national and local H.E.A.L. publications, keeping a diary and learning from every setback helps maintain an upward course toward wellness.

Bitter Through Chemistry?

So are we "better through chemistry" as the advertisement says? And are those of us who developed chemical sensitivity as a result, BITTER through chemistry? Absolutely not. For as you will see if you plough through the other 7 books, it has forced us to become expert in healing. The result: it has taught us so bloody much that it has brought us full cycle and enabled us to heal the impossible, including cancers. All the while the rest of the world still flounders in the misconception that a headache is a darvon deficiency, that drugs are the answer to all medical
problems.

SECTION VI
NUTRITION

WHAT COMES FIRST - DEFICIENCY OF DISEASE?

This article is reprinted with kind permission from the editors of **Let's Live** magazine, Los Angeles, CA 90014, March 1984 issue, pg. 34 (article author is S.A. Rogers, M.D.).

In August of 1965, I was sitting in the auditorium of our medical school receiving freshman orientation; I vividly remember the doctor telling us that a third of what we were about to learn would be pertinent in our lives as practicing physicians, a third of it would be outdated before we graduated and a third of it was not even true. However, because no one had a crystal ball to be able to weed out that which was unnecessary, we would have to learn everything.

One of the non-truths that we were taught in medical school was that no one in the United States needs vitamins. There is no such thing as a vitamin deficiency because all of the foods are vitamin fortified. What they did not know was that the foods are fortified because the original nutrients have been destroyed by artificial chemical fertilizers, insecticides and processing.

The food manufacturing industry has stripped the food of so many natural nutrients and they could not possibly put all of them back. So, they put a token of vitamins back hoping that we would never know the difference. Do you ever see vitamin E added to a box of cereal? Of course not. They put back the easy, cheap things to put in such as thiamine and iron. Vitamin E is irreplaceable. The bleaching and strong chemicals that are used to break down the grains for cereals and breads, for example, remove vitamin E and many other essential vitamins and minerals, some of which have not even been isolated yet, so we don't know of their significance. There are many studies showing the difference between animals fed bleached white flour bread and whole grain stone ground flour bread; there is literally no comparison. The animals receiving the whole grain were much healthier. (Read Dr. Price's **Nutrition and Degenerative Disease.**)

We did not realize that vitamin E (which prevents arteriosclerosis) was removed from grains and oils. By removing vitamin E, they were able to prevent rancidity and then improve the shelf life of the product. That partly explains the current boom in cardiac surgery and deaths. They didn't realize that due to our heightened chemical load in food, water and air that we needed extra vitamins C, E, A and selenium for detoxification.

For example, we do need far more C than the Food and Drug Administration recommends. Most people need several thousand milligrams a day and many need as much as ten to fifteen grams (1 gram = 1000 mg) a day. The reason for this is that Vitamin C is very active in the biochemical cycle of the body to detoxify chemicals. And unfortunately, we have a much higher and more constant chemical assaults against our bodies than our forbearers had.

We are constantly plagued with chemicals in our food, such as additives, anti-oxidants, insecticides, herbicides, chemical fertilizer residues, hydrocarbon dyes, etc. Also, we breathe a much more highly chemicalized air. Our forbearers wore natural fiber clothes; we wear synthetics (polyester or permanent press wrinkle- resistant clothes) containing formaldehyde. We sleep on formaldehyde mattresses and sheets and acrylic blankets. In fact, we are literally swaddled in formaldehyde when we go to bed. We breathe exhaust fumes and natural gas fumes from heating systems. We live in air-tight houses and fill the wall cavities with formaldehyde insulation. We breathe trichloroethylene, phenol and formaldehyde outgassing from all of the myriad of plastic articles in our home and office environments. Is it any wonder we have more cancer? Is it any wonder that we have a higher vitamin C requirement?

In addition, the 1 ppm of chlorine that is mandated for municipal drinking waters and chlorine has a destructive effect on vitamin E. Nor did they realize that vitamin A are destroyed by cold medications and nitrates and vitamin B, if not heat-destroyed, is often thrown out with the cooking water. Vitamin B6 is another B vitamin that is removed from white flour and is not replaced. It, too, has a large role to play in preventing arteriosclerosis and in detoxifying chemicals.

Also, we were not aware of all the trace nutrients which were being removed or destroyed by processing and were never replaced. Some essential trace minerals and vitamins have not yet been isolated or discovered. These are in unadulterated foods such as wheat germ and brown rice, but not in processed foods or chemical vitamin supplements. Many medications put a strain on the biochemistry and surreptitiously deplete co-factors. Some are known and still not replaced by most physicians. For example, the birth control pill causes a folate deficiency in many women, which can then lead to birth defects once the woman decides to get pregnant. Diuretics deplete magnesium, a deficiency that can cause sudden cardiac death.

If that were not enough, the American diet has a vast amount of hidden sugar in packaged foods, not to mention that ingested intentionally. Sugar is a negative nutrient in that it does not add any vitamins or nutrition to the body. It does use biochemistry and vitamins to metabolize it and convert the calories into energy or fat. Therefore, a person is further behind nutritionally after eating than before ingestion.

Have you ever wondered why your garden tomato tastes so good, but the winter grocery store item looks good but is vapid? It is due to many factors such as being grown on nutrient-depleted soil which has been artificially fertilized with a token of the elements necessary for physical growth. Then they are often picked before natural ripening has had a chance to occur and gassed in box cars so that shipment and ripening can occur simultaneously.

What deleterious effect does this chemical concoction have on the finished product? Certainly taste will not be the only missing factor. Indeed, if the biochemistry has been so distorted as to destroy the deliciousness, many other nutrient factors are missing as well. Many people can, fortunately, function in spite of these deficits, but many of us either because of genetics and/or chronic disease states suffer ill-health as a result of a diet of nutritionally inferior foods.

Medicine does recognize a few deficiency states, but they are all pretty much catastrophic end-stage deficiencies such as scurvy and beri-beri.

My interest in vitamins was particularly piqued when one of my asthma patients dropped off a vitamin book for me to read. In it she had earmarked an article showing that asthmatic children were able to decrease the amount of medication needed for control of their asthma when they increased their pyridoxine or vitamin B6 intake. I was amazed to see that this was published in the **Annals of Allergy** in August, 1975. I immediately went to my files and looked it up. Sure enough, every allergist in the country had read it and all of us had promptly forgotten it.

This led me to start looking at serum vitamin levels experimentally in some patients. As a result, over many months, we drew scores of vitamin levels. We tried to be prudent and cost-conscious and not look at a grab bag of vitamins; we tried to be more or less selective of what we thought might be lacking.

I was amazed at the results. Over 80% of the people were markedly deficient in one or more vitamins that we looked at. The commonest deficiencies we saw were B6, then B12, folic acid and then vitamin A. All of these patients represented a variety of illness, and most of them were just plain tired and had had numerous physicals that revealed no cause. We have no statistical studies on these results because they were not randomized. But, it raises a number of interesting questions that we should strive to find the answers to.

The first problem that comes to my mind is that the normals stated by the lab are most likely no more reliable than the U.S. recommended daily requirements for most vitamins. They do not take into account individual variation and needs. So many people may actually be deficient who now
are told their levels are normal.

The second problem is the question of whether patients, who have specific disease states, such as allergies and environmentally induced illnesses, have special requirements for these biochemical co-factors. Such people may require much higher levels than the "norm."

What comes first, the deficiency or the disease? Are those of us, who have environmentally induced illnesses secondary to inhalant, food and chemical hypersensitivities, biochemically unique and born deficient in certain co-factors? Or does the fact that we constantly have more biochemistry going on in our bodies to produce various symptoms, such as headache, depression tiredness, colitis, asthma, arthritis and the like that we use up or deplete our systems of these important biochemical co-factors?

As if that were not enough to concern us, Beatrice Trumm Hunter, at the recent 16th Advanced Seminar for The Society of Clinical Ecology, held in Banf, Alberta, Canada, presented some very pertinent facts in her lecture entitled, "Shall We Be Eating Irradiated Foods?" Many of you may recognize her as the author of one of my favorite books, **Consumer Beware**. In her lecture, (which is available on tape through Creative Audio, 8751 Osborne, Highland, Indiana 46322) she told us that irradiation is used in various levels. Low level irradiation is used to decrease bacterial growth and to inhibit spoiling and sprouting in root vegetables. Medium level is used for controlling insect casings and parasites. High level is for pasteurization. A very high level sterilizes and destroys all living organisms.

In 1953, the United States Army studied ionizing radiation at medium and high levels to prevent spoiling of foods and negate the need for refrigeration. By 1978 even though they had poured over $50 million into this project, nothing had been perfected or approved. In 1980, the FDA judged that low level irradiated foods were wholesome and safe. This included all sorts of fresh fruits, vegetables and grains. At first, this sounded promising because it eliminated the need for fungicides, insecticides and nitrates in certain foods. Also, it allowed food to be sterilized for cancer patients suffering from impaired immunity and for astronauts.

It does, however, have some serious drawbacks as she later mentions. Some nutrients are also especially sensitive to ionizing radiation such as fats and amino acids, especially cysteine, methionine and tryptophan (a precursor to a "happy hormone" in the brain, serotonin). It also is destructive for vitamin A and its precursor, beta carotene, and many of the B vitamins, such as B1, B6, B12 and the tocopherols (vitamin E).

The vitamins B1 and C are destroyed as much as they would be had the food been subjected to heat. So, an orange would look normal but have a reduced vitamin C level as though it had been boiled. If the foods are to be nutritionally adequate, the appropriate enrichment would be desired. There is no guarantee that the form in which a certain nutrient is put back into the food is bio-available to the human organism. Nor is there any guarantee that this nutrient will be hypoallergenic to people who have various food allergies or that it will restore the original state of balance with other nutrients. Often, minor nutrients such as chromium are totally ignored. Chromium has been recently studied in its beneficial effect in diabetes, arteriosclerosis, and hypoglycemia.

Also, free radicals are formed by food irradiation and these cause chemical reactions in the foods, creating compounds with which we are not familiar and do not know for sure are safe in the human body. Many free radicals cause reactions that we associate with changes of aging and cancer.

The FDA estimates that in the very near future at least 10% of our food will be irradiated, and many are right now. This is a low estimate because daily they are adding to the list of foods that can be irradiated. Since 1968, it has approved low level irradiation for wheat, wheat flour and potatoes. This along comprises 16% of the average American diet. However, this does not mean that all of these foods are now irradiated. Many food handlers have held off irradiating because of the mandatory labeling which states a food must bear a label saying it was treated with gamma radiation or ionizing radiation.

This also is a very expensive high technology process: the foods have to be shipped to and from existing irradiation plants with the extra cost being transferred to the consumer, or manufacturers must undergo expensive installation and operating costs for their own irradiation units.

Irradiation doesn't arrest all processes either. It does not arrest oxidating reactions that go on to cause rancidity nor does it stop proteolytic enzyme degradation.

The thorny problem of informative labeling also does not fill the bill because only the man in the last stage of the food processing must label what he has done to the finished product. In other words, a baker can buy irradiated flour and make it into cookies, breads and rolls and he does not need to state that it is irradiated since he did not do

376

it.

The FDA already admits that some shrimp and froglegs are entering our country from foreign sources that have no label requirements and that these have been irradiated. Ms. Hunter has done a fantastic job in researching all of the above facts and now the public needs to be aware of them. This is not a matter to be legislated by some unknown body of bureaucrats who are puffing on cigarettes as they sit at a table eating donuts and coffee.

The safety needs must be established. For now, your safest bet is still to grow your own foods as organically as possible, to can or freeze them in as fresh a state as possible and to use vitamin supplements.

We have an even higher duty to make sure that irradiated foods are safe before we okay them, because approval in the U.S. automatically extends globally. We are the leaders who are mimicked.

NEGLECTED NUTRIENTS

What comes first, deficiency or disease? That's been a question difficult to answer. In many of our cases, the answers is probably both. Did we succumb to Candida because we were low in folic acid and B6 (the birth control pill) or did we develop multiple deficiencies because of the stress on our system of having chronic Candidiasis? One thing we know for sure, the stress of chronic disease does lead to nutritional deficiency. If you have a person with chronic asthma, headaches and sinusitis making copious amounts of phlegm and undergoing bronchospasm on a daily basis, you have someone who has multiple nutritional deficiencies. For these people, it's like having pneumonia everyday of their lives and they're certainly using up more biochemical cofactors than the average person who breathes normally.

What are the multiple factors that have to do with

why we see so many nutritional deficiencies? One is the gradual depletion of nutrients in our foods. Many steps are taken between the farmer's wheat field and the loaf of bread that ends up on your breakfast table. Studies show that the chromium, manganese, iron, copper, zinc, selenium and molybdenum levels in wheat germ are as much as ten times higher than they are in white enriched bread. Bleaching, so that the flour can look pristine white and also not go bad or deteriorate very quickly, removes many of these essential nutrients. Every food that comes in a bag, box, jar, can or wrapper has had something done to it by some process and the end result of this is a product with inferior nutrition compared with the way the product started out.

Foods also are chemically contaminated at many points along their preparation route. These contaminations with various chemicals add to the burden of the body since it is the duty of the liver and many enzyme systems to detoxify these.

Where do these chemicals come from?

First, in the growing process there are nitrates in the soil from artificial fertilizers and pesticides. Then, in the processing, dyes, additives, and various chemicals are used. This is also the stage where many nutrients are removed. Then there is the storage stage where phenols and plastics contaminate the foods as well as further fungicides and other pesticides. In preparation, the foods may become contaminated with gas, plastic or metals such as aluminum.

WHERE DOES INFERIOR NUTRITION STEM FROM?

The major causes of inferior nutrition include:

1) Extensive food processing as discussed above.

2) Irradiation of foods is just beginning in this decade and we will see progressively more of it. Studies show that irradiation destroys a significant percentage of

many vitamins such as C, A and many of the B's, so that in a few years you will go to the store and pick out oranges to bring home to juice for your family. The only difference is that those oranges will not have to be refrigerated and will last in your pantry for months at a time without spoilage. However, they will not have nearly the amount of vitamin C and B as the original product. This information will not appear on the label. In fact, many food processors are working toward getting legislation where you will not have to be advised at all if irradiation has been used to extend the shelf life of your foods.

3) By having such a fast paced life, more people eat processed foods and eat out and eat fast foods. Thus, we become hooked on fats, salts and sweets, leading further to nutritional deficiencies because our tastes lead us to eat repetitively those things that we like and crave as opposed to having a well rounded died with much variety.

4) The soils are progressively more depleted. We feed nearly the whole world. Billions of tons of crops come out of the U.S. soils every year and farmers dutifully replenish the soil with sodium, potassium and potash, but rarely do they replenish with the trace minerals such as selenium. These are more expensive and they are not deemed necessary because the United States consumers don't know enough to complain.

For example, a tomato from your garden tastes completely different from a tomato from your local grocer. The reason is that yours was not grown on depleted soil and has a complement of trace minerals. The ones grown commercially have been grown on the same soils for years and don't contain all the nutrients. Your taste buds can tell the difference. Likewise, there are studies now showing that people who live in areas of the United States where selenium has become depleted in the soil have a higher rate of cancer, since selenium is one of the important trace minerals necessary to ward off the development of cancer (and allergies).

5) Medications. We, as a nation, are a drugged group of people. It is rare to find a person who has not had a single pill, tablet, capsule, injection, suppository or dermally administered patch type of medication within the last month. We are always popping a pill for something and these medications take their toll on the body. In the 1970's it was the Valium era, now in the 1990's it seems everyone is i on Prozac!

The problem is that every drug drags us further down the tubes. They deplete nutrients.

It takes extra nutrients to detoxify these chemicals. The liver is the main organ of detoxification. It requires a number of trace minerals and vitamins as well as amino acids and essential fatty acids to adequately break these down and excrete them.

6) The Candida bowel is widely prevalent but infrequently recognized. People who have had antibiotics often have silent overgrowth of Candida in the bowel. They have foul smelling gas, frequent gas and bloating; they may have no symptoms at all; they may have the classic unwarranted tiredness and depression. Whatever they have, they also have decreased absorption of nutrients because the bowel is so inflamed. Also, an inflamed bowel tends to allow larger molecules across it, hence potentiating the development of food and chemical allergies (leaky gut syndrome).

7) Chemical pollution of our foods, as mentioned, is another reason for inferior nutrition, as the chemicals not only damage nutrients in the foods, but use up more nutrients in our bodies' work of detoxifying these chemicals.

8) Chemical overload in daily life is another overlooked but very important factor. Everywhere you go you are bombarded by odors that may or may not register in your brain. However, everything that can be smelled ends

up in the bloodstream and must be detoxified. That's how people die from carbon monoxide poisoning. In fact, things that you cannot smell also end up in the bloodstream just as well and these all require extra enzymes for detoxification.

9) Biochemical individuality. The requirements for each one of us is uniquely individual, leading further to inferior nutrition when agencies like the National Academy of Sciences attempt to legislate recommended daily allowances as though we were all identical and never exposed to everyday chemicals and processed foods.

10) Chronic disease is last, but certainly not least, as a cause of chronic malnutrition for it depletes the body daily of many essential factors through the chronic production of symptoms.

There are many examples of patients with abnormally low levels of nutrients in whom we have had "dramatic results." Take the lady, whom we have filmed and shown in about a dozen cities in the United States, who was bedridden with rheumatoid arthritis. Within three minutes, a neutralizing dose of phenol has her dancing down the hall, skipping and waving her arms. When she returns to the room, she can touch her toes and is without pain or limitation of motion

You and I know that even though these double blind studies serve to demonstrate the provocation-neutralization technique to teach physicians, our hypersensitivities to the environment are not that simple. She has to watch her diet, have injections for her food and mold sensitivities and do extensive environmental controls at home in order to be pain- free. Last but not least, we found many nutritional deficiencies. For example, her B6 level was 21. Normal is 30-80 but no one knows what her particular requirement would be. Would we have been so successful in improving the status of her life had we not looked at her nutritional deficiencies along with her environmental hypersensitivities? I really doubt it.

This leads me to discuss the adequacy of serum values. These are arbitrarily defined by measuring the levels of a particular nutrient in a population of people who are supposedly healthy. You and I both know that many people who think they're healthy could actually feel a hundred percent better.

The normal level for a serum B12, for example, is 200-900 mg/dl. Well, how to we determine if my level should be 200 or 900 or how do we determine if your level really shouldn't be 1200? No one has the answers to these yet, for there are no unequivocal biochemical indices for many of the nutrients. And every few years, the requirements for one or more nutrients actually gets lower!

Another question is the RDA, or Recommended Daily Allowance, versus normal versus optimal. The RDA for most nutrients are notoriously substandard. They are much lower than they should be for health in the 1980's. These were established years ago when people did not have the lifestyles that we do now. They didn't have as many chemicals to detoxify, the soils were not as depleted, the foods were not as processed and they didn't have many of the environmental stressors that people are subjected to now.

Also, there is a vast difference between normal and optimal. Normal in the United States means you should have a heart attack or a stroke sometime before you are sixty and be dead by the time you are in your seventies. The optimal life span for the human species turns out to be somewhere around 120 years, but very few people make it that long as medicine is centered on acute care and not preventive care.

Common drugs that can lower nutritional levels are diuretics. These waste potassium, magnesium and zinc, for example. Diuretics, or "fluid pills," are commonly prescribed and doctors assume they know how to check for potassium loss, but rarely do they ever check for magne-

382

sium loss. But they check the worst and least sensitive potassium assay, serum. So they miss over half who are low anyway. As for magnesium, over 90% do not know that a serum magnesium is useless. A better assay is a red cell magnesium or preferably, the loading test, but never a serum value. Unfortunately, the chemical profile used by all docs to screen patients includes the worthless serum magnesium, giving a false sense of security. This is especially important since 90% of docs don't even think of checking either version for magnesium status! (JAMA 6/13/90).

Birth control pills lower folic acid and B6. There is a long list of prescription drugs and the nutrient factors they deplete. Diabetes creates a stress on the system for chromium, manganese and essential fatty acids. The ulcer medications like cimetidine and ranitidine work by turning off the acid secretion in the stomach. However, when they do this, they also turn off the secretion of the intrinsic factor which is necessary for absorbing B12 as well as many minerals. Or worse, they are immunosuppressive and actually turn down normal immunologically mediated necessary biochemistry of the stomach! So, many people, after years of anti-ulcer therapy, have pernicious anemia, very low B12 or multiple mineral levels, and for sure, new diseases that were ushered in by these deficiencies.

To make the problem even worse, when I was in medical school twenty-five years ago, we learned that if one has a low folic acid of B12, he will develop a macrocytosis. In other words, as the cells hang around in the bone marrow waiting for these missing nutrients to show up, the cells get fatter and fatter. Hence, the word "macro" meaning large and "cytosis" meaning cell. When a common complete blood count, or CBC, is drawn, it is noticed that the cells are macrocytic and the physician is supposed to be triggered to look for a B12 or folic acid level.

The astounding fact to me is that in hundreds of patients who have had very low folic or B12 levels that we have seen over the years, very few of them had a macrocytosis. This means that we have been missing many potential nutrient deficiencies for years; we were waiting for the mythical elf, macrocytosis (this was subsequently published in the **New England Journal of Medicine**).

As well, various anti-convulsants deplete folic acid and vitamin D. Digoxin for heart failure depletes magnesium, yet a magnesium deficiency may have been the cause of the heart failure! The list goes on. Many of the anti-inflammatory drugs for muscle and joint pain deplete vitamin C and folic acid, and these are just the tip of the iceberg of what is depleted in many people.

We have photographs of people coming to the office, standing on a chair and holding up a computer printout of all the drugs that were prescribed for them within the last one or two years by physicians whom they had consulted. The effect of all these drugs on the nutrient status and immune system has got to be staggering, and indeed, many of these people turned out to be universal reactors by the time they got to us.

This leads me to the question of what is a hypochondriac? I, personally, think it is a non-entity. It does not exist. It's a term that contradicts itself. A hypochondriac is supposed to be someone who thinks he is sick but is not. The mere fact that someone is complaining means that, indeed, he does have a problem. Just because he doesn't have the correct diagnosis isn't his fault. He didn't go to medical school. He just knows something is wrong or he wouldn't be in the office. So, to label someone as a hypochondriac is the ultimate egocentric cruelty in medicine, I think. Just because the doctor is not able to figure out what is wrong with the person does not mean he is making it up! What a cop-out!

There's another term in medicine that doesn't really have much meaning. It really defines the status of awareness of the examining physician. This term is subclinical.

Subclinical means that a person has symptoms but nobody can pick them out or recognize them. As you know, there is a wide range of recognition and a large variance among physicians in the ability to "hear" your complaints. As a result, often when a lab test is abnormal but the physician has no explanation for it, it is called subclinical and disregarded as unimportant. But what could be more important than correcting it early before more serious problems?

When we first started looking for nutritional deficiencies, because the cost of the lab tests were so high, we started looking for only one or two deficiencies at a time. If something is abnormally low, such as a B6 or a folic acid, it's a pretty good bet that there is a lot more that is deficient in that system. For it is highly unlikely that a person could develop an isolated deficiency.

How can you, with all of your wonderful body chemistry, develop a deficiency in one minute area when all this biochemistry is so intricately entwined? The key to treating these deficiencies becomes even tougher, because we always must maintain the concept of balance. In other words, if someone has a low B6 level, we cannot just put back B6. We know that the B vitamins have to be in balance with one another, and as well, they need to be in balance with the other vitamins, amino acids, essential fatty acids and minerals.

For example, zinc is often written about in health magazines. So, people decide that they article sounds convincing enough and they go out and buy some zinc. For a while they may feel good because they probably were zinc depleted. After a short time, they start feeling worse again. As you take zinc unbalanced with other nutrients, you can lower, for example, the copper or molybdenum and thus create other problems unknowingly. Copper is necessary to counter inflammation. Molybdenum is crucial in an enzyme to break down acetaldehyde produced by Candida and also in metabolizing formaldehyde and other chemicals.

Even something as seemingly harmless as extra vitamin C can lower the calcium or magnesium and create an imbalance leading to an insidious development of osteoporosis.

There is also another concept that must be understood when one embarks on a program to correct nutritional deficiencies. This is the concept of corrective versus maintenance dosages. When deficiencies and symptoms are present, very high levels and very imbalanced levels of nutritional supplements are necessary in order to attempt to correct the disturbance. However, after a period of a few months, maintenance levels should be switched to, which would require far fewer medications and a very different balance. If corrective doses are taken for an extended period of time, secondary nutritional deficiencies will be caused unquestionably because of the excessively high levels of specific factors. Maintenance levels, then, are devised for people who have corrected their deficiencies or feel fine and just want to keep on an even keel and have the assurance that they have the necessary nutrients on board.

VITAMIN A

Vitamin A is a fat soluble vitamin that is stored in the body. Beta-carotene is the precursor to vitamin A. Both have strong properties independent of one another in terms of healing the system from anything from chemical sensitivity to cancer.

Vitamin A has a variable level of toxicity in people. In some, as little as 5,000 international units a day could be the top dose. For others, 25,000 to even 50,000 may be necessary for treatment. However, if one is on over 25,000 I.U. a day, it's wise to check the blood level of vitamin A, as well as a liver function periodically after the first and third months to be sure it is not becoming toxic. For vitamin A can cause irreparable damage in the ventricles of the brain if taken to excess.

Conditions in which vitamin A deficiency are commonly found are eczemas and other skin problems. Food allergies and Candida inflame the bowel and this inflamed skinlike tissue inside the intestines not only has increased turnover but decreased absorption of nutrients. Likewise, colitis cases need vitamin A levels checked as well as people with weight loss, acne and severe E.I.

Correction of the deficiency often will clear the skin or clear the bowel condition or aid in resistance of the bowel to Candida.

Some of the lowest levels we have ever seen have been in people with cancers. In fact, whenever I see very low levels of vitamin A now, I make sure the person returns to the family doctor to have an extensive physical to rule out hidden malignancy.

The intestinal tract has the surface area of a tennis court, therefore, it is the largest organ in continual contact with food and Candida antigens. This leaves a large area for potential inflammation; so replacing it for the daily needs can be a major task. With inflammation much of the surface epithelium and nutrients can be lost in the stool.

Because vitamin A is stored, it can be taken two or three times a week instead of every day with the same beneficial effect. Caution: If you are correcting a zinc deficiency, you may be surprised that you have an uncorrectable vitamin A deficiency as well, since the first breakdown step uses a zinc dependent enzyme alcohol dehydrogenase. So monitor levels. Use caution if you use cod liver oil as the vitamin A source, as cod also contains vitamin D; don't exceed 400 IU (total all sources from all your supplements) of vitamin D a day.

In order to absorb fat soluble vitamins, A, D, E, and K, you need adequate pancreatic enzymes. If you have exhausted your pancreas through overeating or too many sweets, this can impair absorption.

Beta-carotene is the precursor to vitamin A. Unlike vitamin A, you cannot easily overdose on this because there is a limiting mechanism in the biological conversion of the body. It also possesses some unique anti-carcinogenic properties so be sure to include it. In other words, you need a minimum of 5,000 I.U. of vitamin A a day plus a minimum of 25,000 beta-carotene. Taking extra beta-carotene is safer than extra A because the body will regulate, or limit, the conversion so vitamin A toxicity is less likely.

B VITAMINS

B1 (thiamine), B2 (riboflavin) and B3 (niacin) are all important vitamins relating to liver detoxification enzymes for various pollutants.

B6 is the most commonly found B vitamin to be low in the serum. It is destroyed by not only processing of foods, but heating of foods as well. So, unless one eats a good diet of raw fruits and vegetables, he risks having a B6 deficiency.

Also, in order to be utilized by the body, B6 must first be broken down to pyridoxal-5-phosphate. If magnesium is low because of eating foods from depleted soils and processed foods low in magnesium, the body will not have enough magnesium as a necessary cofactor to allow this primary conversion step to take place. Some people lack the ability to do this for other reasons, like zinc deficiency in the converting enzyme, pyridoxine kinase. Pyridoxal-5- phosphate can be purchased as a supplement by itself, thereby bypassing this conversion step.

B6 is lowered by many medications. There are many articles documenting the effectiveness of B6 in correcting the Chinese restaurant syndrome (monosodium glutamate hypersensitivity), carpal tunnel syndrome, PMS, abnormal glucose tolerance test, schizophrenia and stocking-glove type neuropathies (Buist, R., **International Clinical Nutritional Reviews**, 4, 1, Jan. 1984).

B6 deficiency should be looked for in cases of asthma, arthritis, PMS, oral contraceptive use, hydralazine (use for high blood pressure), and other medication use, exhaustion, depression, carpal tunnel, renal stones, high junk food diet, severe E.I., diabetes, monosodium glutamate intolerance and alcoholism. In other words, just about anybody is ripe for developing it. Don't forget it is destroyed by EDTA which is sprayed on frozen foods to retain their bright color.

B12 deficiency should be especially looked for in anyone who has a history of gastritis, ulcers, numbness and tingling, severe asthma, bursitis, and any mental symptoms (NEJM). Some stomach medications and aging lower the intrinsic factor, increasing the vulnerability of developing B12 deficiency.

Dimethylglycine or DMG is vitamin B15. This one is rarely heard about but is extremely important. For example, in the **Journal of Infectious Diseases**, Volume 143, January, 1941, an article by Graber and others showed an interesting response to DMG. Volunteer prisoners were injected with the pneumococcal vaccine. Half of the group was pretreated with 120 mg of DMG before the injection, while the other half was given a placebo. The group that had the DMG made four times as much antibody in response to the vaccine as the untreated group. This provides strong evidence that DMG has a positive modulating effect on our ability to make antibodies, and since most of you are on injections, it behooves us to be sure that you have a good daily source of this important B vitamin.

Folic acid is usually included in B-complex capsules (and depletion follows the use of oral contraceptives and other chronic medications, junk food). Remember, the CBC is virtually useless in deciding whether the test should be drawn.

One interesting case was a gal who was 35-years-old

and came in complaining of headache, dizziness, exhaustion, depression and chronic ear pain. She had just had a complete workup at the medical center and everything was negative. It was suggested that she see a psychiatrist. However, when we saw her, her B6 level was 16 (normal is 30-80), vitamin A was 12 (normal is 20-80), B12 was 90 (normal is 200-900) and her folic acid was 3.4 (normal is 4.20). We tested her and found she was also sensitive to a variety of molds and dust, gave her the injections, corrected the deficiencies and all of her symptoms were totally cleared.

I don't understand it yet, but for some reason big name medical centers all across the United States do a bang up job looking for everything except environmental and nutritional triggers. Actually, it is quite easy to see their rejects, because knowing what they have ruled out, it leaves very little else as the possibility for what could truly be wrong.

VITAMIN C

Vitamin C, or ascorbic acid, is a nutrient about which much has been written. When I lectured in Clearwater, Florida for the American Academy of Environmental Medicine in 1986, I had the opportunity to meet Dr. Linus Pauling, who was lecturing on the same day. This remarkable gentleman looked wonderful and was 85 years old. He used 18 grams (18,000 mgs.) of vitamin C a day. This would sound outrageous to many, but what he advocates is taking your vitamin C up to the top tolerated dose. In other words, when you get to triggering diarrhea, back off.

He maintains the high incidence of cancer of the colon in the United States is partly because we eat foods with many chemicals and additives and the foods are so highly processed that they sit around in the bowel for sometimes two or three days rotting or fermenting. This is potentially carcinogenic. He believes by increasing the bowel turnover time, or having a good healthy bowel movement everyday, which means not having the same foods in the bowel longer than 48 hours, that this will reduce the chances of cancer. But beware: you can create severe deficiencies with this level unless you have it balanced with the nutrients and periodically check your mineral levels, as a high dose of C can severely deplete them.

We know, also, that vitamin C is certainly beneficial in warding off many of our infections. In fact, many of us increase our levels when we feel we are coming down with something. It's interesting that the body's wisdom shows itself very nicely during these situations, because when we are sick we find we can tolerate much higher levels of vitamin C than normal, then as soon as we are well again those very same high levels are no longer tolerated and cause diarrhea.

One interesting gal came in complaining of headache, bald patches in her hair and extreme exhaustion. We found that as a small child she and her friends would weekly run out to play in the spray of a passing truck. This was the DDT truck that was spraying for mosquitoes. Even as an adult, years later, when we measured her DDE (a metabolite of DDT) levels in her body, they were literally off the chart. With five months of high levels of ascorbate and other nutrients, we were able to bring her levels down demonstrably and flush it out of her system.

Remember, rarely is someone unable to take vitamin C in some form or another. There are eight antigenic sources (sago palm, carrot, potato, corn, rice, tapioca, soy, pure synthetic and citrus). This even allows for rotation.

Bioflavinoids are nutrients that accompany vitamin C in the live product. They are anti-inflammatory and have many other beneficial effects. Unfortunately, most have citrus antigens in them, except for rutin and quercitin-C (Ecological Formulas).

VITAMIN D

Vitamin D deficiency can occur in people who are rarely in the sun (that means anybody who lives in Syracuse!) or people who do not drink homogenized milk. There are studies vitamin D is potentially atherogenetic. In other words, it actually can potentiate arteriosclerosis. A safe level is to not exceed 400 I.U. per day, (as in 1 tsp cod liver oil) but remember many foods are fortified with it, like homogenized milk. Periodically your phosphorus, 24-hour urinary calcium and hydroxyproline, rbc calcium, and 1-hydroxy vitamin D levels should be monitored. Also the fatty acids are essential for the intestinal transport of vitamin D.

As with any nutrient, you should keep a running tally of what your daily total is. In other words, check all your supplements for vitamin D and see that it does not exceed 400 I.U. Some calcium compounds have extra D in them; as a rule I rarely recommend those for that reason.

VITAMIN E

Vitamin E is another fat soluble vitamin and, therefore, can be stored.

Vitamin E is essential for people with stasis ulcers or any form of intestinal ulcers as well, severe E.I. and chemical hypersensitivities, mastitis, vascular problems, blood clotting problems, gallbladder problems, chronic vaginitis, menopausal symptoms, oral contraceptives, restless legs syndrome, any type of malabsorption, anemia, cystic fibrosis and sickle cell disease.

Vitamin E is incorporated in the cell membrane of every single cell in your body. Vitamin E serves to grab onto chemicals attempting to damage or penetrate the cell's barrier.

The cell membrane is analogous to the computer

keyboard. This is where all of the directions for function and many of the allergic reactions occur. It is the structure that all chemicals must penetrate before they can cause malfunctioning within out cells and the disease called E.I.

There have been many interesting studies that have shown that one can give a group of rats an evening dose of carbon tetrachloride and in the morning 90 percent of the rats will be dead. One can then pretreat a group of rats with vitamin E and given the same dose of carbon tetrachloride, but in the morning there is now a 100 percent survival in the rats. So, if vitamin E is that protective against chemical damage, it certainly behooves all of us to include at least 400 to 800 I.U.'s of vitamin E in our total daily regimens.

Rarely should 800 I.U. be exceeded, however. You might think if four to eight hundred is good, twelve hundred would be even better. Many studies have shown the vitamin E taken in excess of around 800 I.U.'s starts to have adverse affects and also is not as protective. The best type is d-alpha tocopherol. Avoid the dl-type as this is a synthetic molecule and foreign to the body . . . another instance where you must read and understand the fine print.

Since it is a fat soluble vitamin, you want it with a fatty meal where you will have lots of bile secreted so that it can be appropriately broken down for good absorption.

Each year when I begin preparing my lectures for the Advance Course for Physicians Learning Clinical Ecology Techniques, I am literally overwhelmed by the amount of evidence in the biochemical literature for all of these nutrients in protecting against environmental illness, yet still none of this is taught in medical school. Still, to this day when I teach family practice residents, they are almost insulted when I want to discuss nutrition. They are also embarrassed and don't want to discuss it because they don't know anything about it. They are much more intrigued by all the big gun cardiology drugs than they are about vitamins. However, many people such as myself who were universal reactors and who have made remarkable recoveries, know that one of the many things that we did in order to become "normal" again was to maximize our biochemical response in ever way possible.

As with any good thing, however, you can overdo it with any of the vitamins. For example, too much vitamin E can lead to thrombosis or blood clots, hypertension, severe fatigue, breast development in men, altered hormone metabolism and immunity, increased cholesterol and triglycerides and it can even antagonize the absorption of vitamin A and cause blurred vision.

ESSENTIAL FATTY ACIDS

Most people think they already have enough fat and don't need more. However, fat is one of the most important things in the body. You see, every single cell can only function when it has a cell membrane wrapped around it. If there are leaks or defects in this cell membrane, the cell malfunctions and prematurely dies.

The cell membrane is also likened to the keyboard of a computer, because it is here that informational chemistry determines how the cell will work and what enzymes or proteins it will manufacture.

This membrane is composed primarily of lipids or fats, but the types and amount of lipids in its chemical structure are extremely important for its functioning.

There are two types of essential fatty acids in these membranes. One is from the Omega 3 series, the other is from the Omega 6. These two series are not interchangeable. They require an enzyme called delta-6-desaturase to transform them from the ingested food sources into the biologically active components and they cannot be made in the body so the correct essential fatty acid sources must be ingested.

If these sources are deficient, there are profound metabolic disturbances that occur in the cell. Some of these disturbances occur over a long period of time, very insidiously, like chronic disease and aging and cancer. Others can come about rather abruptly, such as the development of environmental illness or an acute onset of a degenerative disease.

Essential fatty acid deficiencies can cause just about any type of problem you can think of: hypertension, E.I., hyperactivity, eczema, psoriasis, chronic candidiasis, chronic fatigue, vasculitis, neurologic disease, thrombosis, seborrhea, schizophrenia, MS, hyperlipidemia or elevated cholesterol and triglycerides, premenstrual syndrome and E.I.

The scientific literature is absolutely crammed with examples of various conditions that clear once the essential fatty acid deficiency has been corrected; but biochemical individuality reigns.

The omega 6 oils are best obtained from cold pressed sunflower oil, safflower, corn, soy, sesame, almond, walnut, linseed oil and oil of evening primrose (73%). The sources of GLA (a metabolite of omega 6) are evening primrose oil, black currant seed oil (which is twice as strong), and borage oil (4 times as strong), none of which you would cook with. The omega 3 series comes from green leafy vegetables, purslane, linseed oil (do not cook with this) again and marine fish oils such as herring, salmon, anchovy, cod, mackerel and sardines, preferably in sild oil. For (low heat) cooking, unrefined walnut, sesame or olive oil are preferred.

The enzyme D-6-D that transforms these acids into useful forms in the cell membrane are inhibited by many factors. The most common inhibitors of D-6-D are a diet high in saturated fats, processed vegetable oils from the supermarket shelves, diabetes, high sugar diet, alcohol, aging in general, high adrenalin or stress levels, smoking, starvation, steroids, a very low protein diet and ionizing radiation.

Natural cold pressed oils such as sunflower, linseed and soy are pressed and the oil is squeezed out of the seeds. However, in modern times, seeds are instead subjected to extremely high temperatures which not only extract the oil from the seed, but also extract vitamin E, B6, zinc, magnesium and other trace nutrients to slow down rancidity and deterioration.

One major problem is that in subjecting oils to these high temperatures, they have also made a biochemical alteration and the molecule switches to a trans form as opposed to a cis form. These two forms look identical but they are actually more like mirror images or a right and left hand glove. The problem is that the trans form does not fit into a cell membrane the way the cis form does and it acts more like a broken key. It fits in the membrane but blocks the sites for proper cell function and for the right oils to enter.

It is thought that this is one of the main bases for much degenerative disease. The bottom line is that trans form oils are the oils found in the regular supermarket. They are labeled "polyunsaturated," "low in cholesterol," "vegetable" or "hydrogenated." They even go so far as to have a picture of a heart on them. But it really means they are bad for the heart! The only oils you want in your body are cold-pressed oils. These are usually found in health food stores or in the gourmet section of the grocery. They must say "cold-pressed" or you are getting the trans form.

You should only use cold-pressed oils. Linseed is one of the best, but should **not** be heated for cooking. You certainly can rotate the others (safflower, walnut, soy) but you should never use the vegetable oils from the regular part of the grocery (except olive oil) nor should you use margarines. Butter is far better for you than margarine. Besides many modern studies have shown several errors in the old studies on cholesterol and it is known that white sugar is a serious unrecognized contributor toward arterio-sclerosis.

The switch from butter to margarine has been a vast mistake and has helped foster the development of arterio-sclerosis. So, whenever possible, avoid stick margarine, tub margarine, shortening and salad oils. Use only cold-pressed. Olive oil is your best oil for cooking (omega-9 and not easily converted to trans form).

As for the omega 3 oils, flax oil is a good source and unless you eat fish two or three times a week. Sardines in sild oil (1/2 can per day) will heal membranes if meat is limited also to once or twice a week.

It might be said more clearly that "A salmon a day may keep a coronary away." We have several instances of people with severe psoriasis that also cleared when the missing fatty acid was found. One man had psoriasis for 57 years; never clear a day in his life. Putting him on linseed oil from the health food store, his psoriasis melted away. When he ran out of it, the psoriasis returned. As soon as he took it again, it disappeared. What this has demonstrated to us is that that was his biochemical defect. It's not the defect in every person with psoriasis, only in some.

MINERALS

Calcium

Calcium is a major mineral necessary for strong bones and teeth. One of the first bones to go when osteoporosis is slowly developing is the jawbone. Hence, loose teeth, periodontal disease and eventually false teeth. There is a grave error being committed throughout the United States. Many gynecologists, realizing that women develop osteoporosis as they age, have told them to go out and buy some calcium. That is exactly what they do. They go out and buy any old calcium. Four important facts need consideration.

First, if there isn't enough gastric acid in the stomach, they will never absorb the calcium. Many stomach medicines turn off or sop up stomach acid, thus inhibiting calcium use. Many forms in the stores are in such a poorly absorbable form anyway that very little is assimilated.

Second, if they don't take enough magnesium in relation to the calcium, the calcium will never be incorporated into the bone and instead it will lay down in other tissues where it does not belong, such as in the interior of arteries. Calcium should be in a 1:1 ratio with magnesium or at least a 4:3 ratio. Many other minerals are needed also in order to be able to put calcium in the bone. It is criminal to recommend calcium without checking the levels of zinc, copper, chromium, and manganese at least, not to mention the rbc calcium itself! And it is progesterone (in a natural not synthetic form) that inhibits osteoporosis, not estrogen (which can cause cancer).

Third, doctors neglect to tell them that if they have a diet that is high in phosphates, in other words a lot of processed foods, meat or softdrinks, including carbonated waters, that that inhibits calcium absorption and all of their calcium supplementation will be for naught as they will still progress to osteoporosis.

Phosphates are ubiquitous in food processing but phosphates inhibit the absorption of calcium. When any ingredient list says that it has leavening or anything used as a preservative, anything used as a bacteriocidal agent, dough conditioner, flavor vehicle, pH buffer, acid flavor, stabilizer or chemical that increases water holding, decreases phase separation and increases the thickening of products, then it means it probably has phosphates in it.

For example, many meats are injected with a phosphated compound called freeze-guard, so when meats are thawed, they don't drip quite as much. How did we ever do without it?!?

A fourth reason for osteoporosis is that we eat too many acidic foods, like meats and sweets, we use up the body's buffers. When this happens, it then pulls calcium out of the bones to use as a buffer.

Zinc

Zinc, as most people know, is essential to the prostate, for hearing problems, problems of inability to smell things well, arthritis, acne, healing, immune system integrity, detoxifying chemicals and much more.

However, if it's not adequately balanced with copper, it will eventually throw the copper level too low and arteriosclerosis will be potentiated. Therefore, periodic measurements should check the balance between minerals.

If zinc is low, it's place is filled by toxic cadmium from exhaust fumes, foods and cigarettes. Too much iron or copper will displace it also.

There are many cases in the literature of people who had not been able to taste for years and their problems were solved by zinc. This doesn't mean that it always clears it. It means that it is a common deficiency in some people with hypogeusia. Bowel diseases, uncorrectable iron, and vitamin A deficiencies, as well as ulcers, often clear with zinc. It is important in over 80 enzymes. As with most of the minerals, the red blood cell assay is far superior to the serum or plasma.

Selenium

Selenium is a mineral that used to be plentiful in the soils. When I was in China lecturing with Dr.'s Rea and Randolph, we saw in the hospital a young woman in her 20's whose entire chest was filled with a gigantic heart. This massive cardiomyopathy, which eventually kills, is called Keshan disease and stems from a selenium deficiency.

It is widely known that people who eat foods from soils that are selenium deficient have a higher incidence of cancer. This is because selenium is the primary mineral in the enzyme glutathione peroxidase, which is important in attempting to detoxify chemicals from the body. Also, a selenium deficiency will predispose to Candida because the white blood cells can capture, or gobble up, or phago-cytize the Candida, but they cannot kill it once they get it in their claws if they are deficient in selenium.

Copper

Copper has many enzymes which are very depen-dent upon it in the body. However, some people have far too much copper because of copper pipes in their homes. The leaching of copper is facilitated by the chlorine in the water. Always run the water a while before you use it for drinking or cooking so that the copper that was sitting in the pipes and leaching out into the acidic, chlorinated water can be rinsed out of the pipes. If we find toxic levels of copper (or aluminum) in your blood, we flush it out with a special program.

Copper does promote tissue repair and helps chemical sensitivity and some forms of arthritis because it is in the anti-inflammatory enzyme superoxide dismutase (one of its 3 forms). Like many nutrients, there is a fine line between too much (depression) and too little (hypercholesterolemia). We find over 75% of people are grossly deficient in it. One man had 10 years of daily headaches that no one could cure. We found it was 100% correctable as long as we kept his copper up.

Magnesium

Magnesium is an extremely crucial element. It can be low, especially in cases where people have used diuretics or fluid pills.

It can be responsible for irritability, muscle spasms, cardiac arrhythmia, premenstrual symptoms, impotency, neurologic problems, chronic pain, renal stones, E.I., chronic fatigue, depression, hypertension, osteoporosis and periodontal disease and it should be suspected highly in someone who has been on digitalis or has had repeated hospitalizations (all the intravenous solutions really rinse you out and lower the magnesium)

Magnesium is crucial for growth, wound healing, neuromuscular transmission, myocardial integrity and conduction, glucose metabolism and protein synthesis as well as energy synthesis.

Magnesium can be the sole cause of exhaustion or depression and I have seen a number of people improve their E.I. once they had enough magnesium. You see, magnesium is in over 300 enzymes in the body, so if we're deficient in it from a diet of junk foods and a lot of sweets, we can do all the environmental controls in the world but we won't be better until we have our chemistry working.

Magnesium is also crucial in cell membrane function and permeability. It's crucial in the metabolism of the essential fatty acids, vitamin D, B6, insulin, the coagulation

401

process, renal stone inhibition and even in forming the matrix of bone tissue.

Things that will lower magnesium in the body are eating foods from poor soils. Also, acid rain flushes out magnesium and calcium, replacing them with toxic aluminum and cadmium from smokestacks and automobiles.

The more you cook something, the more you can lower the magnesium, especially when you throw away the cooking water. High doses of vitamin C will lower the magnesium. High fat diets will. With aging, magnesium goes down. High calcium diets will lower magnesium as will chronic disease by just plain using up many of the precious enzymes that are magnesium dependent. High phosphate diets, constant use of medications and malabsorption (especially if it's because of hidden food allergy or Candida that constantly inflames the bowel) are common reasons for magnesium deficiency.

Fluoridation of water and inadequate acidity in the stomach also markedly lower magnesium. Low magnesium and food allergy are common in people with mitral valve prolapse and when magnesium is supplemented the arrhythmia often ceases. Manganese levels are critical to utilization of supplemented magnesium.

Molybdenum

I never thought much about molybdenum until I heard the late Dr. Carl Pfeiffer lecture at one of the seminars where I was speaking. So, I went to the medical school library to see what I could learn about molybdenum. I discovered that there is an enzyme in the liver called aldehyde dehydrogenase. The purpose of this enzyme is to break down aldehydes. This was a revelation to me since I was very formaldehyde sensitive as were many of my patients. So it made sense that we should have good, hefty levels of molybdenum and, of course, many of us were probably deficient in it because of our high junk food diets previously.

It's one of the trace minerals that has turned around many people with E.I. It's also necessary in the enzyme sulfite oxidase and some people with sulfite sensitivity can lose this sensitivity once molybdenum (or sometimes B12) levels are corrected.

FREE RADICALS

Free radicals are not hippies or any politically active group of people. Free radicals are naked little electrons in the body jumping around mindlessly destroying tissue.

You see, our bodies are in a constant battle of degeneration versus repair and free radicals are the agents of destruction. They are what facilitate or cause aging, arteriosclerosis, degenerative disease, allergies and cancer. When any chemicals get into the body, they damage it by free radical chemistry.

Free radicals can be good things too; that's how the white blood cells in our bodies destroy invading bacteria. Because free radicals are constantly generated and are a part of being a living organism, we must constantly guard against them. There are enzymes in the body to help us do this, such as superoxide dismutase, glutathione and G6PD.

These free radicals can damage cell membranes and also damage DNA which contains our genetic material. They can alter this genetic set of instructions (as in turning on the message to start reacting to chemicals or foods). These free radicals can also damage lipid membranes changing the way the cell communicates and operates, thus another way to turn on new diseases.

Mitochondria are structures within the cell that also are enveloped by a membrane. Since they are the powerhouses where energy is synthesized, damage to that membrane may produce the indescribable the exhaustion seen in

403

E.I.

Most importantly, we want the outer cell membranes strong, for it's through these that chemicals need to pass in order to disrupt the chemistry of the cell as well as reach the mitochondria, the intracellular regulatory proteins (DNA, RNA) and microsomal detoxification enzymes.

So, if we have strong cell membranes, these chemicals cannot invade. This means we need the right oils such as organic, cold pressed, expiration-dated flax oil and Efamol and vitamin E, since all three of these components are in normal cell membranes.

Free radicals have to attack the cell membrane first in order to get to the rest of the cell. Attacking this lipid membrane is called lipid peroxidation and leads to profound metabolic disturbance, inside and outside the cell.

When lipid peroxidation damages cell membranes, the mediators inside leak out and we have anything from allergic reactions to immune system damage to chronic inflammatory disease, indescribable exhaustion, degenerative disease, chemical intolerance, cancer or cell death.

So, what can we do to slow down free radical damage? We need some sort of sponge to sop up these wild, crazy electrons and fortunately we have it in compounds called anti-oxidants. These compounds protect against free radical damage. The most common of them are vitamins A, C, E and selenium.

There are also minerals that are important in the antioxidant defense system against free radicals. These include selenium, copper, iron, manganese, magnesium, molybdenum and zinc and there are other vitamins such as B2 and B3. However, vitamins A, C, E and selenium are the primary ones and are absolutely crucial to recovery from E.I. For people with E.I. have weaker defense mechanism so that chemicals that normally do not bother other people affect them in many strange and dangerous ways.

As with other components of the neglected nutrients, however, anti-oxidants can be overdone as well. Since they are metal chelaters, they may inhibit the synthesis of metal enzymes and make someone dangerously worse if they are not carefully balanced.

Dimethylglycine (B15) and glutathione are other important anti-oxidants, as is the amino acid alpha cysteine which is synthesized from methionine. There are many other nutrients and mechanisms, complete with scientific references, in our subsequent books.

It is the combination of specific and non-specific free radical defenses or anti-oxidants that allow us to live in this world and the price we pay for trying to adapt in the face of not enough anti-oxidants is the development of chronic disease.

Remember also that in the prostaglandin system in the body, PGE1 is an anti-inflammatory prostanoid. PGE2 is a dangerous pro-inflammatory prostanoid and the only difference between those two is one electron. One electron step or one anti-oxidant step makes the difference between something that does good things for us and something that does bad things for us.

Germanium

Another element of interest that has recently come on the scene is germanium. There are many papers in the Japanese literature showing that germanium is also an excellent anti-oxidant, but it has not been studied much in the United States.

There is germanium on the market, but most forms are in doses which are far too low. If the appropriate dose is used, (I have seen it and experienced it myself), food injections may not be needed because food sensitivities are markedly reduced. However, the only form that I know of at this point in time is Germanium 132 in its purest powder form. It is available from Dr. Steve Levine at Nutricology.

405

The dose is approximately 1/4 of a teaspoon two to three times a day, but the expense prohibits its use.

Other forms are much weaker (and far less expensive) and we have not seen the dramatic response with them that we did with the germanium pure powder. However, the number of people on it have not been as large as they have with many other nutrients due to expense. All of the data is not yet in.

Accessory Nutrients

There are scores of other nutrients that are very beneficial, like proacanthocyanidins, glandulars, probiotics, phosphatidyl choline, quercitin, carnitine, etc. discussed in the other books.

Another forgotten nutrient is lecithin which is important in cell membranes. Studies from M.I.T. show an expensive form, Phos Chol 900 (Adv. Nutr. Technol., Elizabeth, N.J.) has doubled choline levels in Alzheimers. See the doctor for dose.

It's exciting that we have the knowledge to manipulate our chemistry to correct biochemical deficiencies. As I look back I recognize many stumbling blocks at the various stages I passed through in recovering from E.I.

At one point, my B6 levels remained abnormally low because I didn't appreciate that I had a magnesium deficiency to correct before I could convert the B6 to pyridoxal-5- phosphate. At another stage, even I.V. magnesium wouldn't correct severe back spasm until I corrected the manganese deficiency that allowed the chemistry to proceed. Still later, I was grossly deficient in vitamin A in spite of 50,000 I.U. a day. Then I discovered why - I was zinc deficient (alcohol dehydrogenase converts retinol to retinaldehyde, the first breakdown step). It reminds us that we can never lose sight of the entire framework while dealing with the intricacies within it. The best defense is frequent monitoring of biochemical balance and corrections in light of the constant flow of new knowledge. Remember, the key is balance.

We have many new tests popping up for vitamins and minerals. Also, you never know when it may be time to check your levels or balance. So, to be on the safe side, never take any of your supplements on a day that you come to the office to see the doctor or allergy assistant.

ASSESSING NUTRIENT NEEDS

At this point in time, you must be ready to throw up your hands and ask how can we possibly decide what factors might be low in people with suspected nutritional deficiencies.

First, we look at the symptoms they have had for years and the target organs involved. For example, if they had skin disease or chronic diarrhea you know they have lost a lot of skin cells or intestinal cells, so they must be low in A, E and essential fatty acids and they must be low in a number of minerals.

We look at how long they have had symptoms. We look at their diets and whether or not they have yeast problems, chemical sensitivities or if they had many medications. Or, perhaps, they don't make enough bile to break down the fat soluble vitamins and excrete toxins.

We look at their dietary source of essential fatty acids but all the while we must recognize that there is tremendous individual variation. The best way to determine what the needs are is to actually assess them in a blood test.

Some disease states are notorious for certain deficiencies, such as PMS. Common deficiencies in the premenstrual syndrome are B6, magnesium, cis linoleic acid (Oil of Evening Primrose or Black Currant Seed oil), vitamin E and folic acid.

407

Drawbacks to a laboratory nutritional assessment are obviously the cost of the lab tests, but even more important is the availability. Some of these things cannot be measured yet. Others can be measured only by specialty labs that are very expensive and time-consuming to use.

The other problem is the cost of the supplements when we do know what you need and the actual physical bulk of the capsular material and the excipients (the things that hold the pills together). After all, there's a limit to how much of this junk we want in our systems.

We have a very difficult problem with the synergy of action. In other words, how these things all work together and the individual biochemistry of each person. Also, there is the stress of the environment and the stress of chronic disease that further make the requirements all the more individual.

For example, Smith Kline, a common lab used in many doctors offices, in 1986 charged $33 for a vitamin A level, $74 for a B1 level, $83 for a B2 level, $99 for a B6 level, $41 for a B12 level, $37 for a vitamin C level, $126 for a vitamin D3 level, $43 for a vitamin E level and $70 for a folic acid level. There is a grand total of several hundred dollars to just look at the majority of the vitamins but by no means all of them.

We are lucky in that, because I teach at the Advanced Course for physicians learning this specialty, and have become a forefront physician, many labs have vied for our business. We have been able to capitalize on this competition by negotiating for lower rates on package deals and save our patients money.

Some people are so sensitive they can't tolerate vitamins. I couldn't take a single one for two years. There were just a handful of foods I could eat. However, we know more now, so let's proceed.

The minerals are one thing that should be supplemented first. In fact, the hallmark of a mineral-deficient person is often one who takes vitamins and feels worse or who does okay for a while then deteriorates. He is actually pushing his biochemistry faster than it can cope by using vitamins and he's bringing out the mineral deficiencies in a more dramatic way.

As many case examples have shown, the correction in biochemistry has made all the difference. For example, Darlene was referred by a dentist because she had recurrent mouth ulcers. She was unable to wear her partial denture. She said her tongue always felt like it had been cut with a hot knife. She had been exhausted for the last year with headaches, nasal congestion and irregular bleeding for three years from the uterus. When we tested her, she had multiple mold sensitivities. When we looked at a laboratory analysis of her nutrients, her folic acid, B12 and B6 levels were all abysmally low. In two months of the supplements and her injections, all of her symptoms were clear and she was happy to report that she no longer had her back arthritis either.

So, what we see is that if we have the proper tools, we can, indeed, make a dramatic change in the health of many people and that E.I. is indeed a disease of hope.

Jeffery was 27-years-old and has sustained whiplash in an auto accident. Four months later he was still in physical therapy, taking a muscle relaxant daily and was utterly exhausted. He complained of disorientation, chronic diarrhea, muscle weakness and depression and became so sick he was unable to work. He came to us with a list of doctors that he had consulted and tests that had been done; no one had been able to find a cause or effective treatment.

We found that his B6 and B12 levels were practically nonexistent and that he had many dust and mold sensitivities. Within a few months he was back to work and had more energy than he had ever had before. If he's late for his injections, a lot of his tiredness returns. I'm certain that if we had not corrected his B12 level, for example (that was only 8 and the normal is 200-800), or if we had not corrected his B6 level (that was 9 and the normal is 30-80), that no amount of injections would have ever restored this young man to health.

We must bear in mind that chronic symptoms and medications almost always produce secondary nutritional deficiencies and that the longer symptoms persist and the more severe they are, the more likely that there is a host of deficiencies. Some people, like myself, got in such a downward spiral of getting sicker, more depleted and more sensitive, that in spite of numerous deficiencies, I couldn't tolerate one vitamin for two years until I had finished lowering my load with strict environmental controls. You must allow the body to "catch up."

AMINO ACIDS AND TAURINE

Some of the common reasons for people not responding to nutritional supplementation are:
(1) they are mineral depleted
(2) they don't make enough gastric acid or pancreatic enzymes to process the nutrients
(3) they have amino acid disturbances.

A disturbance in amino acids can mimic the Candida Syndrome, food or chemical hypersensitivity. Symptoms of amino acid disturbances can be hypoglycemia, headache, shifting neutralizing doses, someone who can't tolerate any vitamins, or someone who sleeps after eating or who has chronic exhaustion.

Taurine is an exemplary amino acid. Although most physicians have never even heard of it, there are many books on the subject. It is a very exciting amino acid because it is an inhibitory protein in the brain and stabilizes membranes tremendously. It is useful in controlling some seizure disorders and congestive failure and has allowed discontinuing prescribed medications for these conditions.

410

It's a membrane stabilizer, making it much harder for someone to have cardiac arrythmia or E.I. in the face of chemical exposure. It's also important in the synthesis of bile acids, deficiencies of which cause poor absorption of nutrients, poor regulation of overgrowth of pathogenic organisms in the bowel and defective detoxification of chemicals.

Taurine, besides being a neurotransmitter in the brain and pineal gland, is an important anti-oxidant. It is important in modulating and controlling aldehyde excess. You will remember that aldehydes are one of the compounds formed by Candida as well as being related to many air-borne chemicals like formaldehyde and trichloroethylene. They are probably the substances responsible for the brain fog that we all have experienced.

Acetaldehyde is a very potent chemical which disrupts membrane function and alters protein synthesis. It depresses the citric acid cycle in the cell, disrupts collagen production and fatty acid oxidation, is a potent blocker of neuromuscular synapses and is a close cousin to formaldehyde. So taurine is useful in people with recurrent infections, resistant Candida, and chemical sensitivity.

A POSSIBLE MECHANISM FOR E.I.

A common scenario is that a young gal would take birth control pills, which would secondarily lower her B6, which then would inhibit her conversion of taurine from methionine, so she would have a low taurine. Then, maybe she takes a diuretic for premenstrual bloating and this lowers her magnesium which also lowers her synthesis of taurine. Perhaps then she is put on an antibiotic for a sore throat, bladder infection or acne. She also has a sweet tooth. This causes the overgrowth of Candida in the bowel. This Candida forms aldehydes which require taurine for their degradation. Meanwhile, Candida, by inflaming the bowel,

411

causes further malabsorption from the bowel of precious minerals and nutrients necessary for the synthesis of taurine.

Add other aldehydes coming from her new home (formaldehyde) and this further stresses the detoxification mechanism so dependent on taurine. Before you know it, she is a classic case of E.I. and/or Candida hypersensitivity with tremendous brain fog, or toxic brain syndrome, who, with specific environmental controls, injections, diet, minerals, vitamins and taurine, can correct this whole scenario.

Candida nutrition requires, minimum, Super-B complex, vitamins A, C, E and selenium (the anti-oxidants) as well as essential fatty acids, multiple mineral, taurine and a general multiple. There are other factors that are also needed, but once the biochemistry is brought under control, no longer will you ever have to hear again, "It's all in your head."

When looking at the total load of our food, chemical, dust, mold, and pollen sensitivities, toxic levels of chemicals or our reactions to our own hormones or neurotransmitters, we should also bear in mind that we must always look for hidden nutritional deficiencies. There is a very delicate balance between all of the components of the total load in the body. We never know if your problem is going to be 20% Candida, 30% food allergy, 30% inhalant allergy and maybe 20% nutrition; or maybe it will be 90% nutrition and 10% Candida. All bets are off because the symptoms all mimic one another and we're all so uniquely individual.

We do know that by constant reading, learning, assaying the levels of nutrients in our systems and periodically monitoring the effectiveness of our trials, we can't help but create bodies more in tune and in balance with nature's needs, thus initiating the healing process.

In this way, progressively more of us are transformed from E.I. victims to E.I. survivors and able to get on with the business of living.

One crucial element to real healing is detoxification, or more properly, detoxication. This can be accomplished by a variety of means and on various levels. The environmental unit is one way to detox superficial levels of xenobiotics. Sweating is another, interspersed with exercise and a program to correct mineral imbalances that occur profusely.

The safest and best detox is with the macrobiotic diet. And it is the cheapest! This is described in **YOU ARE WHAT YOU ATE**, then **THE CURE IS IN THE KITCHEN**. In any detox program, there is a discharge period of worsening symptoms as old toxins are released from tissues back into the blood and excreted. The best way we have seen to accomplish this and concomitantly correct documented nutritional deficiencies is with macrobiotics, exercise and meditation. This triad takes the longest amount of time, but is the least expensive, the most available to the greatest number of people, and appears to be the most complete way of healing. There are additional detoxication procedures for the more advanced student of environmental medicine in **WELLNESS AGAINST ALL ODDS** and the subsequent books, articles and the ongoing bimonthly subscription **HEALTH LETTER**.

Most of us who did the program, as outlined in **The Cure Is In the Kitchen**, no longer have any symptoms, no medications, no injections, and are healthier than we have ever been in our lives. I'm stronger now at 51 than I was at 13, 19, 29, 39, or 49. I no longer have any injections, medicines or symptoms. And I no longer need to adhere strictly to the diet in order to maintain this state of health. And that's what it is all about.

SHOULD I TAKE VITAMINS?

When you are rotating, it's best to skip your vitamins for a while, testing them just as you would a food, because they contain many food antigens. The excipient of most pills, capsules and tablets is corn or lactose (milk sugar). That's the white substance that makes up the body of the pill. The actual chemicals themselves are a very small part of it and so a vehicle and/or a binder are required. Most pills have a plastic coating, chemical coloring, hydrocarbon ink for printing and other additives to retard spoilage. Also, any B and E vitamins often has yeast (mold) antigens. Oftentimes the C vitamins are derived from citrus and usually there are wheat, milk, corn and soy antigens in many pills as well.

Digestive enzymes play a part in how much nutritive value we absorb from our foods. Some never absorb their vitamins or minerals due to insufficient gastric acid or pancreatic juices.

Because of our individual biochemical requirements, vitamin therapy is a very hit and miss proposition. Add to this the fact that some people read about something and take it, never reading further to be sure they have balanced their nutrition.

For example, when the healing properties of zinc became known, people took large amounts of it. It must be remembered that zinc, like everything else in the body, is in a delicate balance with other micro nutrients, for instance, copper. By taking an abnormal amount of zinc, they upset the zinc/copper ratio and lowered the copper. This lowered copper actually potentiated arteriosclerosis. So, they were doing harm and had no way to monitor it. Also, recall that a serum zinc level is not nearly as indicative of a low level as a red cell or erythrocyte zinc level. There are many fine points that will snag the unknowledgeable. For example, you may add a nutrient and for a while it may make you feel better, but, eventually the imbalance accumulates and you feel worse. Read Dr. Richard Passwater's **Supernutrition**, available at the office, for starters.

It is surmised that if the liver is not healthy it cannot deconjugate or break down the natural body estrogens appropriately. By supplementing the diet with B vitamins (which are lost so readily in processing and cooking), the liver should function better. Having heard this, we put a number of young women on vitamins. Previously, they had all suffered with long heavy periods and much cramping. To our surprise, all experienced a reduction in the amount and duration of flow (six days of heavy flow down to three days of moderate flow) and reduction of cramps; they no longer required medication.

This impressed me with how much we do not know. There have been many people with dandruff, infertility, impotence, PMS and fatigue who were merely vitamin deficient. Finding the culprit and correcting it while maintaining the balance with everything else was the trick. If tolerated, I would suggest natural and whole food sources like fresh wheat germ oil capsules, brewer's yeast and cod liver oil rather than a B-complex from a chemical manufacturer which can't hope to compete with nature. Brewer's yeast will also have chromium, pantothenic acid and who knows what else? Also, these nutrients are in the ratio that Mother Nature devised. Most mold sensitive people, however, need yeast free B vitamins, so we need to (temporarily) use synthetic sources.

It would be desirable to take one type of vitamin each week so that you could see if indeed a particular one caused a beneficial effect. However, the problem is that many do not cause the desired effect until they are combined with the correct amount of several other vitamins. They have a synergistic effect; that is, they only work well together. A common story is that someone felt superlative after they started nutrients. Then after a while, they didn't feel so hot. What they did is reach a level of deficiency for a particular

415

nutrient. So now the pathways are shut down. Here is where an assay of the exact levels is crucial.

The other difficulty lies in the fact that many nutrients take months to restore balance to the body chemistry. It takes about four to six months to replace bad membranes, which came from years of margarine, grocery store corn oils and hydrogenated polyunsaturated oils. To tide you over until you see the doctor, you can cook only with olive oil, use butter on the table and be sure you get one tablespoons of organic flax (linseed oil) a day (put on salad dressing, granola, rice, squash, potato or drink straight).

WHAT VITAMINS SHOULD I TAKE

If you are chemically sensitive, it may be months or years before you can tolerate vitamins (I couldn't for two years). The best vitamin to start with is buffered sago palm vitamin C or powdered pure ascorbic acid, because it helps you get out of reactions. (Everything we recommend can usually be obtained from **N.E.E.D.S., 1- 800-634-1380**). The next step should be to try Anti-ox (three times a day with meals). You may have to dump it out of its beef capsule. If you cannot tolerate this, try Klaire Laboratory's Oxy-guard or Tyler's Oxyperm, or the individual components. A multiple mineral and the magnesium loading test (in **Tired or Toxic?**) would be necessary as well. An individualized program can be adapted for you by the doctor.

People often ask, "What about calcium?" The best test at this time is not a blood test but a dual photon densitometry bone scan and 24-hour urine tests. The Chinese never eat milk or cheese, but neither do they have a high phosphate diet (soda pop, processed foods) that inhibits calcium absorption from vegetables and meats. Many people take calcium and don't know they lack sufficient gastric acid to allow absorption of the calcium! Some forms in discount vitamin pills are not in a form that is absorbable to begin with.

Some common deficiencies I've seen can be supplemented by buffered sago palm vitamin C, B complex, Antiox, flax oil, magnesium, zinc, copper, manganese, d-alpha tocopherol (vitamin E), A emulsion forte, a multiple vitamin-mineral, and an extra multiple mineral. These must be individualized, however, for most.

Of course, if absorption is impeded by gastric acid and digestive enzyme deficiencies, a gut wall infested with Candida or inflamed by unknown food allergies or a lack of acidophilus bacteria, it won't matter how many you take. We can test to determine if you have this leaky gut syndrome (see **Wellness Against All Odds**).

Very food sensitive people should rotate vitamins; if this is impossible because there are no substitutes, then those vitamins should not be taken daily. Vitamin C comes from eight sources. This provides plenty of alternatives for rotating. Vitamins are a highly individual matter. Probably no two people have the exact same requirements The problem is, we don't have foolproof ways to determine these needs yet, but they are being worked on. We do know that certain nutrients are notoriously low due to specific environmental factors. Many nutrient systems are under constant strain in effort to detoxify the influx of chemicals (xenobiotics).

If you want vitamin recommendations, you should see the doctor. Following is a sketchy outline of some of the more commonly required supplements and their usual doses. Again, these are not all required by one person and the doses are individual. After you have had your vitamin and mineral levels drawn, the doctor will prescribe an individualized program based on blood tests, history and symptoms.

All vitamin programs must be monitored for balance as well as liver and kidney function. In other words, you should check back with the doctor every three to six months because some supplements are required in high doses initially, but can become toxic or create a deficiency of another substance in the body through continued use. Also, the doctor teaches nutrition in the Advanced Course for Physicians and there are constant new findings. And you will see that in the subsequent books, especially **Tired or Toxic?** and **Wellness Against All Odds**, there is a great deal more on this biochemistry.

DEFINITION OF NUTRIENTS

RDA levels - recommended daily allowance of nutrients (vitamins, minerals, essential fatty acids and amino acids). These are antiquated and inappropriately low designations, partly out of failure to keep up with biochemical literature and partly out of lobbying pressure of food manufacturers who do not want to have to add further nutrients to their products, thereby increasing production costs. For example a 1993 NEW ENGLAND JOURNAL OF MEDICINE study showed that a paltry 100 I.U. of vitamin E a day cuts cardiovascular disease risk in half. Mind you, this is the number one cause of death and illness in the U.S.. But even though there are no side effects from 100 I.U. the U.S. government recommendation is still 10 I.U. But you can take hundreds of dollars' worth of prescription drugs with bad side effects to correct the disease we could have prevented.

Optimal levels - those specific levels that allow each individual function at his best. Only possible through monitoring levels of nutrients along with symptom improvement.

Corrective levels - those levels prescribed by the doctor for presumed deficiencies from chronic symptoms and for documented deficiencies with laboratory tests. These levels, if taken longer than three to six months, can create dangerous imbalances. That is why it is crucial to check back or discontinue the program after three to six months.

Maintenance levels - those levels that are designed for day to day maintenance of a corrected and healthy, optimally functioning system. They, too, require periodic monitoring to guard against unforeseen imbalances.

The field of nutrition, as in ecology, is in its infancy.

DISCLAIMER

Even when a vitamin program is tailor-made for you, you should never continue on it for more than six to twelve months (three to six months if you don't feel good, twelve months if you feel fine) without consulting with the doctor. To do so is to continue the program at your own risk. There are a couple of reasons for this:

1) Programs that are designed to correct nutritional deficiencies are, by their very nature, highly unbalanced (to compensate for an existing imbalance). As correction occurs, high doses are no longer needed and will cause other imblances. For example, zinc (a deficiency in many patients) is necessary to heal the immune system. After 3 - 6 months, the total program should be assessed by the doctor because it will lower copper, magnesium, manganese or molybdenum and cause depression, worse chemical sensitivity, high cholesterol, and lots more.

2) The field of nutrition is growing very fast and we understand much more every year about potential toxicities, imbalances and other missing nutrients. It's very exciting but also potentially dangerous.

3) We have better monitors of levels of nutrients and there are continual additions to our list of available assays.

Why do we designate certain brands of supplements? Taking vitamins can be as potentially serious and dangerous as prescription medications. Some formulations do not strictly contain what they say they do and some do not contain the nutrients in a form that can be absorbed and utilized by the body. Since I cannot know every manufacturer well, I tend to stick with those I feel I can vouch for. With hundreds of patients coming from all over the country, I need a central source of consistent, top quality supplements.

COMMONLY USED SUPPLEMENTS

Cod liver oil - good source of vitamin A - Antigen: Cod. One tbsp. every 2 - 4 days - obtained anywhere, unflavored -used for low serum level, especially diseases of skin, bowel and nervous system. Caution: use no other vitamins with added vitamin D since it also contains 400 I.U. vitamin D.

A Emulsion forte is preferable, but caution: one drop is 12,500 units.

Vitamin A (tablets) component: variable; antigen: variable. 10,000 to 25,000 I.U. 1 - 2 daily. Obtained anywhere. Used for same as above, but not as good because of preservatives used. Antigens: algae, carrot, fish, glycerine capsule.

Beta-Carotene - safer than vitamin A because it's the precursor and you can't overdose as easily. Also, it has cancer inhibiting effects that vitamin A doesn't. Up to 30,000 I.U. a day is a good dose.

Super B Complex - component: all B vitamins, choline, Paba, folate, biotin, etc.; antigen: beef capsule. 1 - 2 daily. May need additional levels of specific components.

B3 or Niacin - this is a good detoxifier, 25 - 100 mg 3 or 4 times a day is the dose. However, if it's too much for you,

you'll know rapidly. You will get horrendous flushing and itching. Don't worry, Benadryl calms it. Start low and work up slowly. When you start to feel a little prickly, you'll know you should not exceed that dose for several days until you no longer get a symptom. Skipped doses reduce your tolerance level and you must build up again. The doctor or nurse will explain how to achieve super high doses for detox without the side effects. If higher doses are used for detox, you'll need an individualized program to counter the imbalance.

Pyridoxal-5-Phosphate - P-5-P by Vital-Life is the metabolite of B6. Some people cannot convert B6 to its first stage. This error in metabolism can be corrected by starting out with P-5-P, 1 or 2 tablets a day. Usually, magnesium must accompany it as well as other minerals.

Dimethylglycine - 62.5 mgs., 3 a day. This is an antioxidant. It's also B15 and it increases antibody production in response to injections.

Biotin - 300 mcg., 1 a day. Good for discouraging Candida.

Pantothenic - **B5** - **component:** pantothenic acid; antigen: beef capsule, synthetic. 500 mg, 1 - 4 daily. Used for allergy and detoxification.

Folic Acid - 800 mcg. Klaire Labs. A commonly low nutrient necessary in formaldehyde metabolism.

Buffered Sago Palm C - **component:** calcium, magnesium, C; antigen: sago palm prior to 1993 when it was changed to corn antigen without notification. 1/2-2 tsp. three times a day. Used for acute reactions.

Vitamin C - **1000 mg.** No wheat, soy, yeast, corn or

preservatives. Used for acute reactions. Klaire Labs pure powder. Must rinse teeth after, as the acid can dissolve tooth enamel.

Rice C - component: C; antigen: rice. 1,000 - 2,000 mg. three times a day. Used for acute reactions.

Carrot C - component: C; antigen: carrot. 1,000 - 2,000 mg. three times a day. Used for acute reactions.

CAUTION: RINSE MOUTH AFTER USE OF ALL ASCORBIC ACID POWDERS AND LIQUIDS AS THE ACIDITY CAN DISSOLVE TOOTH ENAMEL.

Quercitin C - A bioflavinoid that is citrus free. Has very strong anti-inflammatory properties but has a fine line between too much and too little.

Anti-Ox - component: A, C, E, Se, Zn, cysteine, glutathione, DMG, etc; antigen: beef capsule. Used for Anti-oxidant. Also alternatives are Klaire Labs Oxy-guard and Tyler Labs Oxy-perm.

ARG Multi-vi-min - general multiple. Antigen: beef capsule. 2-6 per day. All purpose multiple devoid of vitamin D. ALternatives: Rebalance, Tyler's Nutrizyme, Klaire, etc.

ARG Multi-mineral - general minerals without the vitamins. For people who know "vitamins always make me feel worse," they need to correct their minerals first. Should be continued indefinitely.

Perna Caps - by DaVinci Labs (1-800-451-5190). A good source of trace minerals for arthritis and other conditions.

Alta Sil-X, Silica gel - good source of silica, for nails, hair, tendons, ligaments.

Germanium Pure Powder - dose is 1/3 tsp., 2 - 4 times a day to abort food reactions.

Pro-fem II - component: GLA, B6, folate, calcium, magnesium, potassium; antigen: herbs. 1 - 3 a day. Used for PMS, Candida.

Efamol - component: gamma linolenic acid and other EFA's; antigen: primrose seeds.

Glanolen - Black Currant Seed Oil. Half as expensive as Efamol because only one capsule, three times a day, is needed to get the same amount of GLA that two capsules of Efamol, three times a day, would provide.

Lecithin - phosphatidyl choline for nerve sheath synthesis and detox and cell membranes. Usually soybean derived. Phos Chol concentrate is best and purest source.

Cal/mag - component: calcium, magnesium; antigen: synthetic. 1 - 2 three or four times a day. 2 provides 1000 mg calcium and 750 mg magnesium. Used for osteoporosis, PMS, heart and blood pressure problems, Candida. Dose very individual; depends on levels in urine and blood, diet and levels of other supplements.

Caprystatin - component: caprylic acid; antigen: synthetic. 1 - 3 three times a day. Used for intolerance to Nystatin (not as good). Capricin (Neesby) is a long-acting form.

Zinc picolinate - component: zinc; antigen: synthetic. 25 mg 1 - 3 a day. Used for hearing, taste, smell, prostate. When taken for prolonged months, can cause serious imbalance in other minerals.

Chromium picolinate or chromate - component: chromium; antigen: synthetic. 200-1000 mcg a day. Used for diabetes, hypoglycemia, sugar cravings, high cholesterol.

Copper - maximum that should be taken is 1 - 4 mgs. (total from all vitamins) a day and usually only if you have a proven need for it. Essential for superoxide dismutase function (anti-inflammatory and negates effects of chemicals). Sometimes tough on stomach. Multiple forms: copper, sebacate, copper sulfate, copper plus, and 2.5 mg chelated copper (the best tolerated usually).

Molybdenum, chelated - 150 mcg., three 1 - 3 times a day depending upon need. In detox enzymes. The picolinate form is 1 mg and may be taken every other day.

Manganese picolinate - 20 mg., one a day. Essential for superoxide dismutase and magnesium function.

Sodium selenite solution - component: Selenium. A drop a day up to a tsp. for highly sensitive non-tolerant patients. Selenomethionine 50-200 mcg is preferable tablet form. **CAUTION: MUST COMPUTE TOTAL SELENIUM FROM ALL SUPPLEMENTS AND NOT EXCEED 400 MCG A DAY AS YOUR HAIR AND NAILS CAN FALL OUT.**

Vital Dophilus - component: lactobacillus. 1/4 - 1 tsp. 1-3 times a day. Used for restoring normal bowel flora, colitis, constipation and Candida. Many acidophilus compounds are dead and won't work. This is most consistent and reliable.

Probionate-C. This form is encapsulated since some people have a stomach acid that kills the acidophilus in powder form. The capsule protects it. Also Probifidonate-C provides an additional type of beneficial flora.

Vital-plex - an even better form of acidophilus than Vital Dophilus because it has three beneficial bowel organisms instead of one to compete with the Candida

Pancreatin - component: stomach and pancreatic enzymes; antigens: animal (non-ferment) or vegetable (ferment). 1-4 daily with meals. Used for colitis, food allergy, leaky gut syndrome, malabsorption, and constipation. Enzymes can dissolve antigen-antibody complexes, arteriosclerosis, inflammation, and cancers. References, explanation, directions in **Wellness Against All Odds**.

Taurine 500 mg. - amino acid for Candida and E.I., detox, cardiac arrhythmia and seizures.

Betaine HCL - a digestive that mimics gastric juices, especially good for people who don't have enough acid to ionize their minerals for absorption. One before meals. **CAUTION: ULCER FLARE. MUST DISCONTINUE IF YOU HAVE ANY ABDOMINAL DISCOMFORT.**

D,L,-Phenylalanine - has been beneficial for reduction of pain (along with aloe-vera juice, glucosamine sulfate, and Bromase). 500 mg. capsules 1 - 6 a day.

L-Tyrosine - has helped in depression. 500 mg. 1 - 4 daily.

L-Lysine - 250 mg. 1 - 8 daily, only when cold sore starting. Also use a high dose of C. Helps fight cold sores in many. Combined with L-proline, L-carnitine and other nutrients it is important for arteriosclerosis (special program).

Klaire Labs Amino Acid Complex IV - 1 - 3 four times a

day. Not only can it be therapeutic but also is diagnostic of an amino acidopathy. If it makes anything worse, more than likely you have an abnormality in the amino acids and this formulation pushes the abnormal pathway so that the symptoms show quicker.

L-Glutathione - 50 mg. A component of anti-ox, need 300 mg/day as detoxification aid.

L-Glutamine - 500 mg. Often useful for increased ability to concentrate, weight loss, as well as healing the leaky gut syndrome (that can be the cause of food and chemical allergies as well as auto-immune diseases like lupus, rheumatoid, MS, thyroiditis, etc).

Tri-Salts - Contains calcium, magnesium and potassium salts in a bicarbonate form. Especially good for people who cannot have sodium but need to neutralize reactions. Can use with vitamin C. Dose: 1/2 - 1 heaping tsp. for reaction.

Vitamin E - be sure it is d-alpha tocopherol, not dl-alpha tocopherol- component E. 200 - 800 I.U. per day. Used as antioxidant in highly sensitive, non-tolerant patients.

Adrenal - component: adrenal; antigen: beef capsule, synthetic. 1 - 3 a day. Used for highly stressed, especially severe Candida and chemically sensitive.

The above list is not exhaustive, but merely briefly describes a sample of some of the supplements used. Each person needs an individualized program.

Most vitamins are better absorbed when taken with meals so digestive enzymes facilitate their absorption. Some supplements precipitate or counteract others and cannot be taken together. Be sure to ask the doctor how to take your supplements when you make your individualized plan. See the Vitamin/Mineral Monograph.

New products, as well as new research and new findings, are always becoming available, so check back yearly for an update.

Taking a large number of vitamins a day can be tricky. One way to simplify it and save time is put your vitamins for the week out in ice cube trays, label them with a crayon and cover with aluminum foil. That way the vitamins will stay fresh and you'll only open the jars once a week.

For those who need a noontime dose away from home, there is another trick I use. Take a large baggy and put your Monday noon vitamins in it, put a twist tie tightly around the bag at the top of the vitamins. Now you have one tiny corner of the bag tied off and the whole rest of the bag left over.

Now, put Tuesday's noon vitamins in the bag and close with a twist tie. Then Wednesday's vitamins and close with a twist tie, etc. What you have left looks like a piece of intestine or an old fashioned sausage and it's easy to store in your car or desk. Just open one unit a day. See, there is a way to solve every problem. In fact, the challenge is fun.

WARNING

Obviously, you can see that you can't take everything and, fortunately, you really don't need everything because you get a lot of your nutrients in organically grown foods from healthy soils.

Another drawback of taking so many supplements is that the excipients (the capsule material, binders, glycerine, preservatives such as methylparaben and other chemicals such, as magnesium stearate, that are put in to make the powders free flowing in the laboratories where they make the capsules) are all materials that we really do not want in our bodies.

We have to be very careful in choosing the most important nutrients for each person because of this. You must be extremely careful to recognize the difference between corrective doses and maintenance doses.

Corrective doses are meant to correct and make better abnormal chemistry. However, if you stay on corrective doses, because of their nature of having high doses for certain nutrients, you will eventually create an imbalance in other nutrients and become more sick than you ever were before. Therefore, it is very important that if you do not follow up in three to six months to check the effectiveness of your program, you should either discontinue it or drop everything to far lower levels, such as one of each supplement two or three times a week.

Maintenance levels are cheaper and they require far fewer supplements and are designed then to attempt to keep the body in balance with all of its necessary elements. Maintenance levels are for those who do not need correction. The stress of living in the polluted world is continually pushing us toward imbalance. In fact even normal people who are not sick are using up a vast amount of nutrients each day in the work of the body detoxifying the myriad of chemicals we are all exposed to everyday.

Don't forget that we can never hope to duplicate or scoop or one-up Mother Nature. And since we are the first generation saddled with the business of correcting abnormal biochemistry, we are undoubtedly going to make a lot of mistakes.

We know if you take too high a dose of vitamin C, you will lower your calcium and magnesium and on and on the list goes. So, periodic assessment is necessary when a large number of supplements is being taken. That doesn't mean to flippantly send me a list of supplements scratched on toilet paper or ask if your program is okay in the last two minutes of your visit. This is serious biochemistry and I can't mash it into a lengthy evaluation of your other problems.

IATROGENIC ILLNESS - HOW WE CREATE DISEASE

Since Marilyn was only 5'3", she had to stand on a stool to unfold the pharmacy's computer printout of the prescription drugs she had used in the last year. Her list of symptoms was nearly as long. Within a couple of weeks on a yeast-free diet and nystatin, she was 50 percent better.

As you have read, the Candida hypersensitivity syndrome can be caused by many prescriptions, such as antibiotics, birth control pills or prednisone. The symptoms, recognized by less than a few hundred physicians in the United States, baffle most doctors. Because the symptoms can be anything you can think of and can cross many specialty lines, it is not uncommon for the victim to have seen a family doctor, internist, pulmonary specialist, ENT specialist, cardiologist, neurologist, allergist and even a psychiatrist as a last resort.

Further testing revealed that Marilyn's remaining symptoms could be brought under control by identifying her dust, mold, food and chemical allergies. When Candida strikes, frequently the immune system breaks down so that many other sensitivities crop up that were never there before.

Long before we could straighten out her environmental sensitivities, we had to get her biochemical machinery in good working order. We had to correct her nutritional deficiencies or any further treatment would be doomed to failure.

Many commonly prescribed drugs deplete the body of vitamins, minerals, amino acids and essential fatty acids. For example, antibiotics, in facilitating a secondary overgrowth of the yeast Candida in the bowel, can help create a bowel so inflamed that nutrients cannot be properly absorbed. In other cases, the resultant diarrhea is the cause of malabsorption.

An esophagus or stomach with Candida overgrowth burns so antacids are prescribed. Antacids in turn can decrease the absorption of calcium and magnesium. If stomach problems persist, then acid inhibitors are prescribed, like cimetidine or ranitidine, but using these cause many people to develop profound B12 and mineral deficiencies. Not only do these drugs do an excellent job at turning off acid secretion in the stomach, they also stifle the intrinsic factor secretion which is necessary so that oral B12 can be absorbed from foods and vitamins. Anyone on these drugs for a few months or longer should routinely have B12 serum levels measured.

Usually a doctor won't check for a B12 deficiency unless the complete blood count (CBC) shows macrocytosis (enlarged, fat red cells) signaling a deficiency. The problem is that in scores of people in whom we have found serious drug-induced B12 and folic acid deficiencies, none had this macrocytosis that we were trained to look for in medical school.

Probably one of the most prolific deficiencies we see is magnesium. In medical school we learned very little about this crucial element, but we are literally seeing an epidemic of people low in intracellular magnesium now. For starters, anyone on blood pressure pills or diuretics (fluid pills) has a very good chance of being low in magnesium. Doctors routinely check serum potassium but rarely think of an rbc potassium that is more sensitive. But as the JOURNAL OF THE AMERICAN MEDICAL ASSOCIATION showed (6/13/90), over 90% of doctors fail to even think of looking for a magnesium deficiency, even when the patients are in the hospital dying of it. Since serum is the very last place to exhibit a magnesium deficiency, an intracellular erythrocyte (red blood cell) is the best level to test in blood. An even superior test, however, is the magnesium loading test.

If you really want to see a low magnesium, look at someone who has been in the hospital for a while on many drugs, intravenous solutions (I.V.'s), perhaps a little surgery and, of course, hospital food. This is a perfect way to make any magnesium deficiency dangerously worse. There is a word in medicine that the public seldom hears; it is **iatrogenic**. It means the patient's symptoms were caused by the treatment. As we become an increasingly more drug oriented society, we can't help but cause more drug induced nutritional deficiencies. The problem is that they occur so insidiously that very few victims and physicians are aware of their cause or existence.

Cheryl had years of serious asthma necessitating prednisone. The prednisone caused diabetes, ulcers and hypertension. She also had a vitamin B6, A, B12 and red cell magnesium deficiency when we first examined her in the office and sent her blood tests off to the lab. She had Candida hypersensitivity as well. Is it any wonder that treating her Candida problem, correcting her nutritional deficiencies and identifying the environmental triggers to her asthma got her off prednisone within one month? This was the first time she had been off prednisone in years. These environmental triggers included the newer molds that we had researched (**Annals of Allergy,** 1982, 1983, 1984) and hidden food and chemical allergies.

Doesn't this all sound a bit complicated? You are right and that is the very reason that a new specialty had to be created. A regular allergist does not look for nutritional deficiencies nor does he look for Candida problems or chemical hypersensitivities. Neither does the lung specialist. So, the field of environmental medicine was created to deal with the entire victim of twentieth century technology, not just one or two of his ailing parts. The causes for symptoms are meticulously sought, not masked with medications.

Twentieth century technology and its many excellently trained medical specialists have given us a medical system unsurpassed by any other world, but now we are creating some of our own diseases and need to carefully explore nutritional deficiencies and environmental triggers, especially when no other answers are found.

With such an advanced medical system in the land of plenty, it's difficult to think of suburbanites as malnourished with hypersensitivities to twentieth century products. Environmental illness seems to be a cruel joke on society. Nutritional deficiencies don't necessarily start with drugs. Acid rain washes magnesium and selenium from the soils and repeated monoculture of crops further deplete the soil. Irradiation of foods destroys some vitamins. Chemical pollution of outdoor air by auto exhaust, industrial effluents and of indoor air by formaldehydes and other hydrocarbons from plastics, building supplies, and furnishings and the pollution of water by industrial wastes, agricultural fertilizers and pesticides are some of the most common culprits. The result can be depletion of nutrients from overuse of adaptive enzymes and anti-oxidant systems.

Not only have these chemicals surged upon society so quickly that many are incompletely tested, but also no agency has considered the problem of synergistic effects and individual susceptibility. In other words, maybe several chemicals are safe in low doses alone, but when they are mixed together as they would be in real life exposures, they may be dangerous. Maybe one in ten persons has a biochemical idiosyncrasy that makes him more susceptible to the chemical than someone else. Remember, one reason we got into such trouble with Thalidomide was that it only caused absence of limbs in humans, not in laboratory rats.

Food processing is ubiquitous, difficult to avoid and removes many essential nutrients. In addition, food additives have undesirable biochemical effects. The highly processed nature of food can be appreciated with one example: phosphates. They are used for leavening, as preservatives, bacteriocidal agents, dough conditioners, flavor vehicles, pH buffers, acid flavor and stabilizers. They increase water holding ability, decrease phase separation and act as freeze guards and thickeners. Because they are ubiquitous in processed foods, they are frequently ingested. Frequent ingestion of phosphates lowers calcium and magnesium in the body making the biochemical machinery less than optimum and ripe for any environmental trigger that happens along.

In short, modern chemicals and medications add to the total body burden; they add to the biochemical stress on the system and cause nutritional deficiencies. These deficiencies in turn further add to our total body burden and create a situation that is ripe for succumbing to further mold, food, chemical and Candida stresses that eventually become hypersensitivities. Coming full circle, chronic disease further stresses the system and depletes nutritional factors.

What can you do? Keep reading articles that emphasize how to keep your lifestyle and diet as chemically clean as possible and maintain your ongoing nutritional education. For, it is only through education that you will have a chance of avoiding iatrogenic illness.

THE CHOLESTEROL HOAX
Are You Due For An Oil Change?

Most people never think of oil in terms of having a need for it in their bodies, but oils or lipids are actually essential for life itself. Every cell membrane and nerve sheath is made up of different kinds of oils or lipids. The brain is the most highly lipid part of the body.

As well as protecting the internal environment of a cell through the creation of a membrane, there are a series of membranes inside cells which have different functions.

433

Mitochondria, for example, are membranous areas within the cell where energy is actually manufactured. Another membrane structure, endoplasmic riticulum or the microsomes, is the site where everyday chemicals are detoxified: chemicals that occur in foods, water and air and that are constantly trying to destroy the body and create disease.

Most people's membranes, whether they are intracellular or extracellular, are made up of the wrong oils. They are made up of what we call trans fatty acids. These are the oils that are in the grocery store, such as polyunsaturated corn oil, other vegetable oils like safflower oils and margarines. Years ago, oils were extracted from seeds with heavy pressure, such as in roller presses. With the discovery of chemical processes, extraction procedures called hydrogenation replaced the roller or cold pressed methods. Hydrogenation exposes the seeds to extremely high temperatures in excess of 500 degrees F. This causes a twist in the fat molecule and creates a (trans) form that is foreign to the body and not only blocks the good chemistry but causes arteriosclerosis. This change from the cis form to a trans form is the form that is in the grocery store, polyunsaturated oils that are supposed to be good for you.

The problem is that the body cannot properly utilize trans forms and when these oils are incorporated into membranes they act much like a broken key. They fit in the slot but they do not function the way they should and they retard other good oils from getting in to function well. It is analogous with trying to cram your right hand into a left-handed bowling ball.

At this juncture, your confusion is understandable. After all, the cardiologists of the country recommend margarines and hydrogenated polyunsaturated oils for reducing cholesterol. True, they will reduce it, but at the time all this cholesterol information was coming out, very few biochemists knew of the deleterious effect of the hydrogenation procedure. They did not know that these trans oils actually accelerated arteriosclerosis and degenerative change and that there were healthier ways to decrease cholesterol.

Furthermore, hydrogenation removes many precious nutrients like vitamin E, B6 and magnesium that are crucial to reducing arteriosclerosis. These are not replaced; only the cheaper B1, B2, B3 and iron are usually replaced. The removal of these lengthens the shelf-life of a product and is inversely proportional to it's beneficial effects on your shelf-life. With the removal of nutrients, microorganisms find the food less nourishing and do not grow in it nor make it turn bad. If the bugs do not want it, why should you?

In the wake of the cholesterol craze, bad press was given to the egg. This is an excellent and inexpensive source of lecithin, necessary to ward off changes like those seen in Alzheimer's presenile dementia. If you are on the correct vitamins, you can most likely tolerate eggs and you can always have your cholesterol level checked to be sure. There are very few places in the country where you can check the adequacy of your brain lecithin levels.

Scientists all over the world are now learning that they can manipulate many inflammatory and allergic conditions by directing the chemistry with the better oils and gradually changing over the cell membranes. They first became interested in this when they learned that Eskimos eat an extremely high fat diet, but do not have early coronary artery disease until they come to the United States and eat our diet. They learned that there was a protective factor in fish oil that lowered cholesterol. Scientists also now know that the trans oils in margarines and regular grocery store oils inhibit an enzyme called delta-6-desaturase (D-6- D) which is important in metabolizing good oils into the chemicals in the membrane that are needed.

At this time, you want to take four months and see what effect changing your oils over to the good form will have. Cook only with olive oil since it is less easily changed to a trans form when heated. Do not ever use margarine or regular grocery store oils, except olive oil. Use butter on the table and be sure to get two tablespoons of cold pressed food grade linseed (flax) oil daily. You can do this by pouring it on granola, potatoes, rice or squash, or you can put it in a blender with garlic, parsley and lemon to make a dressing, or you can just drink it plain. Do not heat the oil. If you are sensitive to linseed (flaxseed) or need to rotate, use cold pressed walnut, soy, safflower, or almond oils. Make sure they are cold pressed, however. Also, to make this program successful, you must reduce red meat to once or twice a week maximum. Half a can of sardines in sild oil per day is also helpful and eating oily ocean fish a couple times a week helps make this change come about.

These oils require many minerals, especially magnesium and zinc, as well as B vitamins to become incorporated in the membranes. In fact, most people with high cholesterol have many nutrient deficiencies anyway, hence their inability to properly metabolize cholesterol.

The hoax is we are creating more arteriosclerosis faster by recommending corn oil and margarines and "plastic" egg substitutes and by not looking at the nutrient deficiencies that cause the problem. Does man actually think he can make a better egg than God?!?

Studies from the **Journal of Rheumatology** are now showing that people with severe arthritis who are put on very high doses of some of these Omega 3 (cold water fish) precursor oils are having no pain. For the moment you want to see what effect just changing your oils over to the correct type has in your body chemistry before doing a program such as that.

With all the research that is coming out, however, it is pretty exciting that we are able to learn to manipulate the body into becoming less reactive to environmental insults. So, isn't it about time that you had your oil changed?

Depressed or Just Allergic
to the Twentieth Century?

The following article is reprinted with kind permission from **Let's Live** magazine, Los Angeles, CA 90004 (Titled: Vitamin E Against Environmental Pollution, April 1986 issue, pg. 50, by S.A. Rogers, M.D.).

On the last leg of our scientific exchange lecture tour in China, I was anxious to stop in a particularly famous silk store in Hong Kong. Dr. William Rea, the cardiovascular surgeon who heads the most comprehensive environmentally controlled hospital unit in the world for victims of environmental illness, Dr. Theron Randolph, author of An Alternative Approach to Allergies and discoverer that people react to chemicals, and I had lectured in six major medical schools from Peking (Beijing) to Canton (Guangzhou).

As we entered the store, I could hear hammers and saws and there was the odor of glue. Determined to ignore my chemical sensitivities, I began to peruse the beautiful silks. After about an hour, my husband wandered over and said, "Well, Bunny, are you ready to go? The tailor looked astonished to see a grown woman huddled in the corner like an animal as I cried with glassy, swollen eyes, "We're the only ones who picked out all the ugly things. Everything we picked out is ugly. Everyone else got all the good stuff!"

"Oops, we'd better get you out of here. Looks like you have had enough glue sniffing for one day!" he chuckled and led me to the street where, within twenty minutes, I was laughing and embarrassed that I had said those things. That's what living with environmental illness is like and we felt fortunate that we could control it. Years back an episode like that would drag on for days and we would be baffled by the cause and helpless in deciphering a reason for the sudden emergency of overwhelming unwarranted negativity, depression and irrationality.

Each year I treat hundreds of people from all over the world, who, like myself, are allergic to twentieth century chemicals. Some of the most common causes are natural gas furnaces and stoves, new construction, paint, cabinet glues, new carpeting and furniture. The most common symptoms are unwarranted depression, exhaustion, sudden unprovoked mood swings, inability to think clearly, dizziness, nausea, body aches, arthritis or abdominal pain. All of these defy any modern doctor untrained in environmental medicine to find a cause and cure.

The classic patient has been to over a dozen doctors, has had every test imaginable and has often been advised as a last resort to see a psychiatrist. So, embarrassment eventually forces this epidemic further into silence.

One dentist became sensitized to a formaldehyde sterilizing solution at work. Over the course of a year, he became progressively more depressed, achey, dizzy, nauseated (with chest pain) and unable to concentrate. A temporary solution was to have him move into his garage with a cotton cot, the doors wide open (in spite of our New York state winters) and only enter the house for use of the bathroom. At work the office was ventilated and as many plastics and chemicals were removed as possible, and he wore a ceramic mask which delivers oxygen to him as he operates on his patients. Sound preposterous? You bet! However, he, I and thousands of others are ecstatic with our progress because we now have control over our unwarranted fatigue and brain fog and depression and other symptoms that baffled so many doctors.

We are the first generation of people exposed to the high levels of chemicals that our industrial society has produced. All the rules of medicine are different. We can no longer approach our health in terms of irradiation (diagnostic x-rays) and drugs (prescribed medications).

Indeed, we look to the environmental (external and

internal) for causes; we attempt to remove as many triggers as necessary to reduce our symptoms and restore the integrity of our damaged immune systems. We should avoid chemically contaminated food, homes, offices, water, bedding, clothes and cosmetics. We should also make sure we get the proper vitamins, minerals, essential fatty acids and amino acids in order that our detoxification systems can function optimally. Just as each of us has a unique set of symptoms and triggers, each has unique biochemical needs.

As if this disease is not lonely enough, it exhibits a phenomenon that makes it tenfold worse - the spreading phenomenon. As the individual continues to be exposed to modern chemicals, his sensitivities spread to chemicals and foods that never bothered him before. He may all of a sudden begin having symptoms when exposed to the chlorine in drinking water; additives in foods; formaldehyde in bedding and clothes; pesticides in foods, mattresses, buildings, shampoos and perfumes; industrial effluents in air and water or traffic exhaust. Everywhere the person turns he is bombarded by chemicals which provoke symptoms in him while everyone else appears to be unaffected. The biochemical mechanisms for this are in Tired or Toxic?

Studies have shown that when radioactively labeled formaldehyde is inhaled, the concentration of formaldehyde in the brain is over five times greater than it is in other tissues of the body. With the brain as the most vulnerable target organ, it's easy to see why the plethora of cerebral symptoms occurs.

Other studies have shown it is metabolized mainly to formate, which is an anion that inhibits the major enzyme systems such as cytochrome C oxidase. Again, the brain is particularly vulnerable.

Formaldehyde vapors also increase cerebral glutathione, an antioxidant, and later it increases the acid proteinosis. Both these pathways reflect increased lipid peroxidation. This means that antioxidants, such as vitamins A, C, E, glutathione and more are needed in increased amounts.

Mary had depression, exhaustion, dizziness, headache and at times felt removed from her body as though she were a viewer of herself. She was triggered two years after she moved into her dream house - brand new with all the trimmings.

Dan, a state trooper, saw thirty-eight doctors in four years for his depression and other symptoms. By the time we saw him, he had sensitivities to not only formaldehyde from the home and car exhaust, but also to many foods and molds. Testing him to an amount of chlorine lower than that found in municipal water systems caused severe muscle spasms that only morphine would terminate.

We have created a monster and don't even know it. We've tightened buildings to conserve energy and simultaneously filled them with 20th century products which outgas formaldehyde, toluene, xylene, benzene, tetrachloroethanes, vinyl chlorides and much more. Now, some people are reacting with depression and usually a half-dozen other symptoms. Common ones are exhaustion, dizziness, recurrent infection, headache, sinusitis, decrease in concentration and recent memory, nausea, muscle spasms, asthma or colitis. Just about any symptom imaginable has occurred, including angina, hypertension, cardiac arrhythmias, prostatitis, cancers, arthritis, pancreatitis, diabetes, thyroiditis, and more.

One vitamin stands out as essential in defending against environmental chemicals and that is vitamin E. For starters, among the anti-oxidants, it is the most powerful. In other words, it has the strongest ability to protect against the damage of chemicals in the cell membrane. In fact, it is part of the lipid sandwich of all membranes, so it can grab on to chemicals as they attempt to enter the cell. It also acts as an immune stimulant and helps modulate inflammation once it has been triggered. Most importantly, vitamin E helps detoxify in ways that are not even yet understood.

For example, two groups of rats can be fed a noxious chemical like carbon tetrachloride. Over ninety percent would normally die. However, if one group is pretreated with a dose of vitamin E, there is a hundred percent survival. Other vitamins which help detoxify are vitamin C and vitamin A. Accessory antioxidant related minerals like selenium and magnesium are equally crucial to an immune system being weakened by 20th century chemicals. Each person is so highly unique biochemically that he would need testing before a program could be elaborated for him.

What can you do if you suspect you have depression, unwarranted mood swings, decreased memory and inability to concentrate that are environmentally induced? First, remove yourself from the suspected triggers. In other words, if you have gone downhill since having new carpeting, new mattress, new furniture or renovations, than get away. Camp outdoors if you need to.

Second, suspect the spreading phenomenon. Once symptoms become triggered by chemicals, often the sensitivities spread to other unrelated substances. Discontinue your normal foods of milk, wheat, sugar, corn, eggs, chocolate, coffee and processed foods. Eat a two-week trial of foods rarely eaten such as broccoli, squash, turkey, sole, almonds, avocados, tahini and rice cakes. Just substitute foods that you normally do not eat every week so that you are on a diet of foods that are unlikely to be the cause of your brain symptoms. Be sure you omit mold antigen containing foods like bread, cheese, alcohol, vinegar, ketchup, mayonnaise, mustard, coffee, tea and chocolate.

Third, observe if your mental symptoms clear with cleaner air and foods. If your depression comes and goes for seemingly no reason and you really don't want a divorce or job change, you should think of investigating the possibility that your depression or cerebral/chemical hypersensitivity

441

may be of environmental origin. Sometimes you can prove this to yourself by going to a new shopping mall or a newly built office or home. These usually have high levels of formaldehyde and other chemicals. Does it trigger depression, achey joints or unwarranted exhaustion? If it does, then you may have chemical hypersensitivities.

If you still are in doubt, you should locate a nutritionally and environmentally trained physician. Then you will be equipped to determine if you are allergic to the twentieth century.

HIGHLIGHTS

*The American diet, as it comes from the grocery store and restaurants, is not adequate in providing chemically less-contaminated foods nor a full complement of nutrients. This becomes more evident when the body is malfunctioning because of disease. We found the reason many people could never get better was because their nutritional deficiencies hadn't been found and corrected.

*The major factors causing depletion of essential nutrients from foods are the repeated commercial growing on depleted soils and the destruction and alteration of nutrients through the processing of foods.

*Factors contributing to chemical contamination of foods are: contaminated ground water supplies, fertilizers, pesticides, herbicides and fungicides used in growing, storage and transport and chemical additives, dyes, stabilizers, flavorings, etc. used in processing and packaging. Studies show organic foods (produced without chemicals) have 2 1/2 times the nutrients as regular grocery foods.

*Don't fall into the simplistic mentality trap that I and many others were in. If we draw an iron level, for example, and found it low, we thought we were doing the patient a big favor by prescribing iron. What we were not taught is very logical. It is extremely difficult to develop a singular deficiency. If you are low in one thing, you are low in many things and we just haven't found them yet. So, correction becomes much trickier. Because if you treat only one when several are low, the others will go lower and the person becomes sicker. For example is you give iron but the person is also low in copper (as are 80% of our patients), the iron drives the copper deficiency even lower. Hence the copper deficiency symptoms get worse and the doctor is stumped.

*Internal factors can further promote deficiencies: the loss of important conversion enzymes, such as D6D (from aging) so that oils cannot be converted to membrane lipids; the loss of gastric intrinsic factor so B12 is no longer absorbed; Candida and food hypersensitivities inflame the bowel and inhibit proper nutrient absorption; and the loss of digestive enzymes, such as lactase, so milk sugars cannot be absorbed. Chronic symptoms cause further deficiencies: loss of digestive bacteria such as Lactobacillus from antibiotics, prednisone, high sugar diets or inability to convert B6 to pyridoxal-5-phosphate (either because of gastric reasons, magnesium or manganese deficiencies or other acquired reasons).

*The bottom line is that nutrition is key to health. We are the first generation exposed to all these chemicals. They must be detoxified or they cause disease. But the work of detoxifying them depletes or uses up nutrients. For example, if you walk into a grocery or office that has been pesticided, for every molecule of pesticide you detoxify, you throw away forever a molecule of glutathione, magnesium, ATP (energy) and much more. But in reality we are detoxifying many chemicals from our air, food, and water at all times.

If this were not enough, we are the first generation to

eat all these processed foods with many nutrients removed. So we are seeing and will continue to see an increase in all sorts of illnesses, because medicine ignores all this chemistry and merely covers up a symptom with a drug, never to fix what is broken.

So we have a double reason for people to have poorer nutrient levels:

(1) the depletion through processed foods

(2) the depletion through overwork of the detox pathways. So no wonder more people are less able to detox the ever increasing numbers of chemicals and are developing the muriad manifestations of chemical sensitivity.

And as you read the subsequent books, you'll learn there are many other reasons why the sick get sicker, and quicker. For example the leaky gut syndrome (in **Wellness Against All Odds**), caused by everyday prescription and over the counter medicines, Candida, food allergies, and intestinal dysbiosis can also lead to poorer nutrient absorption. Education is the only way to health.

Much more information about nutrition and vitamins, minerals, amino acids and fatty acids is in the other books, as new information is constantly surfacing. Suffice it to say, it is more meaningful to your health how much you read and who you have chosen to prepare your food, than it is who you have chosen to be your doctor.

SECTION VII
TOTAL LOAD

THE TOTAL LOAD BOAT

The concept of total load is crucial to the healing of the detoxification and immune system that all people with environmentally-induced illness (E.I.) strive for. Not only was it the cause of our downfalls, but it is basic to our wellness. It also is important for non-ecology oriented physicians to appreciate the total load because the complexity of our treatments frequently mystify them.

I like to think of the total load as being analogous to a boat filled with twelve marked boxes. The victims of E.I. are set adrift in the sea, all in the same type of boats with the same twelve marked boxes. The only difference is the location of the leak. Some of us have a leak up near the gunwale so that we only have to throw one or two heavy boxes overboard in order for the boat to stop taking in water. Others have their leak further down toward the keel and have to throw many boxes overboard before they stop taking in water. Only the very worst people have their leak located along the keel. Even if they throw overboard all twelve boxes and get rid of their entire total load, they still will continue to take in water and proceed to sink unless they are taken to dry dock for a repair job. This dry dock is analogous to the environmental unit.

What's in the twelve mysterious boxes? You guessed it. The total environmental overload.

In the **first box** are the **inhalants**: pollens, dust, dust mites, molds, animal danders and the like. Once this box is thrown overboard, it no longer contributes to the overload. Once a person does the environmental controls and receives immunotherapy (allergy injections) for the inhalant hypersensitivities that they have, this no longer contributes to his symptom overload. Now symptoms caused by inhalant hypersensitivity are controlled. For some people the inhalant box is the heaviest box on board. So once this box is taken care of, all their symptoms are clear.

The **second box** contains **food allergies**. Doug was a 39- year-old man who had seen several psychiatrists for depression over a period of twenty years. He had been on many anti-depressant medications. Within two weeks of food injections and the rotation diet, he was able to discard his Prozac. He was not only very happy but also thinking clearly for the first time in years. Food was one of his major heavy boxes that he had been carrying around in his boat causing him to sink. Some just need to do the diagnostic diet or rare food diet to identify a few culprits to avoid. Others need to rotate and still others need all this plus food injections. For most, hidden food allergy is something they never dreamed they had. But because this box is so heavy until it is dealt with, they will never be 100% well.

The **third box** is **chemical hypersensitivity**. Tamara had one year of severe rheumatoid arthritis with elevated rheumatoid factors and sed rates. When we tested her to phenol, we totally neutralized her out of pain and stiffness. This event was filmed double-blind to teach other physicians. It also served to prove to her that chemical hypersensitivity was at the root of her symptoms and led us to know what chemicals she then had to remove from her home in order to attain a symptom-free state.

This is usually the heaviest box; it accounts for more diseases and is the hardest to throw overboard. Look at the person who finally gets his dream house with new carpet and furniture, then a year or two later he comes down with E.I. Think how unbelievable this seems to the person who has lived in a gas heated house all his life and now has severe E.I. - natural gas being one of the culprits. These are difficult and expensive changes to make and do not come any easier to people who have definite proof than to those who are yet too chemically overloaded in their daily existence to react to chemical tests in the office.

The **fourth box** contains the **newer molds** that have been the result of our research published in the **Annals of Allergy** (July, 1982; January, 1983; and May, 1984). Bob was the chairman of the theology department and he had two years of extreme depression, tiredness and weakness. An evaluation at the medical center, complete with lumbar puncture and CAT scans, could not elicit a cause. Within two weeks of injections to the newer molds, his symptoms were totally cleared. Whenever he is late, they recur; within ten minutes after he has had his injection, they disappear again. Also in this box are the rest of the inhalant mixes that deserve special consideration. For example, if someone is on twice a week injections and still having trouble with grass or tree pollen, we can test and give all the trees and grasses or molds individually rather than as mixes. The mix will be one particular dose, but the individual components often have a large spread in their neutralizing doses. This gives finer tuning that is necessary for some highly sensitive people.

The **fifth box** is labeled **phenol-free**. Some people never stop sinking until they are on phenol-free injections. They react to this preservative that also abounds in all homes and offices. They're just plain too chemically overloaded and sensitized to be able to improve without phenol-free injections. Les was a 27-year-old television engineer from New York City. He prefaced his visit with the fact that all allergists' injections made him worse. I assured him ours wouldn't because we use the individualized end-point serial dilution testing method. When we created a severe asthma reaction, I knew instantly why we all had made him worse. Sure enough, testing to phenol dropped his pulmonary function and giving him phenol-free inhalants left him symptom-free and medication-free for the first time ever. Glycerine-free extracts are also essential for the ultra chemically sensitive individual.

The **sixth box** contains **Candida**. Daniel was a 42-year- old attorney from New York City. He had extreme lethargy, depression, weakness and headaches for two years after a surgical procedure had been performed and antibiotics had been prescribed. Treatment of his Candidiasis improved his well-being markedly. Jennifer was told by pulmonary specialists there was nothing more that could be done for her steroid-dependent asthma. With Nystatin and a ferment-free diet, she was off all medicine and had no asthma.

The **seventh box** is labeled **nutrition**. Sue had eczema for thirteen years. She saw several dermatologists and allergists, but she received no help. We drew her serum vitamin A level, rationalizing that her accelerated turnover of skin must indeed deplete her vitamin A faster than a normal persons. Indeed, it was very low. With one month of dust and mold injections and vitamin A supplementation, her eczema was totally cleared for the first time in thirteen years. Vitamins, minerals, digestive enzymes (which promote the absorption of vitamins and minerals), essential fatty acids and sometimes specific amino acids are often crucial factors in attaining complete health. Jim had psoriasis for fifteen years. He was totally cleared with the correct essential fatty acid supplement that cost $4 from a health food store.

The **eighth box** is **hormone hypersensitivity**. Karen had severe PMS. She was psychotic and extremely depressed for four days before her periods. Progesterone neutralization brought her out of this within three minutes and she used it every four hours for those four days to remain asymptomatic. Estrone, luteinizing hormone, DHEA, and testosterone have also been very crucial.

The **ninth box** is labeled **toxic**. It signifies people who are overloaded with heavy metal poisoning such as cadmium from auto exhaust or with pesticides that have accumulated and been stored for years. Levels of pesticides

448

can now be drawn in the blood and heavy metal toxicity can often be found with hair analysis. We're amazed at the levels and types of pesticides that all people carry as part of their total body burden now that we have the ability to measure them.

Angela was incapacitated by insect sprays at work in the bakery. With blood tests we were able to monitor how vitamins lowered her levels of these toxins. Her symptoms melted away concomitantly.

Technology now allows us to measure blood levels of many chemicals commonly found in businesses and homes - xylene and toluene from plastics, appliance wiring, furniture glues, trichloroethylene from dry cleaning fluids, solvents, etc. Some people are never better until their mercury amalgams are all replaced. Remember, all medicines are chemicals which put an added stress on the already overloaded immune system.

Maggie had every x-ray and scoping available for abdominal cramps and nausea. The gastroenterologist sent me a letter advising that her illness was probably imaginary because she also had headaches, inability to concentrate and numbness on only one-half of her body. When I found out that she was the attendant in a parking garage, I obtained her serum level of carbon monoxide. It was six times higher after a day at work than after a day at home. After I wrote a letter to her manager that she was being poisoned, they ventilated her booth and all the symptoms left.

The **tenth box** contains **stress**. Many people never had E.I. until after the death of a spouse, a divorce or an extremely stressful time. We know the immune system is extremely vulnerable to stress. We have seen that men whose wives were dying of breast cancer had very low T-suppressor cells in their blood streams during the last months of their wives' lives. These cells are crucial in restricting the amount of harmful antigens that are produced and a lack of them make these men ripe for cancer, infection, accelerated aging and allergies.

We also know that the chances of success for a patient are extremely reduced if he does not have a spouse who has read and understood all of the literature and is willing to add physical, financial and emotional support to the E.I. victim. This disease is very difficult. Doing it alone is tough, but trying to cope with a spouse who has never been sick and who thinks all allergy is in the head is like knocking your head on a brick wall. And some people will never heal until they get rid of anger.

The **eleventh box** is labeled **miscellaneous**. Here we see the **new things** that **constantly emerge**, like the leaky gut syndrome that can be the reason that food and chemical sensitivities never go away. In this box we also find the various mediators, such as histamine, serotonin, heparin, GABA, Dopa, acetylcholine, etc. and even viral vaccines that neutralize some symptoms. Ron had brain fog and lethargy which are gone in minutes with a neutralizing dose of serotonin. It is the category into which also goes good basic medicine. DHEA (unconjugated!) deficiency, the flat glucose tolerance curve, the lazy adrenal syndrome, or thyroiditis are standard medical problems that are often ignored in workups you should have had prior to coming. It's exciting! I have never seen another field of medicine grow so steadily.

The last box is called the **mystery box**. The **twelfth box** was a mystery to me for a long time because I thought there was something extremely important in there and indeed there is. It is not nearly as elusive as we all would like to think. We have all been looking for a long time for some magic final ingredient that will turn around our disease and make us totally well and not dependent upon strict environmental and dietary controls. I have finally figured out what the mystery box contains. It is **patient compliance**.

Whenever I see someone who is not improving as I would expect, it is usually because he still has some tremendously potent overload that continues to sink his boat. Maybe he still has a gas heated house; maybe he does not have a safe oasis to escape to; maybe he is cheating on his diet by not properly rotating (I find that this person frequently needs to fast to reduce his overload, he needs tri-salts, ascorbate, frequent oxygen and neutralizing doses to keep things under control). And constant growth in knowledge through reading is at the base of it all. The most successful people who have accomplished the impossible have coincidentally devoured all that we could provide.

Hopefully, by periodically reminding ourselves of the total load and the contents of each box, we will be able to attain a constant upward progress toward total wellness.

This is probably the most crucial checklist to memo rize and to implement, for the "dirty dozen" culprits of the total load are what got us sick to begin with.

ROGER'S RULES OF E.I.
(Environmentally-Induced Illness)

Progress in clinical ecology will continue to be impeded until we can clearly explain to the community how current concepts of medical practice are no longer applicable. At the same time we need to be able to clearly demonstrate, by patient examples, the new ground rules.

The following are the most dangerous current medical concepts or myths:

1) "Most diseases have simple, single causes such as a virus." On the contrary, an ecology patient may find a certain chemical, several food sensitivities, a mineral deficiency, and an inhalant overload all contribute to making his arthritis worse.

2) Diseases can be treated by specialists who concentrate on one organ system at a time." What happens

to the person who has formaldehyde induced headaches, dizziness, nausea, muscle weakness, inability to concentrate and arrhythmia? He can go to his family doctor, internist, ENT specialists, gastroenterologist, neurologist, psychiatrist and cardiologist. Not one of them will diagnose the cause of his symptoms.

3) "In order to be mass applicable, medicine must be practiced in a cookbook fashion with standard doses for all." Ecologic illness strikes in mysterious ways and no two patients are alike. Medicine is clinging to the notion that we are all alike. However, there is increasing evidence that there is tremendous biochemical individuality. As a result, the testing and treatments must be highly individualized and "minor" symptoms paid attention to.

The major concepts of ecology will best be understood by actual case examples.

1) Individuality: In a group of patients with arthritis, each will have his own individual trigger. Likewise, a particular antigen can produce one symptom in one individual and a totally different symptom in another. Remember when the EPA put carpet in their mall office? Out of 2,000 workers, 126 got E.I., but no two people had the exact same symptoms.

2) Individual susceptibility: Many people may be exposed but only those susceptible will develop sensitivity (and each may be uniquely different in target organ and severity). We have learned from people in foam-insulated homes that one family member can have headaches and dizziness; another can have an inability to concentrate, rhinitis and asthma; another can have a rash for only a few weeks and others will appear totally unaffected.

3) Any material that omits ozmols into the air can cause a hypersensitivity. If they are breathed, they are in the bloodstream whether perceived or not by olfactory senses. This is how odorless carbon monoxide kills.

4) The spreading phenomenon can start once a

452

person becomes sensitized; thus, he develops sensitivity to many other compounds. By the time we see some people, they have multiple sensitivities to foods, other chemicals, molds and Candida. In addition, they have a multitude of vitamin deficiencies. It is as though the whole system has broken down.

5) Resetting of the thermostat: Once sensitized, any re-exposure will cause quicker and more frequent violent reactions. Also, he may not require as large an exposure to accomplish this. One nurse, who had nowhere else to go, lived in a trailer for two years in spite of her symptoms. Now she becomes semi-comatose in less than two hours while in our office. (Biochemical mechanisms and scientific references in **Tired or Toxic?**).

6) It must be recognized that the brain is the most commonly affected target organ and that cerebral symptoms do not connote hypochondriasis. Most patients don't dare tell even their spouses and closest friends, much less their consulting physicians, the cerebral symptoms that they experience. They know they would be thought of as looney because conventional, non-ecologic medicine lacks the tools (blood tests or x-ray) to substantiate these symptoms.

7) The immune system is damaged but given a reduced chemical load, the immune system does heal. This is evidenced by the thousands of victims who return to society after being abandoned as hopeless by conventional medicine. However, many are on a delicate lifeline and they must maintain a vigilance against environmental overload to keep symptoms from recurring.

8) This damaged immune system is inseparably entwined with the endocrine and neurologic systems. This damaged immune system can and does heal given the reduced chemical load it requires, but it cannot do so if there is hormonal imbalance or too much psychological stress. Frequently, a hypersensitivity to one's own fluctuating

hormone levels produces symptoms that can be neutralized.

9)   The environment is not constant; it is ever changing and this necessitates an adaptation to it.   A goldfish raised in chlorinated tap water dies. He cannot adapt to that environment. Likewise, some men who are put in boxes called buildings begin sustaining damage to their immune systems by chemicals outgassing from the thousands of untested twentieth century products in these buildings. Some survive longer than others before symptoms appear. (Remember the T.V. documentary where all the mice put in a jar with a new piece of carpet were dead in the morning?)

10) The patient's sensitivities are also changing and his reaction at any particular time is dependent upon the total load.   Thus, symptoms are not totally reproducible because the exact same set of circumstances rarely exists twice.

11)   Some food sensitivities are in a stage called masked. In this stage, the food that causes symptoms is not suspected because it actually makes the person feel better temporarily.   In fact, he craves this food much like a drug addict craves his heroin or an alcoholic craves his alcohol (another actual food allergy-addiction disease). When he starts feeling bad, he has more of the addictive substance. It "picks him up." When the action of the substance wears off, symptoms reappear. This is the phenomenon of masking. It is only when the addiction cycle is broken with abstinence for a week that the food is unmasked. Then, ingestion of it can cause the symptoms. The first cigarette makes one sick. After years of smoking, the victim feels edgy if he doesn't have a cigarette. He's addicted.

Tim had such severe headaches for five years that he was suicidal. They only occurred on Saturdays. Although he had lived in three different houses, they always occurred on Saturday mornings.   The cause was coffee.   He had several cups all day at work but never drank it at home. Since he left work early on Friday and did not have any more coffee, he then had withdrawal headaches on Saturday morning.

12) A patient will not improve until the total load has been addressed. This includes inhalants (with emphasis on molds), foods, chemicals, Candida, nutritional deficiencies, phenol-free extracts, reducing the toxic body overload of pesticides, heavy metals and volatile organic hydrocarbons, endocrine imbalance and a psychological support system. I can flare my eczema by missing my inhalant or food injections, going off the rotation diet for several days, eating certain foods, riding on a tractor in a moldy corn field, working in a barn for several hours, being in a chemically contaminated office, etc. For most victims of E.I., chemicals are the hardest to control; foods are a close second. And the biochemical defects in terms of nutrient deficiencies are crucial if the body is ever going to detox chemicals normally again.

More importantly, people can and do get better as they learn to do whatever is necessary to allow the immune and detoxification systems to heal. I don't recall seeing anyone recover fully who did not have understanding and loving people around him. I believe, beyond all doubt, that our H.E.A.L. support groups and a loving and involved spouse or friend are crucial to a healthy, recovering immune system.

HORMONES

Frequently, people come to the office with a history of bouts of manic or "hyper" periods, interspersed with chronic fatigue. They have had thyroid function tests which are all normal, but they rarely have had thyroid autoantibodies tested. They have periodic hyper and hypothyroidism triggered by the thyroid gland become one of the allergic target organs. They actually make varying amounts of undesirable antibody against the thyroid. When I and others are chemically overloaded, we have elevated anti- thyroid antibody titers, which return to normal as we reduce our loads. By controlling the total load, some victims of thyroiditis have become normal and stopped producing autoantibodies.

Many who are especially fatigued need special thyroid supplementation even though the thyroid tests are normal. Others hasve deficiencies of DHEA contributing to chronic symptoms. Others have a lazy adrenal gland and need the cortrosyn stimulation test. Much more can be found on these in **Tired or Toxic?, Wellness Against All Odds, The Scientific Basis for Selected Environmental Medicine Techniques** and subsequent books.

Another potentially autoimmune hormone disorder is PMS. Many women have terrible PMS symptoms. Symptoms can last anywhere from a couple of days to two weeks before the period. The worst are characterized by total personality change, lack of self-esteem, crying and depression for no reason, flying off the handle over nothing, intense negativity, worsening of allergies and more. Some of these women are "allergic" to or hyperreactive toward their own hormones. The most common culprits are progesterone, estrone, testosterone and luteinizing hormone.

For example, we have videos of how one miniscule dose, 0.004 mg of progesterone, duplicates the PMS symptoms within minutes. A five-fold weaker dose turns it off within minutes. We then teach the victim to give this by injection or sublingually as needed to keep the reaction controlled. She gets far more relief than most do from dangerously higher levels of hormones (400 -800 mgs of Progesterone) prescribed by the gynecologist.

Most have concomitant nutritional deficiencies, multiple hidden allergies and Candida hypersensitivity. As these are addressed, the PMS symptoms simmer down.

Many don't even need to test hormones if they take Pro-fem II three times a day with meals, 400 IU vitamin E daily and treat their allergies. An excellent book on much you can do for yourself outside of neutralizing doses is, **The PMS Solution**, by Nazzaro and Lombard. In fact, Dr. Lombard is a psychiatrist who has training in E.I., so you know he appreciates that PMS is not "all in the mind."

As a rule, gynecologists treat PMS with macro doses of hormones; for example, 200 mg or 400 mg of progesterone by suppository or injection. No one knows the long term effects of these large doses. This method is not usually effective for the PMS victim who also has allergies and it is, of course, not nearly as safe and harmless as the miniscule doses we use to neutralize. When you explain the neutralizing doses to these doctors, they are confused and don't understand how it works because we're using a dose that is often 1/1,000th of a milligram of a hormone.

The normal female hormonal cycle starts producing progesterone at midcycle in a small amount. It increases gradually and reaches its maximum premenstrually. Some women are only sensitive (experience symptoms) to the high dose end; hence the need for neutralizing a few days before the period. Others exhibit just as strong "underdose" symptoms. In other words, just as too low a dose of thyroid produces symptoms, too low a dose of progesterone produces symptoms at midcycle. They have a peak of symptoms midcycle and premenstrually. Sometimes progesterone or luteinizing hormone neutralize this midcycle symptomatology. Progesterone, estrone and testosterone have neutralized symptoms anywhere along the cycle in various women.

That is why we usually ask you to come in when you are having your symptoms and we check all four hormones to find the one that lessens your symptoms right then and there. Then, the proof of the pudding comes when it reliably works every cycle. As you may be aware, in some women the cycle is not the same and some months there is no PMS; so, just don't use your treatment until it's needed.

In summary, if you have bad PMS, first get your dust, mold, Candida and food sensitivities better. Use one 400 I.U. of d-alpha tocopherol a day and Pro Fem II three times a day with meals. See the doctor for levels to find nutrient deficiencies and an individualized nutritional program. Be especially certain you have the magnesium loading test (in **Tired or Toxic?**). If after 2-4 months you are not totally clear, schedule hormone testing when you will be having your symptoms. Pay close attention to your body as you test. We are looking for the hormone and dose that makes you feel good again. We usually test progesterone, estrone, luteinizing hormone and testosterone first. The last two are tested in men, also. If this doesn't help, it often pays to look at thyroid, serotonin, histamine and some other neurotransmitters or mediators. For many women, it's crucial to get the yeast (Candida) problem licked first. See the doctor if you have problems. Many think they have Candida, but when we test, it is really another organism in the gut like Klebsiella or Citrobacter.

Once you find the mediator or hormone and its dose, schedule for the nurse to show you how to give it and order a ten dose vial. At the first sign of trouble, give yourself an injection. Some of us need one every 2-4 hours during the bad days and once a day during others. As your total load is addressed, you will need less and less; eventually, none at all. We rarely see anyone needing it over a year. Usually, you will not need it every month, but only every other month.

Once you have established that it works for you, you can give it sublingually. Simply squirt the whole dose under your tongue and don't swallow or drink or eat for five minutes. It works by this route for about 80% of the victims.

Lest you think this is a panacea, let me remind you

that you and I are the experimental generation from whom we are constantly learning.

Provocation-Neutralization Patient Spectrum

1)   Some rare people are actually worse with any injections. Many probably react to the preservative in the extracts. Sometimes the total environmental load is so high that we can only get them settled down by a trip to the unit.

2)   Some don't get better. I suspect they have sensitivities we cannot measure and have no idea of their existence. For example, one gal gets a tight chest, stuffy nose and mental confusion after two hours at her office. Outdoors, she is fine. The formaldehyde level was less than 0.02 ppm (low) and the mold growth is ordinary and a desk electrostatic precipitator doesn't help. What is it that we can't measure - plastics outgassing, sulfur dioxide, carbon monoxide, positive ion overload, electro-magnetic fields, xenobiotics?

3) Some are improved but can never go off injections (I erroneously thought I was one of these).

4) Some are improved and are still good after they stop injections. Is it that they made enough blocking antibody, they have less stress in their lives or did so well with environmental changes that they no longer have T-cell suppression of IgE induction? Or is it something we are totally unaware of?

5) Some are even better without treatment. Did they unknowingly lower their load somehow?

The fact is there are enough people (the vast majority) who have benefitted to make it necessary that we let these techniques be known. Hopefully, in getting smarter we can learn how to help those that we have been unable to help thus far. I certainly am grateful to them all. They have helped us learn a great deal. Provocation-neutralization is the technique by which all of these hormones, neurotransmitters, chemicals and foods are tested.

I must warn there are no medical schools in the country that offer a course in provocation-neutralization that has adequate personalized instruction. It cannot be learned in a classroom, but is a hands-on technique. It would be like trying to teach a surgeon to operate in a classroom and never giving him years of operating room experience. I must emphasize that you ought to be sure that the person you are considering going to has learned the technique in some office that is known to be proficient in it, such as Dr. J.B. Miller's, Dr. Rea's, Dr. Randolph's, Dr. Rapp's, etc. I worked will all of them and owe each one a tremendous debt of gratitude. Also we teach in annual courses through the AAEM and have a certifying exam. You want a physician board certified by the International or American Academy of Environmental Medicine.

In some cases when people are exquisitely sensitive to inhalants and have multiple chemical problems, all of their antigens including the inhalants have to be tested one by one by the provocation-neutralization technique.

For example, Dr. Rapp was testing a young boy to mold when I was visiting her office. Suddenly, he began viciously biting and hitting his mother. He was much too old and big to be carrying on like this. He looked as though he was 8 or 9 years old. When they put on the next neutralizing dose, he simmered right down and was his sweet docile self. The mother exclaimed that this was the way that he often behaved and for no reason at all. It makes me wonder what would have happened to this young man had his parents not been intelligent enough to take him to Dr. Rapp's office for testing. Surely he would have become a young sociopath and been in and out of juvenile institutions until he was old enough for jail.

The most difficult task of any ecologist is getting her patient to appreciate the total antigenic load and to realize

460

that the more severe of us will not improve without strict comprehensive environmental controls.

For example, Kevin's presenting dermatitis was one of the worst any physician will ever see. His entire body was white crusted scales, overlying an oozing eczematous dermatitis from cheeks to ankles. He had seen many doctors in the preceding ten years, including a recent evaluation at the Massachusetts General Hospital. He too, like others and myself, had a change in allergic target organ from asthma of the lungs to eczema or atopic dermatitis of the legs. His IgE was astronomically high at 33,088 (normal 14). He was so disfigured by the total body scales and so socially ostracized that he lived alone and laminated winter skis for a living.

Within two weeks he was markedly clearing and in four weeks he was totally cleared. He's a good example of how important the total load is. He has to have injections to the inhalants he reacted to, the foods, rotate his diet, totally avoid certain ones and lower his chemical load. Without all five parameters covered, he cannot remain clear and starts to flare again. When I sneaked and replaced his mold injections with water, the eczema returned. I did this to be sure he still needed them. If I just ask him to stop them and find out if his symptoms return, many doctors would say he became worse just out of worry! So, we do it more scientifically, or double-blind. Neither the nurses nor he knew of the change. The happy part is that 10 years later now, he is well, only has an injection every month (12 a year) and no longer has to be strict on the diet. He tolerates normal environments and has gone to school and become a computer whiz.

I don't mention the same cases over and over for lack of cases, but to drive home a point. For lack of appreciating the principles of environmental medicine can cause many a patient and allergist to fail and then acclaim these principles as useless: the total antigenic load must be covered.

This entails a very comprehensive allergy or, more accurately, environmental program. For us universal reactors of the allergy world, it is easier for most of us to tell people what we are not allergic to than enumerate what we are sensitive to.

Chemicals and hormones are tested like foods with the provocation-neutralization method, one needle every ten minutes, watching skin reactions and patient symptoms. Jenny had bouts of uncontrollable movements and was thought to be schizophrenic. Testing with chlorine (common sources are drinking water and in cleaning chemicals), knotted her whole body in such cramps she nearly fell out of the chair. The cramps started in her neck, like torticollis, and progressed to the rest of her body. A neutralizing dose restored her to normal. During the reaction, our attempts to open her cramped hands amazed us with cracking sounds.

We also know that various of the body's hormones and hormone receptors are target organs for allergic reactions and we can find neutralizing doses for these as well. One fellow had seen several endocrinologists and internists for a vague feeling that he was always going to be passing out. He just felt extremely dizzy and "removed" and so lethargic and tired. He also had sensations of chilling. Whenever he would get chilled then he knew that his symptoms were going to be worse. He had numerous endocrine studies including several glucose tolerance tests. Having exhausted the medical center's endocrinologists, he then visited some private endocrinologists, then eventually came to our office.

He had concomitant sinusitis and headaches and we worked him up and found that he was sensitive to numerous inhalants as well as foods. After explaining environmental controls, the diet and receiving injections, he was improved but still was not as good as he would like to be. Histamine is a chemical that is released by the body during allergic reactions; hence the reason we take antihistamines in attempt to control them. When we tested Stan to histamine, he sat up within a few minutes and said, "Whatever that was, I feel wonderful, I feel normal again." In fact, he gives himself histamine injections every few days as his body's needs dictate. No one understands precisely how this works. All we know is that it very definitely does work because we can replace them with placebo or water and these patients call us up and tell us that the injections are suddenly not working. Don't worry - we no longer do these placebo studies.

Some people have a particular problem with chilling. Whenever they get chilled, their other allergic symptoms are worse whether it's headache, body ache, tiredness, etc. These people are particularly helped by histamine. When it is injected underneath the skin, we can usually duplicate the symptom that the person has with chilling and then neutralize it when we put on the next dose that is found to be negative.

Serotonin, likewise, is a chemical that is released during allergic reactions. Only this tends to be more responsible for headaches and depression. Sometimes it is related to symptoms that occur with weather change.

Various hormones such as estrone, progesterone and luteinizing hormone produce a variety of symptoms in people who become sensitive to their own hormones. Many women had the onset of their multiple symptomatologies after a pregnancy or hysterectomy and have an exacerbation premenstrually. Science can concede that people can have auto immune disorders and be allergic to their own thyroid, but seems baffled that they can be sensitive to extra levels of progesterone, for example premenstrually, that cause headache, depression, lethargy, irritability, swelling, breast tenderness and cramps. Yet, it is so logical and indeed many of these people are able to obtain benefit from neutralizing doses to the particular hormone that is giving

463

them problems during this period.

Likewise, men have cleared cerebral symptoms with testosterone and luteinizing hormone, but many more have responded to neurotransmitters like serotonin for control of their toxic brain syndrome. The miniscule amounts of hormones and mediators that bring about dramatic results are fascinating.

Priscilla had the severest form of ecologic illness, with multiple food, inhalant and chemical reactions. She went to the Chicago unit and was vastly improved. However, with so many severe problems being addressed there, she overlooked the years of premenstrual depression that she had had. For four days before a period she was transformed. She had a cockeyed view of the world and the slightest benign comment would send her into a screaming, crying rage. She would be exhausted and sleep for hours, awakening unrested. It was difficult to conceive of this because before me was seated one of the sweetest, loveliest and most talented young ladies I had ever known.

We proceded to test her and put on a minute dose of progesterone - nothing happened. We put on the next weaker dose and she burst into a rage. It was an uninhibited, wide open-mouthed cry like a baby. We watched her, thinking it would soon abate, but instead she was becoming exhausted from it. We put on the next weaker dose and within three minutes she was her adorable, smiling self, asking politely for a tissue.

We brought her back in and tested her single blind; some of the needles were water, some were the dose to turn her on and some the dose to turn her off. We filmed it for teaching doctors about this phenomenon.

She uses her neutralizing dose sublingually every four hours for those four days premenstrually and has beautiful results. The amount of progesterone that is calculated to be in the dose that causes her symptoms is 0.1 mg (1/1,000 of a normal therapeutic medical dose) and the treatment dose is 0.01 mg. The body is truly an amazing work of art whose mysteries we have yet to fathom!

Some women have been carried in by their husbands because of symptoms, only to be able to walk out smiling once a neutralizing dose was found. These show us that we have only to let our imaginations run wild and we may be able to control many more hormone malfunctions of the body. And interestingly these doses are not needed forever. As the total load is addressed symptoms usually melt away and these special hormone and neurotransmitter doses are no longer needed.

So, there you have the food provocation-neutralization testing technique which also enables us to test chemicals, hormones and neurotransmitters. For the scientific evidence, explanations and medical journal quotes that people have used to guide them in small claims courts against inconsistant insurance companies, see **The Scientific Basis for Selected Environmental Medicine Techniques**. It is regularly updated and new evidence also is often in the subscription bimonthly newsletter, **HEALTH LETTER**.

NEGATIVE AIR IONS

We are constantly learning about other aspects of our synthetic environment. Ionization is one area that needs further study.

Awareness of ionization came about when a scientist noticed that a generator that he was working next to made him feel optimistic, happy and exuberant on the days it was turned on. On the days it was turned off he felt dull, depressed and tired. It was here that the work began that elucidated the knowledge about ionization. Some people are particularly ion sensitive. Before a storm they ache, feel lousy or have a flare-up of some old arthritis or in a closed stuffy room they feel particularly tense, edgey or irritable.

They oftentimes blame it on barometric pressure but they could prove whether this was really the culprit. An elevator ride in a tall building gives a dramatic chance in barometric pressure, but it usually does not cause an arthritis flare. Positive ions are abundant in large buildings, air conditioned buildings, places where the air is recirculated and the windows sealed, where there is an abundance of synthetic fabric, fluorescent lights, decreased windows and fresh air, many electrical machines, smoke and electrostatic precipitators. Positive ions are also heavy in traffic and even on the inside of the car. A buildup of positive ions is dangerous to one's alertness. An abundance of healthful negative ions is found in the vicinity of such places as a waterfall, fast rumbling brook, ocean, just after a storm or in a country field.

Medicine is just barely beginning to scratch the surface and realize that ionization decreases mold and bacterial growth, infection and the healing time in burn units for patients. Likewise, it increases the productivity, happiness and alertness of people working in offices. The mechanism by which it does this is that it decreases the amount of serotonin or 5-hydroxy-tryptamine in the brain.

This is also one of the neurohormones associated with allergic or hypersensitivity reactions. Negative ions decrease one's irritability, increase tranquillity and increase learning ability. There is much to learn about ionization. I, for one, would not be cooped up in an office all day without having an ionizer on my desk as a bare minimum. Then I am also one who is susceptible to large positive ion factors with changes in the brain leading to irritability, hostility and violent temper.

At first I was super-skeptical about ions. After all, ionization is an insensible factor - it is not able to be perceived by our five senses. Yet it turns out that many people with ecologic illness when presented with an imbalance of the natural electrical charge of the air, feel anxious, feel a peculiar type of draining tension, feel depressed, feel below par or sometimes feel even suicidal.

The normal level of ionization is between 1000 and 2000 per cubic centimeter. This is what it is in an open field on a clear day. Negative ions are in part responsible for why people feel great at the beach or hiking along a stream. The ratio of positive ions to negative ions should be about five to four. However, most of us spend a majority of our time indoors where there is a vast decrease in the number of negative ions and a large increase in positive ions. This is partly due to the presence of electrical equipment, wiring, polyester clothing and many other factors (synthetics).

Studies of animals show a dramatic change in behavior and in even such physiologic parameters as fertility. Once certain people are affected by a positive ion excess, they manifest an increase in their serotonin (a stress neurohormone) and consequently experience depression.

People who are especially helped by ionizers are those who are sensitive to weather changes and chilling and who have exacerbation of symptoms with either of these.

Thanks to Dr. William Rea, I have come to appreciate ionization. For years I had increasingly severe problems

467

traveling in planes. The fumes from the diesel exhaust, especially when we were on the runway sitting behind other planes waiting for takeoff, always gave me extreme headaches, burning eyes, nausea, depression and mental dullness. Usually I had saved immunology readings for these trips, but I was barely able to read the simplest magazine in front of me at a speed 1/10th my normal reading speed.

In hotels I have the same problem (but to a lesser degree) caused by the recirculated fumes from all of the outgassing and cleaning solutions. On a plane, if someone should sit next to me wearing a heavy amount of perfume, I really become wiped out for the entire duration and sometimes for several hours to days afterwards.

We found that by carrying a small ionizer with me and holding it just under my nose the entire duration, I was less affected by the chemicals. As soon as I took it a few inches away from my face, I could start smelling all of the noxious diesel exhaust and perfumes. As long as I held it very close to my nose, I was able to just smell clean air.

What happens is that the machine puts out a field of negative ions which repel the heavy positive ions that carry dust and various odors. This cloud of negative ions is very small and only surrounds the head of the person holding the ionizer. This small cloud of negative ions is enough to repel the ambient positive ones that carry noxious gases and odors.

A book, **The Ion Effect,** by Fred Sroyka, plus handheld ionizers available at **N.E.E.D.S. (1-800-634- 1380).**

EMF

Electro-magnetic force or field (EMF) is another physical entity that we must become more aware of. It is necessary but difficult to become enthused about short and long range effects of electrical fields that are not easily measured or perceived, but that range from irritability to cancer.

It is not exciting to me (even as a general class amateur "ham" radio operator (K2RRU) of over thirty five years) to study electricity. Let me simplify this so you can see why it is so important. If we have a 60 amp circuit at 120 volts and another circuit of 600 amps at 120 volts, the latter requires a heavier wire. They both have the same electric field, but the latter has a stronger EMF. Magnetic fields are proportional to the amount of current flowing in a wire.

In our society, EMF's are difficult to escape. There is definite evidence from multiple sources that EMF does accelerate the growth of malignant cells through enhancement of DNA production. No one knows what phase of the growth cycle is being stimulated nor whether pre-malignant cells are equally stimulated. The cell cycle time could be shortened or we may be recruiting more cells. However, the government so far will not call it carcinogenic but only cancer- enhancing. But voluminous data, especially from countries not dictated to by the FDA confirm it is carcinogenic.

EMF produces varying immediate effects in people such as irritability, undue fatigue and photophobia. As with other ecologic illnesses, we will probably find that we can find any symptom imaginable in someone. There are highly sensitive people who can even "hear" EMF and complain of the feel of or noise in a house until the power is shut off. They are very rare.

There is evidence of profound personality changes as well. Mary Patterson reported in **Omni** magazine of the use of acupuncture needles placed behind the ears of heroin addicts. A small current was run through these needles, creating an EMF. As a result, the patients obtained complete freedom from their heroin addictions and there were no withdrawal symptoms. After a few weeks this was stopped and a two-year follow-up revealed continued success. So, a couple of milli- amps of current at a low frequency have produced a profound and long-lasting change for which we have no explanation.

What are the places with high EMF exposure and what can be done about it?

1) Offices provide the most common heavy exposure (outside of living near a high-voltage line). The wiring usually encircles the building creating one giant EMF. No one has measured these or done studies to see what the long-term effects are. We are the experiemental generation. In the **Journal of Epidemiology,** 1978, N. Werdheimer has outlined how certain wiring configurations can produce higher EMF's. Studies in the U.S. and Sweden have shown higher leukemia rates with elevated EMF.

2) Fluorescent lights are a common source as well and we are often in close proximity to them. It is not known if these two fields have a synergistic effect. There are meters on the market for a lay person to detect and measure this (N.E.E.D.S. or the American Environmental Health Foundation of Dallas, 1-800-428-2343). There is no effective grid that shields against it, but new products keep emerging. It would have to be a very fine mesh and well grounded. Full spectrum incandescent lights or vita-lites are an alternative. Studies are needed.

3) Large video display terminals (not small desk top models) in Canada have already caused miscarriages and stillbirths. Now, by law, pregnant Canadian women have a choice of another job without loss of pay and seniority.

4) Microwave ovens also produce a higher type frequency radiation that has not been adequately studied.

5) Electric blankets and heating pads are definitely not advised.

6) Ionizers are not a source of much EMF (nor ozone); in fact, they are very inefficient ways to produce ozone.

An orthopedic surgeon, Dr. Robert Becker, has authored over 150 papers on the biological effects of EMF. He pioneered the research on accelerated healing of non-union fractures with electric currents. He also testified about the effects of high voltage power lines; and later, mysteriously had his government research grants withdrawn. The TV program, **60 Minutes**, did a superb show on him a few years ago. Fortunately, he has written a book titled, **Electromagnetism and Life**, (S.U.N.Y. Press, P.O. Box 978, Edison, NJ 08818). This book contains voluminous references. He was kind enough to discuss all of this with me. At this point he recommends that each person try to lower his EMF as much as possible through the above recommendations and try to push for funding of studies that are needed to further study the biological effects of electro-magnetic fields on human organisms. His second book, **The Body Electric**, is also recommended if you want in depth information.

The reason we are concerned is two-fold:

(1) EMF can cause serious symptoms, and

(2) It can be part of the total load that needs addressing before wellness can be achieved.

CHECKLIST FOR GETTING OUT OF A REACTION

1) Identify that you are reacting and leave the area.

2) Try to learn from the experience.

Also identify the immediate culprits of the last few days that have contributed to your vulnerability. Write this up in your notebook for future reference. Make it explicit, so if your reaction makes you depressed or confused, you can in the future diagnose the problem and follow the directions you have left yourself. Then you can get out of future problems much quicker.

3) Take neutralizing doses. Have you been delinquent in any doses of anything? Maybe your inhalants

471

should be back on twice weekly or your foods on daily.

4) Empty the gastrointestinal tract with two tablespoons of milk of magnesia. Start a fast until your reaction is totally gone or you will add to your overload.

5) Shower (it removes smoke and chemicals from your hair and body to reduce overload).

6) Take six alka-aid tablets (or one teaspoon Tri-Salts or two Alka-Seltzer in gold foil) followed by a quart of water. Have this 1/2 hour after the milk of magnesia. This may be repeated every two to four hours; maximum four to six times a week.

7) Have a heaping 1-3 teaspoons of buffered sago palm vitamin C (or pure ascorbic acid) a half hour after the alka- aid and repeat every few hours to help detoxify.

8) Begin fasting, except for safe water; alka-aid and buffered C may be repeated in a couple of hours if needed. They should be spaced one/half to one hour apart from each other for best absorption.

9) Go to an oasis. Stay there until you clear.

10) Go on oxygen with a ceramic mask.

Everyone eventually figures out what is best for himself or herself to terminate reactions quickly. Don't panic; it only adds to your stress (part of the total load).

Whatever you do, don't feel the day is a loss and use this as an excuse to pig out on your favorite food or you will be in deeper trouble. Always fast immediately if you are even just suspicious that you are going to be headed for trouble.

Above all, remember that an inadvertent exposure which causes a reaction greatly raises your total load. Therefore, you have to be super careful for several days or weeks afterwards. For example, as we were cruising down the Yangtze River in China, Dr. Rea became overloaded with the coal smoke from the riverbank towns and with diesel fumes and pesticides from the boat and who knows what else. One of the important things he did was to fast for three days until the reaction had stopped.

If you become overloaded, I would suggest you fast or at least back up to one or two extremely safe foods a day like raw carrots and raw cabbage. I would suggest a food injection daily and an inhalant injection twice a week. As you simmer down, you can resume your former intervals and diet.

CAUTION: Six alka-aid are equivalent to two Alka-seltzer in gold foil. In fact, they are better. You don't need to wait for them to fizz in a glass; you can pop tablets with water from a bottle anywhere you happen to be. Also, it avoids the citric acid which bothers some people because it is synthesized by mold fermentation. Too much salt can harm kidneys, heart and liver; so, try to use it sparingly and avoid reactions in the first place. Don't use it more than two to three times in a day nor more than two days a week or you may get into electrolyte imbalance and create a cardiac arrhythmia or kidney failure. Always follow the "salts" with a quart of tolerated water to keep flushing toxins from your system.

Some people need oxygen at home to clear out rapidly; some need portable oxygen for work or shopping. Another use for oxygen is the person who hasn't yet done enough environmental controls and can't afford a trip to the unit. Temporarily, he can go on oxygen at home for eight hours a day. He'll probably not totally clear with this temporary measure. It simply unloads the system a notch or two. It's better to make a safe, tolerable, temporary oasis in the garage, as several have done, than to resort to oxygen. Most insurance companies won't pay for it unless you have abnormally low blood gases (they think emphysema is the only reason for home oxygen).

473

PROTOCOL FOR OXYGEN USE
IN CHEMICALLY SENSITIVE PATIENTS

Acquire oxygen in tanks. The flow should be 2 - 8 liters per minute and maximum of eight hours a day. Portable tanks are available. The yellow pages provides many oxygen dealers. Find out who will give the best rates, service and understands chemically sensitive people.

Tygon tubing is necessary and can be obtained through the oxygen dealer or at a large medical supply type pharmacy. However, it is not chemically acceptable for most chemically sensitive people until the following procedure has been performed:

In a large bowl, mix 1/2 cup of baking soda for every two quarts of water. Soak the tubing for one to two weeks. Daily rinse the tubing out and fill it again with the baking soda solution. When the plastic fumes are no longer perceivable, the plastic is ready to be used. If, after three weeks the fumes still bother you, stainless steel tubing can be purchased from:

Environmental Purification Systems
P.O. Box 81
Blain, NB 68008
Phone (402) 426-9398
OR
Human Ecology Research Foundation
(aka American Environmental Health Foundation)
8345 Walnut Hill Lane
Suite 205
Dallas, TX 75231
Phone 1-800-428-2343
They also have porcelain masks and tygon tubing.

Making Your Own Mask

A portable filtering mask can be inexpensively made with barrier cloth which can be purchased from:

The Janice Corporation
(1-800-JANICE'S)

It can be filled with activated charcoal of coconut source purchased from:

E.L. Foust Co., Inc.
P.O. Box 105
Elmhurst, IL 60126
Phone (312) 834-4952

You can also make a wire frame to support the mask on so it is handier than the bean bag configuration. Many of us always carry a charcoal filter pollen type mask at all times for inadvertent exposures. It is easier to be safe than sick! Charcoal masks are available at our office. And cloth masks are available from Dallas (above).

Surgery in the E.I. Patient

Sooner or later you may need hospitalization. In order to facilitate your doctor's understanding of E.I., I prepared the following prototype letter. Schedule an appointment so that we can tailor-make additions, subtractions and comments so it suits your needs. We may also map out a pre-hospital nutrition program to assure that you get through in the best condition. This is not something that can be left until the last week before surgery. Some of us are too sensitive to do well in an ordinary hospital. Such people should be scheduled for any type of surgery or evaluations they need at the Dallas Environmental Unit. There they can receive surgery and have clean air, water and food. These surgeons and hospital personnel specialize in E.I.

Dear Doctor:

I have a condition called Environmentally Induced Illness, or E.I. When exposed to certain places, chemicals, foods and other substances, I usually have the reactions which I have stated below:

Trigger (allergen)   Symptom (reaction)   Avg. Duration

1.
2.
3.
4.
5.
6.

The severity of a reaction is dependent upon the total load to my immune system at any one time. I know it sounds bizarre and even hypochondriacal. As no medical schools yet teach E.I., I have spent thousands of dollars with many physicians before I learned what I have and how to control it.

I would like to explore some requests with you that will help you and me through my surgery with minimal complications. Before I even come to the hospital, I will reduce the total antigenic load to my immune system as much as possible by eating a diet free of allergenic foods and keeping my chemical exposures to a minimum.

If you feel I will need a blood transfusion, I would rather store my own blood three weeks prior to surgery than have someone else's blood.

For the hospital admission, I will bring my own cotton bedding, pillow, aluminum foil, clothes, chemically less contaminated and rotated foods, clean water, ionizer, room air depollution device, soap and towels. I will see that the room is prewashed with water or provide borax or Neolife. I will see that as much as possible, such as plastic mattress covers, foam pillows, nonmetallic cabinets, carpeting and synthetics are gone, including the curtain dividers.

I would request from you that you write in my orders that I have a room with no one entering who wears perfume, cologne, aftershave, deodorant, hair tonic or hair spray, scented cosmetics or who has the odor of tobacco on their clothes, fabric softener, fresh shoe polish or freshly dry cleaned clothes. I will also put a sign to that effect on my door.

I would like to be able to have a window that opens but not toward a heavily trafficked street, parking lot, incinerator or truck delivery area.

I would like to have oxygen available but I will have to bring my own ceramic mask and low outgas tubing.

We can test my tolerance to the surgical scrub (Betadine) that will be used, the tape that will be used and the suture material. All we need do is put the scrub on one area of my forearm, the tape that will be used in another area and one small suture. These three test areas can be left in place for forty-eight hours to see if there is any adverse reaction.

If there are going to be any metals or acrylics used, I should test these as well.

One of the major problems with E.I. is that it can get dramatically or even irreversibly worse, especially if I have gas anesthetics. If there are adverse effects because of the gas anesthetic, my recovery can be delayed days or even weeks. I would like to request that the surgeon and the anesthesiologist wear no hair tonic, preshave, aftershave, cologne or deodorants and that they wash in Ivory soap and unscented Almay shampoo. I will bring a gift of these to each of the people involved. Please let me know the number of people who will be close to me during surgery.

I will bring my own inhalant, food, mediator, chemical and hormone extracts that I may need. I will have a charcoal mask, alka-aid and baking soda drops; I will maintain a high level of vitamin C for two days prior to surgery and all through the hospitalization. One to four grams every four hours usually helps me tolerate chemical overload. However I will have none 8 hours prior to surgery (since it accelerates the cytochrome P-450 enzymes and would make me require extra anesthetic, which would be contraindicated).

Five to ten grams of IV vitamin C, run in over an hour will help me come out of anesthesia if I have a prolonged reaction to it. An I.V. of bicarbonate also helps me rebound.

I would need a list of all anticipated I.V.'s. It should go to the hospital pharmacist so that he can get as many of the I.V.'s in glass bottles as possible. Plastic I.V. bags leak pthalates or plasticizers and cause symptoms in people sensitive to it (Remember the latex allergy?).

Preoperatively, I will take no oral medication. I can take Benadryl if you feel I need it and an injection of 0.4 to 0.6 mg of I.M. Atropine should be okay to prevent excess secretions.

During surgery, regional anesthetics would be preferable whenever possible. If I need Xylocaine, I prefer cardiac or single-unit dose vials of Xylocaine without preservatives. Multi-dose vials have preservatives to which I can react. I should not have Carbocaine nor halogenated or fluorinated hydrocarbons (Fluothane, Ethrane, Penthrane). As little nitrous oxide as possible should be used.

The basis for anesthesia that works well is a bolus of thiopental sodium (Pentothal) or Brevital to induce me, preceded by 100 percent oxygen for five minutes; then succinyl choline chloride (Anectine) or curare to paralyze me. Sublimaze can be used to obliterate memory and

Innovar, Demerol or alphaprodine (Nisentil), a shorter acting narcotic than Demerol (2 hours) is usually well tolerated.

If you feel I should alkalinize the stomach contents to reduce problems with aspiration pneumonitis, Alka-Seltzer in gold foil (without aspirin) or my alka-aid is a preferable antacid for me. I will bring these.

Ad lib hyperventilation is used. I should not test these anesthetic drugs prior to use. I.V. (half normal saline) in glass, not plastic bottles, works best for me. I can have D5W if I am not corn sensitive. There are fructose and invert sugars, and I realize I must contact the company that makes them beforehand because they frequently change their formulations and sugar sources without making it known on the bottle.

For shorter procedures, a Brevitol drip, and/or regional anesthesia would be better for me.

I realize all of this takes a great deal of extra skill and time and if you feel that you are not qualified, I would appreciate your recommendation to someone whom you feel is.

I also want to have you help me figure out some way to compensate you for the extra efforts that are necessary in a patient with E.I. I don't expect you to do it for nothing. I know this disease is bizarre and that it places extra stress on all medical personnel because it breaks all the rules of medicine.

Post surgery, I would like to try to use a Tens unit for pain control. I will keep my charcoal mask handy for inadvertent exposure to personnel that visit, since I know I can't begin to control the sixty or more people who enter my room on a daily basis. I do try to control as much as I can, however, like the people who will be having close, prolonged, intimate contact with me. I should be allowed to take the nutrients prescribed by my ecologist to speed the detoxification of the anesthetic and speed healing.

I cannot express how much gratitude I have for your willingness to work with me. I know much of this sounds utterly impossible; unfortunately, only the people who have lived through this illness know how devastatingly ill they can be made by seemingly innocuous exposures that cause other people absolutely no harm.

I look forward to having an uneventful recovery.

Very appreciatively,

CAVEAT - Under no circumstances should this letter be copied and used without a consultation with your ecologist. To do so only confuses and antagonizes most anesthesiologists. It is meant as a tentative guideline worked out with Dr. Rea, a cardiovascular surgeon. It is not intended to be a blanket prescription and does not serve that purpose.

Some of us cannot smell the things that make us react. Our reactions are sometimes delayed; by the time we're in a reaction we are too illogical to know it. We don't know enough at that point to get out of the area and if you suggest to us we might be reacting, you risk getting your head bitten off in protest. These times make it imperative that a loving and observant spouse intervene and get you to safety. Also, analyzing the situation calmly together later helps the victim realize that well-meaning warnings by the spouse must be heeded.

HOW TO TRAVEL

Many people ask me how I ever managed to lecture

all over the country each year when I had so many chemical, food and inhalant (pollen, dust and mold) allergies. Credit for most of what I have learned about travel must go to my two most trusted advisors, my husband Rob ("Luscious") and Dr. Bill Rea.

It's discouraging to travel and get sick from chemical overload. At a time when you should be excited and happy in anticipation of seeing old friends and learning new things, it's very inconvenient to have a flare of migraine, colitis, brain fog, asthma, arthritis, nausea or any of a host of other symptoms. Since the brain is the commonest allergic target organ, many of us develop a deep depression or become disoriented and hostile. More than once I've arrived in tears and locked myself in a hotel room when I was supposed to be delivering a lecture.

It becomes imperative that we plan for our trips far in advance to reduce our total load as much as possible and to get in as good shape as possible. The week before, start making your lists so you don't leave anything at home. Go down to one to five foods a day (very safe foods) and get plenty of rest and fresh air.

The day of the trip, fast. Pack a teaspoonful of buffered sago palm vitamin C in your carry-on bag. In addition, your bag should contain bottled water, a couple charcoal masks, Alka-aid, a battery operated ionizer, any neutralizing doses that work for you and your aluminum foil seat wrapped in cotton. Nowadays you can purchase a very smart and comfortable easy to carry leather seat from Dallas which is far superior. Even though I am well, I still travel with this. If you must eat, then include very safe organic foods. Include also your food and inhalant extracts in case your luggage gets lost. Bring a good outgased book.

Your auto should be older; it should have cloth seats and no exhaust leaks. It should be equipped with an ionizer and/or air purification system. When you get to the airport, don't linger in areas with smoke, perfumes or bad smells any longer than necessary. Try to sit in the best ventilated spot and away from anyone else.

On the plane, get midway between smokers and first class, preferably an aisle seat, as the more stagnant air is at the sides. Use your aluminum foil seat wrapped in cotton and keep your mask on for take-offs, landings and anytime in between that it is needed. The small ionizer can be propped on your shoulder or in a sling made by a neck scarf so that a cloud of ions surrounds your head. Planes have the worst air quality and the attendants are loathe to let you use oxygen or allow you to bring your own. With education, this may change in the future. But I'm not encouraged when I just had a flight in a new American plane which was the first one I ever saw with no individually-operated air vents over each seat! Talk about regression!

In the hotel, get an older, non-renovated room with a window that opens. If you can, call ahead and reserve one that was not previously occupied by a smoker and specify that no cleaning supplies be used on the day of your arrival.

The bed should be stripped down to the sheets and five layers of extra heavy duty aluminum foil should be put down, shiny side up. Use your own cotton sheets, blankets and pillow. If I was too limited with packing space, I put a cotton towel over their pillow. Have your head away from the wall and headboard, which usually contain more chemicals and EMF. Sleep at the foot of the bed. Sometimes I have had to put my mattress on the floor so my nose is near the patio door which is chained open as far as possible. I have also slept in the bathtub. If the place is really bad, you can rent portable oxygen, which I have done on occasion. Unplug the TV set since it offgasses phenols from the wires leading to a part that keeps the tube in partial readiness to minimize warm-up time when the set is turned on. Bring enough food and water or order as safe a meal from room service as you dare. Sometimes you can find an organic restaurant or health food store and stock up locally. I used to have to cook all my meals in my room or a portable hot plate!

Watch out for gas smells in restaurants with poor ventilation. Do not let them light your table candle. If they are lit when you arrive, tell them not to extinguish it in your presence, but carry it away from the table before doing so.

I know this all sounds incredibly ludicrous and cumbersome, but we know why it works. Before I was well, I tried to skimp and cheat many times, only to get abysmally ill. The worse your pollution exposure is, the more careful you will need to be. If you are outside in good air all day, you can probably eat in a few restaurants. If you are trapped in a meeting, you will need to try to find good air in the evening. I know people who have slept outdoors at the hotel. Everything is relative to how bad you know you have been in the past.

HOW TO GO TO THE DENTIST

Fortunately, most dental hygienists don't wear a lot of makeup or perfume. You might request one in particular. I like to go early in the morning to be the first one in and out. Get to know them. If you scare the dentist with your sensitivities, he's only going to call me and ask what he can and cannot use. We do not test for something you have not used to see if you can tolerate it. The reason is because you may tolerate it a few times before you lose your tolerance. So, why waste one exposure on testing when you could have at least gotten some dental work done with it?

Do not take your buffered vitamin C before you leave, as it revs up your detox system so much that you might (as I did) require 12 injections versus one. It was not fun! Fast and take your own water. For anesthetic, try to avoid gas. The best and most often tolerated is xylocaine 1% or 2% injectable anesthetic. However, if you use this, you will need to get a prescription from him beforehand. When having the prescription filled, don't forget to get your own needles. Be sure he writes it for individual 2 ml glass ampules and not the unit dose vial. The former has no chemical preservative while the latter does. You and he can negotiate whether he wants it with adrenalin or not. If he uses his own adrenalin, it has sulfites in it.

Packing for root canals contains many chemicals, usually phenol or formaldehyde. The rest is hit or miss, but remember to return to your oasis if you suspect a reaction brewing. The rest is highly individual. If you discover any tips be sure to let us know so we can share them with others.

The Toxic Time Bomb and **It's Not All In Your Head** describe the many people whose E.I. symptoms have cleared once their mercury amalgams were replaced with gold. I recently lectured at the same seminar as Dr. Hal Huggins and Dr. Guy Fasciana and they both agree that with the onslaught of people who have had their amalgams removed but have not recovered, new facts are apparent. Foremost is the fact that for many, this is just plain not the most important part of their total load. Or, the total load is so high, that removal of amalgams is equivalent to only removing 1 of 5 nails from the shoe; it doesn't appreciably affect the overall symptoms until the total load is addressed.

You're getting the idea now. People with this disease are desperate. They fly by the seat of their pants and listen to their bodies. They must be good at learning from their mistakes to survive. They are inventive and resourceful. I know a woman who slept outdoors in Buffalo for a year. I know a dentist who slept in his garage in Albany. I know people who have gutted, renovated or moved to obtain a tolerable environment. Whole families have lived for a year on their front porch or moved to the attic while they got their oasis ready. Whatever you do, don't let denial and procrastination take the place of action.

CAUTION: You know when you feel lousy; the only thing to do is get away from the molds, foods and chemicals that are triggering you. Fasting in your oasis can bring the most welcomed and unimaginable relief. But if you have not had your nutrient levels done and are sorely deficient in nutrients that are crucial to the detox paths, fasting can push you over the edge and make you many times worse. So you are playing Russian roulette to fast and not have addressed the rest of you total load, namely nutrient corrections.

You've spent years ignoring your symptoms because medicine had no answers and so intimidated you from voicing them with the threat of hypochondriasis. Now you must change your tack and heed every single symptom. They are there to warn you, so that you don't return to worse symptom levels.

RISING TO THE CHALLENGE

Having environmental illness (E.I.) is not as easy as other diseases for a number of reasons:

1) Very few lay people or even doctors have ever heard of it. Since it is a product of our technological advancement, it is a recent epidemic.

2) Even those who have heard of it have such a poor comprehension of how it changes all the rules of medicine (see Rules of E.I. article) that there is often doubt as to the victim's psychological integrity

3) Since it is not easily treated with drugs or surgery, many doctors don't want to know about it. Unlike other diseases, there is less sympathy and more isolation and loneliness felt.

4) The diet and necessary environmental controls can further serve to isolate one from society and family ties. It is potentially a very lonely disease.

5) Many victims of E.I. don't know they have it. The symptoms can accumulate slowly and quietly until one or

many parts of the system break down. Once a label is given, such as arthritis, colitis or depression, then it is assumed that no cause should be sought; only drugs and surgery should be used.

Environmental illness can produce a lonely, guilt-ridden and self-hating patient who is asking "Why me?" As Richard Bach (author of **Jonathan Livingston Seagull**) said in **Illusions**, "There is no such thing as a problem without a gift." For one thing, those of us who are now reacting to the twentieth century most likely have not only staved off chronic incapacitating disease with our diets and environmental controls but we have most assuredly set back the hands of time for ourselves and our spouses in terms of when our biological time clocks would strike heart attack, stroke or cancer.

Remember, in contrast to the average cancer victim, this is a disease of hope - not hopelessness and helplessness. Studies of patients succumbing to illness show far greater survival and recovery rates when the victims have these three C's:

1) They feel in control of their lives; not helpless.

2) They are committed to a goal of wellness and act accordingly.

3) They view each change as a challenge to be met and conquered. They read and study voraciously.

These three C's constitute mental hardiness as opposed to the common distortions practiced by those who succumb to mental and physical deterioration. These distortions include exaggerating the problem, ignoring the positive aspects and personalizing (making oneself feel guilty and responsible for what has happened).

Another common distortion is to think that there is no in between - a situation is either impossible and dreadful or it is wonderful. Another is to over-generalize and jump to conclusions (the wrong ones) with ease.

486

Having E.I. involves breaking habits. Addictions are one aspect of E.I. to overcome. It's easier once you recognize they represent non-growth by our robot-like adaptations. Addictions also represent an attachment to something that allows us to temporarily forget who we are. They represent postponement of meaningful growth-related actions, for real transformation only occurs in the now, not tomorrow.

Having any disease first takes owning up to it. How often have we all wallowed in denial and tried to pretend we could tolerate what everyone else does, only to pay for our indiscretion with two days in bed!

Another healthy quality of survivors (versus victims) that is essential to develop includes altruism. Helping others has always been an essential emotional nutrient, but it cannot be freely utilized until you first love yourself.

With more attention to detail, a childlike enthusiasm or romanticism for life can emerge with a renewed appreciation and joy from many of nature's previously unseen gifts. As Richard Bach said in The Bridge Across Forever, "Change our thoughts and the world around us changes." Start noticing how much you have to be thankful for. Let us not forget the importance of a sense of humor. Not only does it help in maintaining perspective, but laughter is actually healthful for the immune system.

Norman Cousins, formerly editor of **Saturday Review**, was struck in 1964 with a genetically-linked, incurable, progressively debilitating form of arthritis called ankylosing spondylitis. By now, he should have a boat-shaped spine, so fused with arthritis as to leave him bedridden. Instead, he decided to put himself on an excellent nutritional program, physically and mentally. Each day was structured so it would be filled with laughter and positive feelings. He cured himself and wrote his story, **Anatomy of an Illness**. Nearly twenty years later he had a heart attack. The doctors, knowing of his fame said, "This is more serious. You won't be able to laugh yourself out of this. You need surgery." He completely recovered without surgery and wrote his second book, **The Healing Heart**. After that he was laughing all the way to the bank.

Much success is also being seen now with patients who practice positive imagery. It is the opposite of negative imagery (worrying) where you constantly practice or mentally rehearse for the worst to materialize. Studies show if you practice positive imagery and imagine yourself getting better and stronger, if you mentally rehearse what you're going to do when you are better and how life will be, you will facilitate healing. The presence of positive good feelings (acting somehow through the psychoneuroimmune system) have a beneficial and healing effect.

Spiritual healing is an essential component of our physical healing. Whether it is religion, meditation, yoga, self-hypnosis or whatever you prefer, get some aspect of this going in your life. Like exercise, we tend to feel we are too busy to make a place for it in our lives. Taking time for meditation can be easier than you realize. It has many benefits since it can refresh and fortify you for the day, relax you for sleep and help you over the hurdles of addictions, cravings and emotional upsets. (See Spirituality chapter in **Wellness Against All Odds.**)

Primary positive goals to set for yourself are to increase your self-esteem and self-love, mobilize your altruism and enthusiasm, maintain a sense of humor and practice positive imagery and meditation.

For some, E.I. is like a double edged sword with guilt on both sides. On one side is guilt for the burdens we place on our loved ones - we spend money that could be used by other members of the family, we cause changes to be made in the home so that it no longer conforms to the Jones's, we impose sacrifice on spouses who would prefer to go to restaurants, dances and parties and we add to their tasks and responsibilities. In addition, we have self-imposed embarrassment and guilt for being a prisoner in our homes and for being different when we are in public, whether it is for wearing a mask, eating strange foods or sitting on foil.

On the other side of the sword is the guilt for failing to rotate our diets or to do the necessary environmental controls. We set ourselves up in a no-win situation. If we do what we should, we are guilty of depriving our families. If we don't do what we should, we are guilty of non-compliance which is the twelfth mystery box in the total load boat (see The Total Load). In fact, 50% of non-compliance stems from guilt.

One start at overcoming guilt is to realize that at the root of all guilt is poor self-esteem and lack of self-love. Remember the hair coloring advertisement, "This product may be a little more expensive, but I'm worth it!" Victims of E.I. do not believe they are worth it, whereas survivors of E.I. all believe they are worth it. It is the only way they can direct their energies sufficiently to succeed. Remember, survivors of E.I. believe they are worth every effort.

One part of E.I. that has always excited me is that the mechanism for wellness is within us. All the machinery is there. We just need to find the magic combination of total load that allows it to function again. How can I say wellness is present? Easily. Look at all the times we will be testing someone to a particular substance and it will suddenly turn off a symptom he has had for years. We have merely unblocked a mechanism somewhere with our neutralizing doses. The machinery was there ready to work all the time - we just didn't have the right key. The tricky part is many of us require several different keys at once (see Total Load section).

Some psychologists worry that people with specific diagnoses learn to identify with their diagnoses and would feel naked without them or would not get as much attention or sympathy (called secondary gain). They are concerned that there are people who fear getting better because they will no longer "belong" to a group and will have to share more responsibility and work. I have never feared these problems in the people I meet, but it does help us to remember that we need to concentrate on wellness as opposed to illness. Wouldn't it be a good idea for every H.E.A.L. meeting to start with people getting up and announcing positive aspects of their illness that they have overcome? Or for that matter, it would be a good idea to start each day by reminding yourself what you have accomplished.

Having E.I. means your very best efforts are constantly being thwarted. It goes with the territory. You may have every intention of planning a day with no chemical hits only to find twentieth century chemicals looming up from unexpected places. That's life with E.I. However, every hit teaches us something useful about our bodies, so don't waste precious psychic energy on depression and anger, but see the humor and begin to accept the challenge in devising ways to overcome these temporary obstacles.

Let us oust those deprecating and purposeless draining emotions of panic, fear, rage, frustration and depression and let us nurture our positive emotions of hope, faith, love and laughter.

In essence you have every opportunity to grab the bull by the horns and begin to heal yourself now. Set your goals to become a truly healed person within the next year or two, maximum.

If you prefer, wallow in self-pity, anger, guilt, self-hate, procrastination and denial. You can steadily go downhill and continually reset your thermostat at each stage which overloads you, getting a little deeper into the hole until you really do have irreversible illness. Many of us, including myself, wish we knew years ago what we know now about E.I. We could have prevented ourselves from getting as affected as we are. That is one reason we contribute our energies to our H.E.A.L. groups.

You can recognize a shot in the arm when it is needed (pun intended) and accept control of your health which really only you have. By committing yourself to wellness, you can optimistically embrace the disease as a challenge to be controlled and conquered. We are admittedly pioneers in this disease and pioneers never had it easy.

Are you ready to rise to the challenge?

VERY HELPFUL READING

Padus, Emrika, et al, **The Complete Guide to Your Emotions and Your Health**, Rodale Press, Emmaus, Pennsylvania, 1986.

Cousins, Norman, **Anatomy of an Illness**, Avon Books, Department FP, 190 Broadway, NY 10019, 1979.

Benson, Herbert, **The Relaxation Response**, Morrow Press, New York 1975.

Jampolsky, Gerald, **Good-Bye to Guilt**, Bantam Books, New York, 1985.

Jampolsky, Gerald, **Love is Letting Go of Fear**, Celestial Arts, P.O. Box 7327, Berkley, CA 94707, 1979.

Simonton, C.O., et al, **Getting Well Again**, Bamtam Books, New York, 1978.

Laurie, S.G., Tucker, M.J., **Centering: A Guide to Inner Growth**, Destiny Books, 377 Park Avenue South, New York 10016, 1978.

Krieger, Dolores, **The Therapeutic Touch**, Prentice-Hall, Englewood Cliffs, New Jersey, 10732, 1979.

My Triumph Over Cancer, Beata Bishop, Keats Publishing, 27 Grove Street, New Canaan, CT.

Lakein, Alan, Getting Control of Your Time and Your Life, The best and most concise little paperback for time management. If you don't have the time to make the changes for wellness, read this.

The Holy Bible.

SUMMARY

Multiple illnesses may be due to environmental exposures that need to be identified on an individual basis. The key is to look for someone with chronic symptoms that no amount of medicine can make better. This disease is only controlled by total re-education of the victim. We can provide the specialized diagnostic tools to determine which of your symptoms are due to inhalants, foods, chemicals, hormones, Candida sensitivity, nutritional deficiencies, pesticides, heavy metal toxicities, etc. It is up to you to follow through with identifying your total load and consult with the doctor when you get stuck, discouraged or confused. This disease breaks all the rules of medicine by which we were trained (see Rules of E.I.). The tremendous individuality is just one of the many idiosyncracies of the disease.

Each of us needs to whittle away at the total load. Only then can we tell which symptoms get better when we start inhalant injections, diet, anti-Candida treatment, etc. Then, when we get an unavoidable exposure, we are not clobbered as ruthlessly as we would have been in the past.

Chemicals cause chronic diseases. Any target organ can be involved; usually multiple ones are involved and there is a tremendously large individual variation. Since we are living organisms in a constant state of change and our surrounding environments are constantly changing as well, we rarely have the same set of circumstances twice. Therefore, our reactions may seem mysteriously different and unpredictable.

One very strong deterrent to wellness is the occasional person who emanates anger, hostility and an exaggerated need to dominate. I have never seen this type heal until they dealt with these powerful emotions and their underlying causes. This may require specialized help far beyond my capabilities, but I will be happy to help try to match you with the most compatible experts.

HIGHLIGHTS

*It is not easy having E.I., but unlike any other disease, whether we accept it or not, we possess nearly total control over the amount of symptoms we have.

*Each person has a unique total load that must be addressed before he heals.

*This total load is in a constant state of flux, due to fluctuations in our own internal and external environments.

*The two most common reasons for failure to get well are not addressing the diet and denying the chemical overload. The third most common reason is lack of a knowledgeable, compassionate support system.

*Never underestimate the potency of prayer which reflects a true faith. I have seen many medical miracles.

SECTION VIII - POTPOURRI

A Second Chance at Life
by
JoAnn, Registered Nurse

On August 10, 1984, I was told by Dr. Rogers that I could no longer receive allergy extracts. (I had been having reactions to my regular inhalant injections and also my food injections). It had been determined that I could no longer tolerate the minute amount of glycerin present in the allergy extracts. The doctor advised me that I should go to the Environmental Unit in Dallas, Texas, and be titrated to Dr. Rea's extracts.

This information did not surprise me. I knew she was going to tell me this, but I also knew that I couldn't go, not in the near future anyway. Too many things were happening in my life to just pick up and go. I had a husband and a three-year-old at home. I was on my summer break from nursing school and I was gearing up for my last semester which was to start in approximately three weeks. I would be graduating in December and taking my RN state boards in February. I had worked too long and hard to postpone that. I also had no idea if our medical insurance would cover something like that (later on they did refuse to). So, I explained all this to Dr. Rogers and she calmly looked at me and said, "JoAnn, when you get sick enough, call me. I'll get you in the next day." She then advised me to write to the unit and "set things up just in case."

Well, I was devastated. Dr. Rogers had been my physician for fourteen years at that point and she had always been able to "fix" whatever went wrong. Now she was telling me there was nothing else she could do. Never before had I felt so alone. I told her I felt like an outcast. She half-grinned and said "We are outcasts." She gave me a few names of patients who had been to Rea's unit and told me

494

to give one or two of them a call to find out about their experiences. So ended my last allergy consultation with Dr. Rogers - after fourteen years!

On my way home I wondered how I would get through life without my injections. I had been on them for fourteen years. They had controlled my symptoms so well that I looked forward to getting them. In all that time I had missed only one. I thought maybe after all that time my symptoms wouldn't be as bad as they had been in the past, that is before I had been on any immunotherapy treatment.

Well, it didn't take me long to find out. The next day I awoke with a severe headache, stuffy nose, blocked up ears, sore throat, runny red eyes, tight chest and severe dizziness (and I hadn't even sat up yet). My legs were cramping (reminiscent of the days when as a child I was told it was "growing pains"). My whole body shook and I also felt nauseous. I honestly couldn't remember a time when I had felt so bad. I wondered how I was ever going to drag myself out of bed to take care of a 3-year-old while my husband worked. How was I ever going to attend classes, absorb new information, and learn and practice nursing techniques on patients in the hospital? Then, if I got to that point, how in the world was I going to cope with the chemically- contaminated hospital? I knew I couldn't use antihistamines; the doctor had stressed that with my chemical sensitivities I shouldn't use any systemic medications. Furthermore, if I had I would have been way too drowsy to be good for anything.

On August 13th (just two days late for my allergy injection) I had all of the above symptoms but they were much more severe. I honestly felt like I was dying. I remember calling Frank (an RN at Dr. Rogers' office) and begging him to see if there wasn't anything that could be done to get me at least half-way on my feet. They had me come in that day to see if I could tolerate two antigens (mold mixes A and B). Within five minutes after that injection, I felt like a new person. To this day, I don't think anyone knows how thankful I was to have received those two antigens. By the way, I was able to tolerate those two antigens for two more injections. The third brought on my glycerine symptoms again - intense panicky feeling, heart palpitations, my chest felt like it had caved in, I couldn't get any air and everything looked black and very far away. Therefore, glycerinated allergy injections were forever off-limits for me.

So, how did I survive, complete school, be a wife and a mother without any medications or allergy injections? To say that it was difficult is an understatement; to say that I felt good during that time is a gross lie. Many times I had thought that my only way "out" was through death, and I can honestly understand how someone can feel so desperate for any kind of relief that he might take his own life.

One thing for certain - I couldn't have done it without my family, friends and new environmentally ill friends I had just made through the office and H.E.A.L. group. I contacted Rosalie who put me in touch with Mary and Carla. (Carla was chemically sensitive, but had not been to the unit). These three people (who had never met me before) stayed on the phone with me for hours. They explained how they coped with their illnesses, they told of their experiences at the environmental unit in Dallas, and they told me where they obtained their chemically less contaminated organic foods. They were and are still a great support and they encouraged me not to give up. Carla came to my home after our phone conversation with a cooler filled with organic meats, vegetables and fruits.

My husband, mom, dad, mother-in-law and father-in-law helped me obtain a Micronaire filter, cotton pillows and organic foods. They helped me store my foods as we didn't have a freezer big enough then. They came over to visit me, which helped a lot with my feelings of isolation. I hardly left my home. Whenever I went outside, my symptoms came back in full force - all those molds and pollens during August!

After doing stricter environmental controls at home, I finally started feeling better inside my home. If I went outside, the pollens and molds made me feel so miserable I wasn't good for anything. My symptoms of headache, nausea, sore throat, blocked up ears, extreme tiredness, stuffiness and wheezing came on within minutes of being exposed to the outside air. Within ten minutes of being outside my hands and fingers swelled so badly that they split open, bled and oozed. My old eczema had returned as well.

The stricter environmental controls I had done involved the chemicals that until this time had never before bothered me. I never realized they were an unseen part of my total load. I soon discovered that my symptoms seemed to worsen in two rooms: the bathroom and the kitchen.

My husband was very patient when I threw out all of his aftershave, shaving cream, deodorant, soap and when I ordered him never to bring any of it back in again. I discovered that a certain corner in my kitchen caused my headache to increase in severity. I finally made the connection between this and the tupperware I had stored in those cupboards. I threw it all in the basement and my headache eased up. I then spotted all of my daughter's plastic toys in the living room. I knew I couldn't throw them all out and so explained to her that her plastic toys would have to be kept in her bedroom and her door closed. Janine was very good about this and to this day, if I have a headache or am not feeling well, she will look around for plastics and either put them away or throw them out. Our windows had always been open in the summer and my husband enjoyed sleeping with the windows open. I now have them all shut tight with the air conditioner and Micronaire running continuously.

In addition to all of this, a lot of work had to be done.

In order for me to wake up feeling somewhat well, the floors and walls of my bedroom had to be damp dusted at least twice a week and my bedding washed every two weeks. The filter on the air conditioner had to be cleaned at least once a week, or I was soon sneezing and had a runny nose and watery, burning eyes. The Micronaire filters had to be cleaned every two weeks or I noticed a bad smell. Newsprint was a big problem. It caused headache and dizziness and its smell made me nauseous. When my husband brought home a newspaper to read, it was read quickly in a room away from me and then thrown outside immediately.

I had always used baking soda, vinegar and borax for cleaning purposes before stopping my allergy injections. I also had used a regular (what I had thought then to be not highly scented) dishwashing liquid. I now was reacting to it. The scent was overpowering and with just standing at the sink to wash a few dishes, I would become very dizzy - so much so that I would have to get clean air quickly and sit down. The headaches soon returned and muscles in my legs would begin cramping. I contacted a Shaklee representative and bought Basic H for dishwashing and had no further problems in that area.

While cleaning my room (any room, air conditioner and Micronaire filters, etc.) I had to wear a charcoal mask, cotton gloves and rubber gloves. I had to make sure none of my skin was exposed or I would break out in eczema from the dust and mold. My husband helped me immensely with all of this and many times I asked him if he thought I was crazy. He always answered, "No, I know you are not crazy."

My next big problem was foods. I had done great on my food injections, but now they were gone too. That eliminated a lot of food that I could eat, such as most nuts, fish, milk, wheat, corn, lettuce, carrots, soy, sunflower seeds, peanuts, all legumes, tomato, cucumber, peaches, sugar and others. I had to eat foods that were "safer." Since there weren't enough "safe" ones, I tried to rotate longer than my usual four day rotation.

I ate three different foods a day. I tried a lot of new foods, such as goat's milk and venison. I tried other foods that I had rarely eaten before, such as cherries, macadamia nuts, cranberries, turkey, etc. When I had been on my food allergy injections, I had been using organic grains and dried fruits because the insecticide spray caused my fingers and hands to swell and break out. Now I needed organic meats and produce.

To say that I was symptom-free from the foods I ate was not true. Many symptoms that I had had as a child now returned - abdominal cramping, bloating, swelling and weight gain. My eczema flared and I was broken out in places where I hadn't been broken out since my immuno-therapy treatments began fourteen years ago.

The insides of my arms and elbows, hands, feet, backs of knees and legs, abdomen and face were all broken out again. Once again my sleep was disturbed by incessant itching and I would wake up exhausted and sore. It is really strange and sad how familiar all of these symptoms were and how much they reminded me of being a kid.

I kept looking forward to the first frost which would kill off the ragweed, goldenrod and most of the molds so my total load would be lowered, thereby alleviating some symptoms. Until that time, I used a charcoal mask while outside and I only went out when I absolutely had to. I used the mask in the car, on the street, in classes and in the hospital. (The nursing staff smoked cigarettes during morning report and tobacco smoke now caused me to have asthma attacks.)

I wore the mask during classes because other students wore perfume or wool and I often sat near an open window. I would much rather battle the pollens and molds than the chemicals. Some of my friends in school were quite familiar with my symptoms and "saved me" special places to sit and looked out for me. They were very encouraging and helped me with environmental controls in class and in the hospital. They helped me find a few new places to obtain chemically- less contaminated foods. I will always be thankful for their surveillance and help. It got me through school.

When I had been well, I wore contact lenses. Now, since my eyes were red, swollen and watery, I wore my glasses. On my good days, I would put my contacts in. I used sterile normal saline solution as a wetting agent and Basic H as a cleanser because I reacted to the commercial brands.

A lot of my family and friends asked me what I thought about being so severely allergic, especially since I had already spent thousands of dollars on testing and injections. (Now that I couldn't tolerate the injections I was worse than ever.) They asked if I felt it had all been a waste of time, money and energy. The answer to that was and still is "no."

A person cannot associate symptoms with a cause without first being clear (feeling completely well.) In my case, the only way I could ever be clear was to be on inhalant and food injections. In order to receive these injections, I had to be tested. While testing, I had a few whopping reactions and some very familiar, vague, subtle sensations which I had always thought of as being "normal." Knowing what was being tested enabled me to know what foods, inhalants or chemicals caused symptoms. With my injections I became clear. Lengthening intervals between injections caused some symptoms, but I was able to associate the symptoms with the cause by paying close attention to the foods I ate and the inhalants and chemicals I was exposed to.

In fact, if I had not gone through all of the testing in the first place, I wouldn't have been able to have made a "safe" home. I would not have been able to figure out that plastics caused terrific headaches; newsprint caused red, itchy eyes, a spacey feeling, inability to concentrate and sleepiness; and that certain foods caused abdominal cramping while others caused eczema and dry skin.

This was also a good lesson for me on the concept of the "total load." When I was on my allergy injections, most of the above problems were not problems. My injections helped lower my total load, thereby enabling me to tolerate much more. Without my injections, my load was so high that everything made me react. Without the injections, I had to lower my own load via environmental controls, diet and very limited chemical exposure. When these were employed, I tolerated my foods much better and I was able to get through the day without napping. I could even fake being "normal" to most people.

I do have a happy ending though. I did finish school, graduate and am currently an R.N. I am now working for Dr. Rogers, am using injections (food and inhalant) and life is again a lot simpler with fewer symptoms to suffer with. It is nice to not be afraid to go outside. I feel more energetic, my skin is usually clear, I can tolerate more foods, my headaches are gone (unless triggered by perfumes or other chemicals) and I can wear my contact lenses every day.

At the time I was hired, Mr. Rogers went to great lengths for me and stepped up the program that had been planned for the next year to make glycerin-free extracts. Because of my need and despite many other matters needing attention at the time, such as a new computer system and several new employees, he got the glycerin-free program rolling. The extracts are many times more difficult and expensive to make which is what makes them so rare.

I still have to do all of the environmental controls I described; I am afraid not to keep up with it. My chemical exposure is very limited. Usually when I go out with friends, I feel like I have run up against a brick wall (perfumes, tobacco smoke, formaldehyde, phenols, gasoline and animals). I always carry my charcoal mask. I feel that I am slowly building myself up with my injections and various vitamin supplements. The extracts I am using are glycerin- free and phenol-free and I am not having a problem with them.

At one time, receiving an injection was taken for granted. Not anymore. They really have given me my life back. I am fully aware of this and especially thankful for my second chance.

A Note From JoAnn's Doctor:

Even though I have known JoAnn since she was an adorable 10-year-old, even though I too have E.I., and even though I treat hundreds of severely involved cases each year, until I read her warm account of how she really felt, I was missing part of reality. I thank her for sharing it with us and heightening my awareness.

Because advances in the field of environmental medicine are barely keeping pace with our most desperate needs, I lecture yearly all over the country with other leaders in the field so that we may all keep communication networks open among us for the in between times. Maybe a dozen physicians have phenol-free extracts now, but there are less than a half-dozen of us in the world who have made phenol-free, glycerin-free extracts which are the current lifeline for courageous pioneers of this twentieth century maladaptation like JoAnn.

We got the idea for her to put her story in writing as she accompanied me to Atlanta where I was giving a lecture for the American Academy of Otolaryngic Allergy. We thought it would help the newcomer to E.I. to get a glimpse of how difficult this disease is for all of us.

Anyway, after JoAnn and I registered at the hotel, we went upstairs to see our rooms. As we got off the elevator, we were greeted with signs apologizing for the new paint job! While we were fumbling with our keys, a housekeeper came down the hall spraying a big cloud of "Heaven Scent." We quickly jumped inside and had a big laugh as we donned our masks. The world is constantly out to get us! We did change to a non-painted floor and asked for no maid service while we were registered. There is always a solution and keeping a good sense of humor helps the overall balance.

And now 8 years later, she is still on injections, works full time as a loving oncology nurse and needs much less strict environmental and dietary controls, having gone macrobiotic for a period of time.

> "We are all continuously faced with a series of great opportunities, brilliantly disguised as insoluble problems."
> **W. B. Prescott**

Painfree and Drugfree Arthritis

The stiffness and pain were indescribable. For three months Tamara barely made it from the bed to the bathroom. This abrupt change in her life during this last year was still like a nightmare. How could she have gone from a healthy 48-year-old mother, wife and teacher to a victim of crippling rheumatoid arthritis within a few months?

The ineffectiveness of her response to the plethora of medications prescribed by the three rheumatologists left her with nothing but the time-worn advice, "You'll have to learn to live with it." Even though she rarely gave in to it, eventually depression crept in. Life was over for her since each day offered only more pain on top of being able to accomplish nothing. She was an invalid, a total burden on the family with no hope for recovery.

It is no wonder that months later she and her English

professor husband were brought to tears when within three minutes of an injection she had no pain and vastly decreased limitation of motion. That morning she had been unable to peel a banana with her swollen, crippled hands. Her husband had to help her up the one step to the office. Squatting and touching her toes were not possible since it took every effort to just hoist herself out of the chair. She couldn't even comb her own hair because her stiff, swollen shoulders wouldn't allow the necessary arm motion.

Within three minutes of her injection, she was laughing through tears of unbelievable joy and flapping her arms as though they were wings that would make her airborne. She squatted, touched her toes and bounced in and out of her chair. For her the relief lasted two days.

What was in the injection? A miniscule (but very specific) dose of a chemical called phenol.

In the next room was Rita who walked like a retired lumberjack, swaying from side-to-side. X-rays of her hips confirmed what all the doctors had told her - degenerative arthritis of both hips with barely any lubricating joint space remaining. Every forward motion of the legs produced intense pain in these poorly lubricated, weight bearing joints. It was easier to sway from side-to-side and sort of pivot forward. Medications could not help her pain and she was advised to have artificial hip joint replacements.

Within three minutes of an injection, Rita was walking normally about the room without any pain. What was in her injection? A minute (but specific) dose of formaldehyde.

How could miniscule amounts of such toxic chemicals as phenol and formaldehyde produce instantaneous relief from the pain and limitation of motion caused by different types of arthritis? No one understands the biological mechanism yet. We do know that many of these people are victims of the twentieth century environment; they have an environmental illness. For instance, five years before the onset of her rheumatoid arthritis, Tamara unknowingly overloaded her home with phenol and formaldehyde - the very substances that relieved the arthritis.

Tamara built a new bedroom using plywood. There were new carpets throughout the house and new upholstery. We have found that new furniture, new carpets, building materials (especially indoor plywood and particleboard), new mattresses, plastics and most of the products of our twentieth century living give off small amounts of "new smell" or gases which contain phenols, formaldehydes and many other chemicals. Some people have an immune system that becomes weakened by these chemicals creating a situation that can be thought of as an allergy. Instead of reacting with sneezing, their target organs can be their joints.

Frequently, the joint affected is one that has already been weakened by polio or an accident. For example, as a physician, I had my share of exposure to formaldehyde-pickled cadavers. I was also exposed to many other chemicals through renovation and new offices. I have no disc in my lower back; only two worn out arthritic bones that grind on each other. If I stay in a shopping mall for more than an hour-and-a- quarter, I get such severe pain in that area I don't know if I am going to throw up or pass out. An hour outside in fresh air and you are certain I must be the biggest hypochondriac ever as I'm back to normal without one bit of medication - only a change of air. Shopping malls, because of all the new polyester fabrics, plastics, papers and synthetic materials constantly being introduced, have higher than normal levels of chemical off-gassing.

Unfortunately, for people like Tamara, Rita and myself, once the immune system has been damaged by chemical overloads, it doesn't stop at that. The reactivity snowballs as we become reactive to a host of other environmental agents, predominantly foods. In other words, foods that we have enjoyed all our lives now cause a flare of arthritis. Because the reaction is dose-dependent and slow in occurring, because there are several foods that cause reaction and because we are fairly repetitious in our diets, food is rarely suspected. Only a specially prescribed diet will enable detection of these now allergenic foods (rare food rotation).

As with any disease, there is a spectrum of involvement from person to person. Tamara avoids certain foods that she has found through the diet flare her arthritis. Amy gives herself an allergy injection of her neutralizing dose to each food. She has had crippling rheumatoid arthritis for twenty years. No stranger to surgery, she has had many prosthetic joints placed in her hands to maintain function. At 39, she walked stiffly with a cane as if she had a stick up her spine. One month after we started her on the diet and food injections, she walked with a bounce and reduced her medication from twelve aspirin a day to two. This is a first for her and she has maintained this for over two years now.

Joyce had twenty-eight years of rheumatoid arthritis and the classic gnarled hand deformities as well. The only difference now is, after two months of injections for foods, she no longer has to take any pain medication. Before this, she was on two anti-inflammatory drugs a day. Now she takes nothing and has returned to work outside of her home for the first time in eighteen years.

Don't let me lead you to think that treating environmental illness (E.I.) is as simple as getting an injection and following a diet. Tamara can vouch for the amount of work and education required to get better. Her injections of a neutralizing dose would only work in our office; they would not work in her home because the chemical overload there was too great for her. She has a great deal of work ahead of her. Some people are never better until all natural gas utilities and appliances, all carpets, all furniture fifteen years or younger and all plastics are removed from the home.

These people must become experts in E.I. They must know more than any conventional physician because E.I. is not yet taught in medical schools. Some doctors have even disputed the validity of the testing methods used in E.I. This prompted us to demonstrate these methods in a non-hypochondriacal model, so we used horses with heaves (like human asthma) and turned their asthma on and off with the appropriate doses of mold and Timothy (hay).

Besides ridding their homes of as many offgassing twentieth century materials as possible and using a restricted diet, these chemical victims have other needs. Tamara was found to have very low levels of iron, B6 and vitamin A in her blood. It is not surprising that she should have multiple deficiencies since her body was working overtime producing joint swelling and pain. Also, she needs good levels of anti-oxidants (A, C, E, dimethyl glycine, magnesium, selenium, glutathione, etc.) now to help ward off future damage to the immune system by chemicals in her air, food and water.

Addendum - We have made tremendous advances with arthritis. If you are a sufferer, read **Tired or Toxic?**, **You Are What You Ate, The Cure Is In the Kitchen**, then **Wellness Against All Odds**. It is highly unlikely you will still have arthritis of any form if you do these recommendations. For example, many were plagued with years of back pain in old injury sites or in old arthritis sites just because they did not know the nightshade story.

The Irony of E.I.

There are few diseases more ironic than E.I. Think about it. Medicine is stagnating in an era where drugs, especially antibiotics, are the mainstay and infection is one of the few recognizable causes of disease. The majority is chalked up to chronic disease. If drugs are ineffective, irradiation or surgery are all that remain.

In spite of scientific papers, the majority of "medical experts" are unaware of the tremendous impact the chemical environment, our nutritional status and the food we eat has on chronic disease. The evidence is staggering, but there are just too many journals to read. Many still cling to the notion that organisms cause everything and keep searching for the one "virus" that causes cancer. Meanwhile evidence continues to mount that it is a multi-factorial problem - chemicals, environment, individual chemical adaptability or genetics, diet, state of nutrition, attitude, stress...you got it! It also involves the total load.

The billions of dollars in advertising by the food, construction and chemical industries is more than able to offset the avalanche of scientific data that we now have. So, you take your strange and frustrating symptoms to an already overloaded doctor. His easiest way to save face or still feel good about his abilities is to label you neurotic.

Fortunately, control of this disease is now within the grasp of the victim. You are no longer powerless. If you choose, you can create an internal and external environment where you are able to return to your normal function. It is not easy being your own doctor, but that is what is required. I am really your consultant. The real progress in this disease is totally dependent upon the knowledge and effort expended by you, the patient.

That included me! Sure I knew a great deal about the causes of E.I., but all that knowledge didn't help my back pain. What did help were the constant reminders by Dr. Rea to clean up my environment (and diet and nutritional deficiencies) and my husband's extraordinary and herculean accomplishment of this. Also, getting off the "pity pot" of "Woe is me" and doing some intense soul searching. There were over a dozen facets to my total load and superior health wasn't possible without all of them.

Luckily, feeling good is addicting. Once you find the

magic key and understand the causes, there isn't much you won't do to maintain your state of newly discovered health.

Yes, we get hooked on feeling good and that is our salvation. After years of ignoring symptoms we have done an about face. For instance, realizing that symptoms are God- given, if I have the slightest negative or black thought or the slightest ache or pain, I say to myself, "Time out! Hold everything until you find out what you are reacting to. What are you eating, breathing or touching that may be causing this?" I correct it. For, I never want to go back to the mountains of symptoms I endured for so long.

Many would call this hypochondria. That reflects the brain washing by a medicine that is excellent in treating acute, end-stage symptoms because it knows very little about health, wellness, prevention and environmental medicine. In order to "save face", people are intimidated into not complaining about "minor" early symptoms which medicine is powerless to diagnose and treat. So, the term hypochondriac is used to squash you into a guilt-ridden silence.

To compound matters, here you are a person who has not felt well for years. Now, all of a sudden, it seems to your friends that you are really losing it. You think you are reacting to foods you have eaten all your life and chemicals that don't bother them. In fact, they can't even smell what you are talking about. Heaven forbid you should be snowballing while you are unmasking, because you will be reacting to more things than ever before and quicker. They'll logically try to intimidate you further by suggesting the program is ridiculous and without scientific basis. Hopefully you are too smart to ever fall for any intimidation again. Get hooked on feeling good and stay well! You will look better and have more energy than they ever dreamed of once you get yourself committed to wellness and decide to leave sickness to someone else.

An excellent book I would suggest you read if you

start to get blocked at any stage or facet of your unloading is, **Love, Medicine and Miracles,** by Bernie Siegel, M.D. (Harper and Row, NY, 10 East 53rd Street, NY 10022, 1986).

The rules for success are simple: good clean God-given food, air, and water. But like religion, it is thought of as too simple to be true. If we got into trouble by violating God's environment, it is only logical what we need to do to reverse this.

What To Do for Your Colitis - After Your Doctor Gives Up

Amanda, at thirty-nine, had the figure that most women desire - thin. No one would envy the way that she got that way. She had Crohn's disease and she was a veteran with the town's gastroenterologist having endured many x-rays and succumbed to many drugs. She had to plan every outing around being able to quickly locate a bathroom, for some days she had as many as a dozen bloody bowel movements replete with cramps.

As with any disease, there is a spectrum of severity. On the more fortunate end of the scale are those with periodic gas, cramps, bloating and diarrhea alternating with periods of constipation and normalcy. Many are told they have a spastic colon due to nerves. On the other end of the spectrum are Amanda and others with severe, incapacitating symptoms and various labels such as chronic ulcerative colitis or regional enteritis. It is an embarrassing disease without much sympathy, interfering with work and social activities.

As specialists in environmental medicine, we see people after they have exhausted all that medicine has to offer. For the colitis victim, this usually entails many prescriptions of anti-spasmodics or anti-cholinergics, full bowel x-rays, colonoscopy by a gastroenterologist and further prescriptions of more potent and potentially dangerous medications, such as sulfasalazine, cortisone enemas, opiate antispasmodics and prednisone. Surgery is a dreaded outcome, for eventually, when enough bowel segments have been removed, a colostomy bag must be used.

Most victims will tell you, "As long as I don't eat, I am fine." This has led ecologists to search for causes in the eating habits of the patients. Let me discuss some of the more common dietary causes.

Milk is the most common cause. Lactase is an intestinal enzyme that helps break down and digest milk sugar called lactose. A deficiency of this enzyme can occur at any time in anyone and can produce any intestinal symptom one can think of such as gas, bloating, cramps, severe pain, diarrhea or constipation. Many people will say, "Oh, I never drink milk, so it can't be that." They forget that milk occurs in cheese, ice cream, butter, sour cream, sauces, etc. Sometimes it is disguised on labels as casein. A simple test is to have no milk products for two weeks and then load up. Your body will tell you the answer.

Some people with milder forms of the deficiency (but not milk allergy) can tolerate yogurt or milks with an enzyme added (you can add your own or buy it that way) that partially digests the lactose for you.

The next most common cause we see is general food allergy. We frequently encounter patients who tell us that they had formula changes as an infant because of milk allergy, but now they no longer have problems with milk - or so they think. One theory is that the milk allergy persists in a different form inflaming the bowel wall and allowing other food proteins premature access into the intestinal blood stream. As a result, this predisposes the patient to the development of multiple food hypersensitivities.

Another cause of bowel inflammation leading to systemic absorption of large food antigens and predisposing to the development of food allergy is Candida overgrowth. Candida is a yeast that is normally in happy balance with other yeast and bacteria in the bowel. When antibiotics, a high sugar diet, prednisone and other agents are used, the intestinal flora becomes imbalanced since these stimulate wild, uncontrolled growth of the yeast. This yeast can inflame the bowel so badly it mimics irritable colon, spastic bowel and colitis of many forms. If yeast overgrowth is the problem, a three month trial of the Candida program will leave no doubt and it is used thereafter as needed.

Along with restoring the flora, the use of acidophilous is important in recolonizing the bowel with proper bacterial flora. In other words, putting back some "good" bacteria to aid in assimilation of food as well as compete with Candida has often been of major help with these bowel problems.

The same is true of pancreatic and digestive enzymes. For some individuals the difference with and without these is dramatic. It is logical that there may be a defective secretion of gastric and pancreatic enzymes to aid digestion; however, these enzymes are rarely prescribed. Sometimes it is as simple as a lack of acid secretion in the stomach or biocarbonate from the pancreas.

Giardia lamblia is a protozoa infection that is endemic in the United States. It is easy to get and difficult to diagnose. Therefore, a trial of metronidazole prescribed by your doctor is worth a therapeutic trial.

Next, some have vitamin deficiencies, which are reflected in inflamed tissues with the GI tract as the target organ. Some of the most common deficiencies I see are vitamin A, C, B6, B5, folic acid, intracellular magnesium and zinc, and essential fatty acids. If taurine, an amino acid crucial to bile formation and also integral in stabilizing the cell membrane against the effects of Candida, is deficient, the symptoms remain recalcitrant.

And a hyperpermeable gut or the leaky gut syndrome can be the sole cause (see **THE LEAKY GUT SYNDROME**). Until the hyperpermeable gut is healed, most forms of colitis are considered "incurable". But as we have repeatedly witnessed, "incurable" merely means that that doctor is unfamiliar with the total load. A nutritionally oriented ecologist can guide the patient through this maze.

Usually, when a patient arrives at this point and is no better, I have a fairly good idea that usually injections to the foods will simmer him down.

Peter was a 27-year-old who had fourteen bloody bowel movements a day for eleven years. He had had two small bowel resections when he had severe bouts of bleeding. Within two weeks of food injections, he was down to two to three bowel movements a day unless he cheated on his diet or forgot his injections.

Usually we have to cover the total inhalant load with injections to dust, molds and pollens as well. These patients often have hidden inhalant allergies anyway in the form of chronic sinusitis, headache or asthma. In fact, in some, colitis is no different from asthma. The latter is a smooth muscle spasm in response to inhaled antigens. Any other target organ, for instance, the bowel, can have the same smooth muscle spasm in response to a stimulus.

Ramond was a 39-year-old printer whose wife caught on quickly to what I was leading up to and exclaimed, "You know, your proctitis is always worse every fall!" Putting him on the diet and giving inhalant injections has left him happy as a lark with the freedom he now enjoys. He rapidly healed his rectal ulcers and fistulaes much to the amazement of his proctologist. He has remained clear for four years.

The unlucky ones are what we call universal reactors because they not only have food and inhalant sensitivities, but they also have chemical allergies. When they are exposed to natural gas or specific levels of formaldehyde, they suffer bowel spasms (just like the bronchi of the lungs do in asthmatics). Strict environmental controls as explained in Dr. Theron Randolph's, An Alternative Approach to Allergy, are necessary for these patients to be clear of symptoms. Some require a workup in an environmental unit to get clear.

Chemical hypersensitivity is particularly difficult for many to conceive of, yet it is the basis of much chronic disease. You know if you breathe carbon monoxide, even though you don't smell it, you can die of poisoning since any gas you breathe can pass from the lungs into the bloodstream. One person can breathe natural gas from the oven and get severely depressed; another can breath formaldehyde emitted from new office interior and become dizzy, nauseated and unable to concentrate. Someone else can breath phenol from plastics and have arthritis. These are common reactions.

For Lydia, one night in a newly refurbished hotel room (containing much formaldehyde) can kick up her severe leg phlebitis, which she cleared with diet, environmental controls and inhalant injections. She has multiple sensitivities and chemicals are included.

Inhaled chemical vapors can cause contractions of the smooth muscle of the bronchus causing asthma; of the smooth muscle of the cerebral vessels causing migraine; of the smooth muscle of the intestine causing relentless cramps and diarrhea.

Of course, no person with any bowel problem should forget to have a trial of a yeast-free, sugar-free diet, Nizoral and pure Nystatin powder for three months. Yeast overgrowth, especially after antibiotics, prednisone, pregnancy, surgery or with diabetics can be the mysterious culprit, or at least part of it. Read Dr. William Crook's, The Yeast Connection.

However complicated this may seem, once you have identified the triggers of your colitis, life is a great deal more pleasurable. You may be hesitating before embarking on trying to pinpoint the causes, but remember, you have your whole life to have colitis and its resultant, mutilating surgeries. So, why not see if you can discover in a few short weeks what you need to know to have complete control over your bowel?

Pamela came accompanied by an enthusiastic and supportive spouse. Since the birth of her last child six years ago, life had been a nightmare with her colitis and she was being pressured by the gastroenterologist to have her colon removed and wear a colostomy bag.

Her symptoms? Twelve bloody bowel movements a day. Her medications? An incredible 40 mg. of prednisone, cortisone enemas, Azulfidine four times a day and an opiate derivative to try to control the spasm and pain. Her age? Thirty-two.

When I say enthusiastic, I mean more than that. They were far too intelligent to waste time in stages of denial or procrastination. They never once tried to bargain for foods. They knew I wasn't Dr. Claire Voyant. Instead, they dug in, tested, started inhalant and food injections, the Candida program, corrected nutritional deficiencies and cleaned up the house. The payoff? Within two months she was on no_medication for the first time in six years and she now had two normally formed, bloodless, painless bowel movements a day. They were ecstatic and have remained so for twelve years.

We don't have all the answers yet and we certainly don't know if all colitis victims have ecologic triggers. We are not able to help all comers. All we know is we have a few tools that mainstream medicine should become well-versed in, because of the starling improvement in the majority of peoples lives that we have had the privilege of helping. The beauty of it all is that not only have these modalities totally cleared many colitis victims, but they are far safer than the barrage of medications that is currently required that doesn't provide nearly the relief. So, what are you waiting for?

ARE CHIROPRACTORS QUACKS?

"All chiropractors are quacks." At least that is what they told us in medical school. We were told, "They claim to move bones around, but how incredible! Bones are so firmly attached by ligaments and tendons, it would be impossible to move them." In addition, these chiropractors further claim that these magical adjustments of bones cause certain medical problems to disappear. Over the years, many patients would come in the office and confide in me that they had been to a chiropractor and that it really helped them. I always said to myself, "I wish I had a back problem so that I could go to a chiropractor and see what they do." Finally, one day I got my "wish." When I did get my back problem, I hurt so much that I didn't dare go to a chiropractor because I was sure that they would injure me further.

I damaged my back with many horseback riding falls while trying to learn to train and jump horses. (They call it "breaking" a horse - but I know which one of us was broken). As the pain increased, I just took more and more medication and tried to ignore it (especially since I already had all my other E.I. symptoms in addition to this gift!). Over the years, the pain got so bad that I would slide in and out of bed on my stomach; I would get up an hour early so that I could work through the pain and stiffness, to be able to get into my panty hose and arrive at the office walking normally.

After a while, it hurt so much that I found myself riding less and less, crawling in on my hands and knees from weekend gardening and living on pain drugs. Finally, I went to an orthopedic surgeon and had x-rays, suspecting that I would probably need disc surgery. He just laughed and said that I didn't even have a disc anymore. What I had were two raw bones grinding on each other and pinching the nerves that ran down my legs, giving me the severe back and leg pain and numbness that I constantly endured to varying degrees for the last few years.

He said that there was nothing I could do except wear a special corset and continue taking the medication. I was in tears when I left his office, not only because I was in such pain but also because now I was left with no hope. I was to see this same theme repeated many times in medicine: the attempts to strip people who are desperate of all hope. I consulted another orthopedic surgeon who was a great deal more knowledgeable. He had me enroll in a physical therapy program to strengthen my back muscles to support these rickety old bones. Indeed, after several months of two hours of physical therapy exercises every single day with eight pound leg weights on my ankles, my back was improving. I was so religious about the exercise that if I calculated the next day provided no time for them, I got up at 4 am to do them. I could get in and out of the car without bursting into tears from the pain. I also was fitted with a fiberglass cast that I strapped on whenever I did any riding or gardening or water skiing. It was terribly uncomfortable but allowed me to get some activity that I desperately needed. If I attempted to do anything physical without the cast, I was laid up for several days with severe pain. But I felt I would go mad without exercise.

After six months of daily exercises, I had definite improvement, but still I had daily pain and was taking so many Darvons I was worried that I was going to become a drug addict. Periodically once a week I would make sure that I took no medications so that I could be sure that I was not having withdrawal symptoms. Indeed, nothing happened except I just plain hurt.

After four years of this, I must have gotten too muscular since I was not taught to do any stretching exercises. As a result, the exercises started making me worse and I would have more severe pain with the exercises and had to stop them.

In about the sixth year of chronic daily medication,

I was in Texas giving an allergy lecture. My back was extremely painful at that time. One of my fellow lecturers and partner of Dr. Rea, Dr. Alfred Johnson, happened to have a D.O. degree and he told me he could fix my back. I lay down on a table and he did a manipulation. In less than half-a-minute, the stabbing pain in my left sacro-iliac joint was completely relieved. I felt naked without the daily pain that had become a part of me for years! I enthusiastically inquired how I could find someone to do this at home. When I got back home, I found a chiropractor who would do manipulations fairly similar to what I had experienced. Within a short time, I found that I was progressively getting more and more relief from these twice a week manipulations. Within a few weeks, I was off medication for the first time in ten years.

Whenever I had that stabbing, knife-like pain in the left side, I merely had to have a manipulation and it was gone in seconds. Indeed, our teachers in medical school have done a disservice to us by incorrectly bad-mouthing chiropractors. Also, they have done us a disservice by not teaching us chiropractic manipulations. Look at all the medications we could have spared people over the years had we known how to "crack backs." By attempting to discredit chiropractors (question motive; economic greed), doctors have marred their own credibility.

I was further shocked to learn that chiropractors prescribed vitamins and natural foods and are generally more aware of nutrition than medical doctors.

There is another interesting aspect of back pain and that is that many people have severe muscle spasm, pain and muscle weakness in areas of former injuries and former polio. And this pain is commonly caused by chemical and food hypersensitivities. For example, if I am in a shopping mall more than an hour-and-a-half, I have severe back pain and I don't know if I'm going to throw up or pass out. However, there is no physical limitation. I can bend and twist and move every way possible, but I am hunched over form the severe pain. After an hour outside in the fresh air, I am laughing. Most people would think I was the biggest hypochondriac they had every seen. What has happened is I have aired out my system.

In airplanes, I get painful muscle spasms across my upper back and neck that last two days. It can be precipitated by someone applying nail polish behind me and last for four days.

Formaldehyde and other chemicals tend to give people who are susceptible to them severe muscle spasm and pain. Natural gas in a tightly closed home is a common culprit. Some people only have chemically induced symptoms in foam-insulated houses or in their office buildings. Others get pain as their reaction to specific foods: beef, tomatos, potatos, peppers and chocolate are common causes of arthritic pain. Likewise is formaldehyde in mattresses and seat cushions. That is why we use our aluminum foil covers.

The causes are specifically different from person to person. Of course, anti-oxidants, such as vitamin C, E, A, zinc, magnesium, cysteine, zinc, B6, DMG and selenium are only a sample of those necessary in helping the detox system cope with chemical pollutants.

Thanks to the great teachings that osteopaths, like Dr. Alfred Johnson of the Dallas Environmental Unit and chiropractors, like Dr. Jean Cohen, Dr. Dale Cohen, and Dr. Steve Wechsler of Syracuse have exposed me to, and thanks to the knowledge of ecologic illness that I have gained from Dr. William Rea of the Environmental Unit in Dallas, I have been able to improve musculoskeletal disorders which were resistant to medications.

ADDENDUM: I recently read that in 1966 the A.M.A. publically spoke out so strongly against chiropractors that they threatened to oust any doctor who referred to them.

Twenty years later, many knowledgeable physicians refer to them and insurances cover their services. In fact, it is well-known that injured people are able to return to work more quickly with the aid of chiropractic manipulations.

We have found that the frequent need for adjustment on a chronic basis is a sign of environmental, especially chemical, overload. Many chiropractors are aware of this also and appropriately refer these people for ecologic management. When someone requires frequent adjustments, that is a sure sign of environmental overload. As an example we might find chemical and food triggers as well as nutrient deficiencies. For example, my back x-ray still looks horrid with now 2 missing discs, bone on bone, and many arthritic spurs. But I have no problem, water ski backwards, slalom, horseback ride, golf, and wind surf in the middle of the ocean. But if I wanted I could be bed ridden within a week. The trigger? Eat any of the night shades (white potato, any peppers (red, green, yellow, jalapeno, chili), cayenne, tomato, eggplant, paprika, curry, MSG, modified food starch, potato water in breads, commercial soups, foods with hidden "spices"), get over exposed to formaldehyde or natural gas, or become deficient again in magnesium and manganese.

Many people we have seen who were signed up for disc surgery. But with these techniques they, like me, became pain free and never had surgery. (For details, and special detoxification procedures necessary in order to get free of pain, see **Wellness Against All Odds**.) In the meantime, however, the manipulations certainly give tremendous relief and save us from many drugs. It is fascinating and uplifting to discover there are so many alternative therapies that offer new levels of wellness.

SECTION IX
THE NUTS AND BOLTS OF IMMUNOLOGY

How to Choose an Allergist

In the early 1900's, it was discovered that an extract of ragweed pollen could be made by grinding up the ragweed and mixing it with a little bit of water. A superficial scratch was then made on the skin of the person to be tested and a drop of this solution (extract) was placed on the skin. If the person had antibodies to ragweed, (that is, was allergic to ragweed) the area surrounding the nick soon became red and itchy or it might even wheal (that is, create a lump like a hive). From this rudimentary knowledge, the sophisticated extracts and testing procedures that we have come to know today were derived.

The Prausnitz-Kustner test was also used for awhile, especially for testing babies. If a baby was thought to be allergic, but his skin was so diseased that it was difficult to find a clear space on which to test him or he was just too tiny, the following method could be used: some of the baby's serum was injected under his mother's skin, and then she was tested in that same spot to determine if the baby was allergic.

A tube of his blood was drawn and the serum was extracted (separated from) by high speed spinning of the tube (centrifugation). A tiny amount of this serum was injected just under the skin (intradermally) of his mother. Then, in this same site, an extract of dust, for example, could be injected. It would also be injected in another site on the mother's skin where the baby's serum had not been injected. Then, if the site of the baby's serum and house dust reacted (but the site of dust alone on the mother did not react), it would be assumed that the baby was allergic to house dust and the mother was not. This is also called a passive transfer test.

521

Although these tests are a very clever way of demonstrating the presence of an allergic antibody in another patient, they are very time-consuming and there is always the risk of spreading serum disease, such as hepatitis or syphilis. As the years went on, the extracts got more sophisticated. It was found that as the extracts were kept over a period of time, they lost their potency and did not react as well. So, chemicals were added to maintain the potency of the extracts as well as their sterility. As things sit around, they tend to develop bacterial and fungal contamination and have to be thrown out because they are no longer fit for injecting into humans. So, antibacterial agents were added.

Gradually, the field of conventional allergy as it is known today evolved where allergy extracts are made with additives like phenol, glycerin and human serum albumin. Usually, after a history is taken, the allergist can tell just how sensitive the patient is going to be and he will screen with a prick test method. Just a prick of the skin is made under the drop of testing extract. When the amount of reactivity of the patient is determined this way, then further tests are done with intradermal testing where a small amount of the testing extract is actually injected under the first layer of skin to form a little bleb or bump. In five, ten and twenty minutes, it is looked at to see if the bleb or bump has grown into a **hive (wheal)** and if there is surrounding **redness (erythema or flare)**. It is this wheal and flare reaction that tells us that antibodies are being made against that substance. This is taken as a sign of positive reaction to that extract. It suggests that this substance should be avoided in the environment and probably included in the final allergy injection mixture.

The value of this method is that many people can be tested quickly and easily by the allergist's technicians. The problem with it is that it is not highly individualized. It is sort of like the panty hose commercial where "one size fits all" because one dose strength is used for testing most people. If there is a reaction under that intradermal injection (redness, swelling, hive or erythema), then it is considered positive and the patient is given this extract along with all the other positives. Likewise, the dosage schedule is not highly individualized since everyone starts at a low dose and gradually builds up to a predetermined high dose. If they start having reactions, they stop where they are and cannot go to higher doses.

Anyway, in the nine years of practicing this type of conventional allergy, we would frequently see people with classic allergic stories (chronic headache, sinusitis, asthma, recurrent respiratory infections with constant sore throats and recurrent ear infections) who would be negative to all the tests! We still to this day see many people who say they were tested by a conventional allergist only to be told they weren't allergic enough to receive injections. Their stories tell us they are obviously allergic!

Therefore, we started doing nasal provocations. On the end of a toothpick we placed a small amount of dust, mold or pollen and we had the person sniff it. Usually the patient would get stuffy or wheezy and say, "This is the headache I've been trying to tell the neurologist about!" If we gave a placebo, no symptom was produced. In this way, we could show that the symptoms were triggered by inhaled antigens and that the conventional testing route was not adequate to diagnose them.

Allergists got even lazier a few years ago and jumped on the band wagon of the RAST (radioallergosorpent test). This test was acclaimed to do what the PK test did in a test tube. In other words, it was supposed to show where a person had antibodies to a certain material. The problem with the test is that it is not that sensitive and it is four times more costly. I can show you many people who have wild reactions to certain antigens and their RAST's are negative. In one published study, researchers took many samples of the same serum and sent it all over the country to the best labs for a RAST determination. The values they received varied from 4 to 621 I.U.! So, you can see it is not a dependable test despite its high cost; therefore, it should rarely be used.

Before the middle of this century another method became popular, particularly in the Midwest. It is called the Rinkle method or serial dilution end-point titration (SDET). This method will make more sense to you even though you are not an allergist because it considered individual needs rather than using the same dose for everybody. Let me explain. One strength of house dust is put on the skin and observed. If no reaction, then a second dose which is five times stronger is applied and observed. Again, if no reaction, then another which is five times stronger. When we find a point where you react (that is, you get redness and a hive), then we know that the strength just before that is the highest dose that your body, at this point in time, can tolerate without a reaction. This then is the dose that is chosen for your treatment extract for that particular substance or antigen. If no reaction occurs, no antigen is given, obviously. Controls are also used.

For many people, symptoms can be turned off within a few days or weeks of injections rather than waiting years. For many, the dose never needs to be raised and only the interval between injections needs to be extended as they get better coverage of their symptoms. However, others need to have the dose raised to get relief.

For example, a young girl, 23, was sent here from four hours away by her physician brother. She had headaches for six years. She had all the workups, including CAT scans of her brain. We tested her and found she was very sensitive to many genera of the new molds we had introduced to testing. When she came back for further tests, I examined her and she said her headache was terrible that day. I was glad because we were now going to give her her first injection of her molds. Within ten minutes her headache was gone!

This method is much more individualized; it is a fine- tuning, increase in precision. We let the body of each person tell us the top tolerated dose to every one of his antigens. We do not see nearly the amount of anaphylactic reaction that we did with conventional testing where everyone was receiving the same canned dose. We also see quicker results, usually within the first few months, if environmental controls are incorporated into the program.

When I came back from Kansas City after learning this method, I couldn't help but say to myself, "Wait a minute. If this is so good, how come all the other allergists in my area don't use it?" So, for three-and-a-half years I did every other patient that walked in the door with conventional rather than serial dilution end-point titration. The result: there was no comparison. The serial dilution titration method was far better.

I must add that due to my indoctrination in allergy, I was initially opposed to going to a course to learn this. It was my far more intelligent husband who saw the logic and decided we should be open-minded and investigate this technique.

Since that time, there have been articles in the **Journal of Allergy and Clinical Immunology** and the **New England Journal of Medicine** (August 16, 1988, Jewett D, et al) saying that the serial dilution end-point titration method is no better than placebo or water injections. The fallacy with these studies is that they were carried out at prestigious medical centers where the investigators were well-versed in conventional techniques but not well versed in SDET. It took us months to teach this technique to our staff. No one from the universities ever came to our courses or offices to learn it. They just read about it and did the study! Obviously, if you want a method to fail, give it to someone who is not well-versed in it to test it out. For sure you will have failures. For one study they were so outrageously ignorant of the technique that they used the dose that turns on symptoms for the one to turn them off. The neutralizing doses in the other studies were thirteens. There were many errors in their methodology besides their neutralizing doses being far from "normal" (even given the possibility that they had only exceptionally sensitive patients).

It would be like my reading a book on brain surgery and then saying all brain surgery is fatal because everyone I operated on died. I'm sure they would all die, since I have no neurosurgery training and a four hour crash course wouldn't help much. Likewise, no medical schools, including these, teach SDET. In order for SDET to become accepted gospel, it must emanate from a medical school! Studies are not accepted and in fact are rejected when they are submitted using SDET. Can you believe that adult physicians and "scientists" conduct themselves this way?

If you find it hard to believe as I did, read **Wellness Against All Odds** for documentation of really dishonest "science." Serial dilution titration indeed works well for the inhalant antigens. These are the things that we inhale such as dust, dust mite, molds and all the pollens of the grass, tree and weed family. However, this method does not work for food or chemical allergies. Also, there is a small group of highly sensitive people for whom it cannot be used because they cannot tolerate testing several antigens at a time. They must have only one needle placed on the skin at a time or they will have severe reactions.

Hence, the provocation-neutralization method must be used for foods and chemicals for everyone and for inhalants for the highly sensitive individual. With this method, one dose of the suspected food or chemical is injected intradermally. Then, seven to ten minutes is allowed to pass during which time the patient's symptoms are observed. At the end of this time, the wheal is measured.

If it has not grown, a higher dose can be put on. If it has caused redness and a hive or has produced a symptoms, then the preceding lower dose is the treatment dose to be selected. With this method, people are often provoked to display the very symptoms that they have been seeking relief for.

For example, it is not at all unusual to be testing someone to a food and have him have an asthma attack or a severe migraine or a loss of voice, stuffiness or arthritis pain. Sometimes he may fall asleep right in the middle of testing; only after the neutralizing dose has taken effect will he fully awaken. Of course, this falling asleep (narcolepsy) was one of his symptoms for which no cause was known. Other people burst into tears or have flagrant personality changes. Most of the time we will not trigger reactions, however, because we rarely have a need to make anyone feel any worse than they already do. So we try to stay in a safe range where we do not expect reactions.

When the neutralizing or treatment dose is then applied, the symptoms are relieved. This shows the patient that not only is he sensitive to that antigen, but that the neutralizing dose is able to turn the reaction off.

Some physicians do the provocation with sublingual drops. That is, a drop of the solution under the tongue instead of injections under the skin. With this method, the person opens his mouth and the drop is placed under the tongue. It is allowed to be absorbed just like sublingual nitroglycerin would be and then the patient is observed for symptoms. A problem with this method is that if he doesn't have any symptoms with this test, there is no wheal or skin reaction to watch.

Often, even though a reaction doesn't occur, a sensitivity to that substance exists and we need to use the dose obtained from watching the response of the wheal for treatment. So, you can see why the provocation done intradermally is more preferable. For example, strawberries make me break out within eight hours. If tested sublingually, nothing would happen to me. So, it would be assumed that I was negative to strawberries and they would not have been included in my shot. However, I needed to have them in my shot to be able to eat them.

Some allergists, however, give the treatment dose (after testing intradermally) by sublingual drops instead of having the patient inject it under his skin. I was very skeptical that this would work, so I asked Dr. Doris Rapp, (an excellent pediatric ecologist in Buffalo, New York, whose book, **The Impossible Child**, will be especially appreciated by parents), to test me by intradermal provocation- neutralization, the method we both use, to about twenty of my foods and make up sublingual drops so that I could see if they were as efficacious as the intradermal injections. Sure enough, they worked just as well. If I didn't use either method, I was broken out within a few days with eczematous dermatitis on my face. If I used the drops and ate the foods that were in the drops, I was clear. If I ate foods that were not in the drops, then I had problems. I had to use the drops after every meal. The injections I only needed every few days.

Dr. Rea tells me, however, that drops are only effective for about 80% of the people; the other 20% must have intradermal injections. Therefore, it makes more sense to have intradermal injections unless you have a pediatric practice such as Dr. Rapp has. I am sure her little patients appreciate the lack of needles in their treatment.

There are other tests, such as cytotoxic tests, which, like the RAST, can never give as much information as the patient's actual body can. There are too many other variables inside that test tube which can cause many people to have negative cytotoxic tests even though they are actually sensitive in real life to a particular antigen.

So, being the guinea pig that I am, I tested the various methods on myself: the serial dilution titration or Rinkle method, Dr. Miller's (derived from Dr. C. Lee) provocation-neutralization methods for foods and for chemicals and Dr. Rapp's sublingual methods. This enabled me to evaluate these methods personally without using my patients as guinea pigs.

One of the problems is that as environmental medicine becomes more popular, there are going to be more and more "overnight specialists." These are people who think that they know how to do the serial dilution end-point titration and provocation-neutralization methods because they have taken some quickie courses.

Unfortunately, the young American Academy of Environmental Medicine (A.A.E.M.), formerly the Society for Clinical Ecology, is slow in formulating its accreditation procedures. This is to be expected with any new discipline. So, it is going to be very difficult for the person with an environmental illness to find an appropriately trained physician. But the highest certification available now is Board certification by the A.A.E.M.. Drs. Rapp, Rea, and others of us write and administer the courses and tests along with others and we are continually trying to upgrade the courses and exams.

It is interesting that since 1951 when Dr. Randolph discovered chemical sensitivity, not one single thing that we have talked about has been disproven. In fact just the opposite. Everything we have talked about at first was not believed, and then was eventually proven. Think about it: Chemicals in our drinking water, formaldehyde in our homes, radon in our basements, etc.

A conventional allergist will be unable to help you in terms of food and chemical allergies and he may or may not be able to help you with inhalant allergies. However, there are still many of our patients who are on the old conventional methods and there is no question it helps many with their inhalant allergies. In fact, my asthma, headaches and sinusitis were all cleared with conventional allergy techniques. However, now I would not do well with them because the conventional doses cause reactions in me. I became very sensitive to the phenol preservative that is in all of them. The problem was that after years of conventional injections, I was developing sore and swollen arms, (about the size of an orange) after injections and this persisted for three or four days. If I lowered the dose, I didn't have as much symptom relief. However, when I switched myself over to the individually titrated serial dilution titration (Rinkle method) I had better relief from my symptoms and I no longer had the sore swollen arms. I had even better control of symptoms than I had had prior. We have since seen this with many patients.

So, how does the conventional allergist go about expanding his repertoire to the treatment of all environmental allergies? Not very quickly nor very easily. After having taken several courses and observed in offices, it takes about three years of experience in one's own office to become proficient in Rinkle titration to inhalants. Meanwhile, he should also learn the provocation- neutralization technique which will take another two or three years to become proficient in. It is going to take him about one to six years to train his personnel and himself and become proficient in these newer techniques. Remember, there is no one in his office to show him what he is doing wrong and correct him as he goes along. He must learn by himself since there is no residency. So, he must be in constant communication with those who do it well.

He must also completely change the physical nature of his office, making it safer for chemically sensitive people. He must develop a tremendous stockpile of resources for the many needs of E.I. patients. He will find he is spending about ten times more time with each individual patient than he did with the conventional approach. The history-taking, patient instruction and education will be very time consuming. He will shortly learn that as well as having to work harder, he will be making less money. Also, he will have to spend a great deal of time dealing with the anger, hostility and distrust that these patients carry with them, many have been labelled neurotic when no diagnosis could be found and loathe doctors.

I think some of the hallmarks that would be useful in determining whether your doctor is proficient are whether he has studied with any of the leading ecologists and how long and whether he has preservative-free extracts. Preservative- free extracts, or at least phenol-free extracts, are presently available in probably no more than a dozen offices around the country. They are truly the hallmark of a serious ecologist. It will increase as time goes by because we realize the need for them.

However, without having chemicals in the extracts, there are a great number of difficult and very expensive problems that arise for the allergist. First, his testing and treatment extracts must be destroyed and made up totally fresh every six to eight weeks because they will decrease in potency and lose their sterility. Even unused ones must be thrown out. They must be kept frozen at other times because there is no preservative. This requires a great deal of time, expense and dedication. On the other hand, a conventional allergist's extracts will last years or until they are actually used up.

In Dr. Rea's office, they even go one step further - the foods used for the preparation of the extracts are not purchased in powdered form from a commercial allergy laboratory but are made from organic foods so that the antigens themselves are insecticide and pesticide free. This to me is the ultimate in allergy extracts and I don't see how it can be improved upon in the future. Unfortunately, it is a laborious, expensive and time-consuming technique, but the results are well worth it. We have started it for select patients.

A serious clinical ecologist will have an ever-expanding repertoire of resources for patients and a network of people constantly contributing to it. They most likely will organize a H.E.A.L. group with a newsletter and promote lectures on the subject in the local area. Most importantly, a dedicated physician will want to nourish your mind and mental growth. He will supply books galore. For without knowledge, you can never become a partner in your care. And without being a partner, you have very little hope for recovery.

By now, you realize that you are not looking for a conventional allergist. A conventional allergist does not use the titrated individualized method. He does not use newer mold plates nor test the newer molds. He does not test extensively for foods and chemicals and he does not concern himself with the possibility that you may have a Candida infection or nutritional deficiencies. In fact, most vehemently deny the existence of Candida and nutritional deficiencies. As of 1993 the American College of Allergy and Immunology gave a full day's course showing doctors that chemical sensitivity was mostly a psychiatric disease.

What you are looking for is a specialist in environmental medicine. Actually, you are lucky if you have one within a four hundred mile radius of your home, for there are only a couple hundred of us in the U.S. But there are doctors in every town who, with a little coaxing from you, could become one, once they see the light and are ready. For the one nearest you, write or call the A.A.E.M. (Resources).

The Immune System

What is the immune system? It consists of different types of cells all with specific functions. Mainly B cells make antibodies to bacteria. Without the immune system we would die, for we would have no antibodies to fight the infectious organisms that abound. If the immune system becomes overactive as it does with leukemia, we die, too.

532

So, as with most things in life, there is a delicate range of function or balance. If we veer on either side too far from the normal balance, bad things happen.

If you are exposed to a Streptococcus, you make antibodies against it. This enables you to fight off the next exposure even quicker. If you are injected with tetanus toxoid, your B cells make antibodies against tetanus toxin so you don't get lockjaw from wounds infected with Clostridia tetanae. If a normal person is exposed to ragweed, nothing happens because the body knows ragweed is harmless. However, if I am exposed to it (or anyone with the right genetics to become allergic) my body makes large numbers of allergic antibodies called IgE, and these antibodies are directed against the ragweed. Then, when I am exposed again, these antibodies attach to cells that then release histamine to cause water, itchy eyes, tremendous exhaustion, sneezing and wheezing.

T cells govern the B cells and tell them when and how many antibodies to make. They also tell them when to stop making antibodies. Exposures to certain chemicals damage T cells and cause them to function aberrantly. When they behave their worst, we have cancer. Less serious problems are types of arthritis, colitis and all the other symptoms of environmentally-induced immune dysfunction. Some of these diseases are called autoimmune because the antibody attacks a part of the body as viciously as it would a streptococcal antibody. It doesn't know any better. Arthritis is an example of this, where antibody and antigen attach to joint synovium or lining and cause the destruction that results in pain and deformity.

In rheumatoid arthritis (RA), the bad antibody is not IgE but IgM. It is directed against our very own antibody IgG! The IgM:IgG immune complex is determined by a blood test called rheumatoid factor. Actually, everyone makes rheumatoid factor (RF). Yes, all normal people make it. But, their T suppressor cells say, "That is enough! Don't

533

make any more than a smidgeon." In people with RA, the T cells were damaged by a virus, chemical, nutrient deficiency, hormone imbalance or hypersensitivity to food or other environmental antigen. So, the body goes wild and creates large amounts of this antibody to cause destructive and painful joint deformity. If the causes are found early, the disease can be turned off or attenuated. When causes are looked for after much damage has been done, obviously the damage cannot be reversed but often the pain and progression of the disease can be arrested.

What is an antigen? An antigen is anything your body reacts to by producing an antibody. It can be the measles virus, tetanus injection, ragweed, poison ivy, strawberries, beef, sugar, natural gas, etc. For some of these antigens we have not found the antibody, and, indeed, the symptoms may be caused by a mechanism other than antibody production (Prostaglandin, T cells, macrophage, DNA or membrane dysregulation, etc.). So, in a more correct sense, they are termed incitants or idosyncratic hypersensitivities.

What is an antibody? An antibody is a protective protein molecule that the body makes when it is exposed to something that it sees as harmful. Normal people make antibodies to Staphylococcus, Streptococcus, tuberculosis and measles. Abnormal ones, like me, make them to dust, molds, foods, etc. When the antibody is made normally to fight infection, it attaches to cells to make them release chemicals that kill the infecting organism. When an antibody is made in abnormal amounts, as in allergic people, it attaches to different cells to cause them to release histamine. This causes our allergic symptoms by making leaks or holes in vessels and tissues. This allows body chemicals and antibodies to leak into areas where they normally do not have access. This is the gatekeeper stage. Being in contact with tissues that are not normally touched by them, these body chemicals and antibodies trigger more chemicals to be released and may in turn trigger more reactions.

What is allergy? Allergy is an abnormal reaction to something. Conventional allergists limit their area of expertise to allergy where an IgE antibody can be demonstrated, as in ragweed allergy. They do not yet acknowledge foods that cause immune complexes or IgG antibodies to be formed, chemical reactions involving prostaglandins and other mechanisms that produce symptoms in response to environmental triggers.

What is the T cell system? It is the system of helper cells (whose function it is to turn on) and suppressor cells (whose function it is to turn off) which regulate (control) what types and amounts of antibodies are made. In allergic people there is damage to the T suppressor cells that are supposed to limit antibody production. Instead, we allergic people make IgE antibodies to a multitude of environmental agents. Basically, cancer and AIDS victims have too many T suppressor cells and literally wipe out their own defenses. We with allergies and autoimmune diseases (arthritis, colitis, etc.) make far too few suppressors and our bodies respond and make antibodies to everything!

In order that you will not be intimidated by doctors who might be tempted to quiet you by using immunologic lingo, I think you need to know some immunology. The problem is that when you are done with this, you will probably know more than most physicians and this will be even more intimidating to them than your knowledge of environmental medicine, which already surpasses theirs. This may only serve to further inflame their fragile egos and make them even more obstinate.
Be kind.

Educate them with compassion and tolerance. Tread delicately. I realize the material is difficult, but, remember now you know how the doctor feels. Plus, he feels intimidated because there seems to be an unwritten rule that he has to know everything about medicine at all times. It doesn't bother them to prescribe daily drugs for which the mechanism of action is unknown. Yet when we get spectacular results with a technique whose mechanism is unknown, it's quackery. Our training and egos don't allow us to say, "I don't understand," or worse, "I don't know." So, skim through and get what you can from this information. Some of you have enough medical knowledge that you will enjoy the insights.

LAB TESTS

In terms of lab tests, when the T suppressor (T-5) cells are phenomenally low, you usually need to be in a unit. There are many types of T-cells. One type that is commonly lacking is NK (natural killer cells). These cells are supposed to be responsible for tumor surveillance. In other words, they are supposed to be on the constant lookout for cancer cells and destroy them immediately upon contact. This is normally an ongoing process in the body. These cells are reduced in number in a surprising number of people with environmentally induced symptoms.

Sometimes we measure the IgE or immunoglobulin E level. This is the level of allergic antibody. If it is high or elevated, we can say fine, you have a high level of allergic antibody. It is usually elevated in people who have mostly inhalant allergies, but there are many people who have the combination of inhalant, food and chemical allergies who have zero or low levels of IgE observed in the blood. This is because IgE may not be responsible for the whole mechanism of their allergic symptom complex and also because IgE is an immunoglobulin which has a tremendous affinity for being in tissue, not floating freely in the bloodstream; floating freely in the bloodstream is the only place where

536

we can measure it. Generally, if the IgE is low then chemical and food problems are probably overriding the inhalants.

The IgE level never, and I repeat, never indicates that you are or are not allergic. Unfortunately, there are many unknowledgeable physicians who tell patients with low IgE levels that they do not have allergies. Many very sensitive people have low or zero levels of IgE. It is a useful adjunct if it is elevated, but it is meaningless if it is low or absent. There is absolutely no blood test that rules out allergy and least of all environmentally-induced illness. So, don't ever let a doctor tell you he did a blood test and found that you are not allergic. Get rid of him fast, for he hasn't the faintest idea of what has gone on in the allergy world in the last fifteen years. If he is not honest with you on this level, how honest will he be on other levels? Also, it shows he does not hold you in high regard and thinks you are dumb enough to believe his authoritative proclamations.

The RAST test is fraught with tremendous insensitivity. It stands to reason that no test-tube test can give as much information as your own body can, but newer versions promise improved sensitivity and we are studying this.

Cytotoxic testing can never be as good as in vivo (testing in the live subject). What happens to cells on a microscope's slide may not parallel what happens to them in your body.

Sometimes we draw formaldehyde levels (formic acid) and these are very helpful, especially in dissuading smokers because these people are usually elevated in smokers.

Analyzing the vitamin level in blood must be approached cautiously because it is highly individual. A normal serum vitamin B-12 level is stated as 200-900 picograms per ml. How was this arrived at? After the test was discovered, readings were taken on about a thousand random people and they found that this is where the "normal" fell. A vitamin B-12 deficiency has serious symptoms - it can cause paralysis and permanent neurologic damage. Yet we don't even know what the normal is for a specific individual. All we can say is if your level falls between 200 and 900 you must be normal. What if you are at 200 but feel best at 900? What if optimal functioning in your sensitive system requires 1200 pg/ml? At this point in time, we can only judge empirically. What if the chronic stress of a disease (such as an allergy or a cold) or a highly chemical diet of junk food causes you to require more? How will we know especially when all the vitamins and minerals require a precise synergistic balance to operate optimally?

In people like myself with inhalant allergies, it has already been proven that an IgE antibody is made. When IgE attaches to the cell membrane, it causes the release from the cell of histamine and other factors which cause our allergic symptoms. Allergy injections stimulate the body to make specific IgG which blocks these so that the IgE cannot attach; therefore, we don't have our symptoms. When IgE attaches to mast cells and causes release of histamine, the result is an opening up of the spaces between cells (gatekeeper phase). Now we get a leakage of fluid which can take many forms - swelling, hives, nasal congestion, bronchial congestion, headache, fluid retention, mood swings, phlebitis and much more.

SRS-A (or leukotriene) is a chemical that is often released with the histamine. It can cause tremendous muscle spasm in the colon, head or chest giving us colitis, vascular migraine or asthma. Other chemicals are released as well, but it appears that the histamine is primarily responsible for the creation of holes in vessels and membranes which cause the fluid leakage and allow reactions to progress to something far more serious than a sneeze or runny nose via the gatekeeper effect.

Conventional allergists only label a condition allergic if the specific IgE (like IgE directed against ragweed) is proven to exist. So, in their strict sense, most food and chemically induced symptomatology is not recognized as an allergy but rather as a hypersensitivity. I don't care what you call it, I just want to do everything in my power to give you control over it. I prefer to use the lay connotation of the word "allergy" which corresponds well with its actual Greek derivation and the dictionary meaning which merely means an altered way of reacting toward something. Very few of the reactions to foods, chemicals, hormones and mediators involve IgE. Conventional allergists tend to restrict themselves to treatment of only IgE allergies. Specialists in Environmental Medicine treat food and chemical sensitivities even though we do not yet know the complete mechanism. The mechanism of most prescription drugs is also unknown, but that doesn't stop anyone.

Things like formaldehyde, natural gas, chlorine and pesticides change cell membranes and wipe out the regulatory parts of the immune and detoxification systems or T cells causing hyper-reactivity or hypersensitivity in those who are genetically predisposed. Chemicals often knock out the T cells that are responsible for telling the B cells to stop making antibody. The T cells that tell B cells to stop making antibody are called T suppressor cells or T-5 cells. When they are injured by chemicals, they don't work well. The B cells go wild and produce all sorts of antibodies that give us allergic symptoms. As well, some chemicals may alter the genetics so that one year you are normal and the next year you have E.I.

The target organ can be anywhere. It may be in the brain where it manifests itself as perception problems. The individual may have difficulty remembering and thinking. It may be in the uterus where it manifests itself as hemorrhaging; the uterus is a smooth muscle that can become inflamed just as easily as the bronchus or the colon. These reactions can be triggered by seasonal antigens, such as ragweed, or perennial antigens, such as foods, causing stomach aches, abortion and menorrhagia (unusually heavy menstrual flow).

When we treat a patient with hormone injections, the treatment is not directed at the organ in supra-physiologic doses as conventional medicine does. It is directed at the immune system where the tiny neutralizing dose for some reason blocks the effect of the exaggerated symptom of the hormone on a receptor. The hormone receptor on the cell is a spot where the hormone normally attaches to direct the cell to respond appropriately to insulin, thyroid, progesterone, etc. If there is an antibody blocking this receptor, no amount of hormone can make the cell work correctly. These people may have symptoms of hypothyroidism, but blood tests leave the doctor saying, "Your thyroid level is normal."

The antibody blocking the hormone receptor site may have been initially directed toward natural gas, cane sugar or a mold. Recall the case of Priscilla who had severe premenstrual depression. She cleared with a neutralizing dose of progesterone that is about 1/1,000th of a therapeutic medical dose.

Although it may sound as though I am knocking conventional medicine, I am not. If it were not for the many miracles of conventional medicine, many of us would not be here. I am only trying to lift the barriers so that the growth of knowledge of ecologic illness is not quite as slow as that of the germ theory in the past. Many life-saving ideas in medicine took decades to become accepted, while people suffered needlessly or died.

Medicine is guilty of blaming the patient for the cause of symptoms if the diagnosis cannot be figured out. Look at all the people with lupus, arthritis, migraines, allergies, colitis, etc., who have been told that it is due to their nerves and that they should see a psychiatrist. When a cause for devastating diseases cannot be found, the patient is told that his disease is either caused by something

540

outside of him like a virus, or nerves. They never consider the possibility of a food, chemical or inhalant that can do the same thing or by the reaction to his own tissues. In other words, the patient must be reacting to himself in the form of an autoimmune disease. These minds are so close and yet so far away from comprehending!

They have only to look one step further beyond the virus and see the multitude of chemicals in the environment that are indeed causing this symptom complex. What impedes their seeing that chemicals are distorting the way the immune system responds to its own tissues and environmental incitants, especially when there are over 5,000 articles in the scientific literature supporting this?

Only you can help yourselves at this point in time because no one else is going to suggest this diagnosis to you and test you for foods and chemicals unless you are fortunate enough to go to one of the few environmental medicine specialists around the country. How many times have you been told, "Whatever you have Mrs. Jones, it is not in my field."

In self-defense, you must know more about politics in medicine than most doctors do. They are too busy in their own fields keeping up with all the new developments (mainly drugs). Little do they know that the diseases of their specialty encroach on a field vastly larger than they ever imagined -that of environmental illness. Frankly, many don't want to know. It is very comfortable knowing all there is to know in one narrow field. How devastatingly inadequate they would feel if suddenly they had to know not only all this new immunology that has come about since they graduated from medical school, but also the ramifications in other parts of the body outside their specialty area. What gastroenterologist wants to hear about your migraines, asthma and depression?

Some relish the newness and ability to expand their usefulness to other areas. All we require at this stage is

541

honesty. State your position up front, Doc. Don't knock a field that has saved thousands of lives just because you haven't read all the supporting literature. Don't mouth interest and then be inadequately trained and poorly motivated. To practice environmental medicine well requires a great deal of effort. To practice it poorly deprives, frustrates and cheats the patient. It gives bad press and slows down the development of the field. Little did I ever suspect years ago that people with severe headaches could get marked relief from histamine, others from serotonin injections and still others from Candida treatment. We are not so far removed from the time when blood letting was the treatment for most illnesses. I still would not believe a bit of this if it hadn't happened to me and if I hadn't been able to turn on and off hundreds of people's symptoms in single- and double-blinded scientific trials. So, I would be the last one to blame doubting doctors for not understanding because I was one of the non-believers once.

There are no medical centers that test for ethanol, formaldehyde or natural gas sensitivity. Patients who do not respond to foods should look to chemical hypersensitivity, nutrition and psychoneuroimmunology for the possible answers. The key for many failures is cleaning up the house and the immediate environment. If you can go anywhere (camping) and get relief, you have gone a long way in making your own diagnosis of maladaptation to the environment as the cause of immune dysregulation. Then, the work is nearly half done. The unfortunate ones require weeks in a meticulously controlled unit to clear and even then not without a stormy course.

So, if you have reached the end of your rope, what do you have to lose? Make a few environmental changes and some dietary changes and go for it. It is immaterial whether you have been labeled neurotic, psychotic, depressed or retarded. What difference is the label? The causes can be toxicities, reactions to certain foods, chemicals, inhalants or nutritional deficiencies. Learn to turn off with no drugs. Diagnose and treat problems through identification and avoidance of environmental incitants.

There were studies at the Banff meeting (17th Advanced Seminar for Clinical Ecology) showing that glomerulonephritis can be triggered in people by hydrocarbon (auto exhaust) exposures. Certainly, it is more economical to find that a person is sensitive to hydrocarbons than to give him a lifetime of expensive renal dialysis at $30,000 a year or involve him in a renal transplant program. After all, most of our governmental medical funds are becoming bankrupt as it is. There are studies to show that hypertension is really ecologic illness caused by the lead and cadmium found in auto exhaust. One study from Pakistan showed that blood pressure could be lowered 15 points by simply getting patients totally out of synthetic fabrics and into natural cotton! (C.E., 1987)

We certainly don't intend to say that the environment is the cause in every disease, but if there is a chance that something I have has such a cause, I sure want to find it!

The Candida problem is, likewise, difficult for those untrained to comprehend. They know that normally Candida is harmless. They know it can be fatal to some with a damaged immune system, as with AIDS or Cancer. They know there is voluminous evidence that many chemicals damage the immune system.

For example, benzene is known to cause leukemia. We know after gassing up your car you have measurable levels of benzene in your bloodstream for several hours. (Laseter)

What they fail to see is the very next step. Chemicals in some of us have damaged another part of the immune system. They haven't damaged the part that causes AIDS or leukemia; they have damaged the part that allows us to control Candida normally. You see, they are correct. Can-

543

dida is harmless, normally. The problem is we are not normal. We are not playing with a full deck. We remain sensitive to Candida, foods or chemicals until each of us lowers our total load sufficiently to bring about the healing that is necessary to again be non-reactive.

You might ask why I did not show before and after photos of myself and that is a good question. When I was as bad as I was, I was so depressed and looked so bad I wouldn't let anyone see me. I took large doses of steroids so that I could be presentable in the office. When I was good (which wasn't too great), I was still red and broken out. I had much denial and I did not want to even think of the disease coming back. I had seriously thought of stopping my shots, environmental controls and the diet in order to get bad for a photo, but frankly, it wouldn't have been worth it. If someone doesn't believe my account, he won't believe a couple of ugly photographs.

I have included a token of Dr. Rea's vascular references. Other than that, the other books that I have mentioned are loaded with references. Doctors love to say, "Well, if this is true, show me the references." The problem is that when you do, they never look them up or read them; they still don't change their ways. If you do need the references, they are available in our subsequent books.

For example, we now know the biochemical mechanism of brain fog (difficulty concentrating, spacey, dopey, depressed, dizzy, nauseous). When a chemical is to be detoxified by the body, there are multiple pathways it can take, depending on the number of other chemicals you are currently detoxing and the availability of nutrients in the detox system. One of the intermediaries that common chemicals break down to is chloral hydrate. Yes, the old Mickey Finn or "knock-out drops" with the exact same symptoms. The acetaldehyde produced by alcohol, Candida and airborne chemicals produces many of these effects as well as strange body aches and the other symptoms of E.I.

that bewilder the unkowledgeable.

Basically, if a chemical can be smelled, then it (osmols) is able to get into your blood stream and cause an immune dysfunction. That is how carbon monoxide gas kills. It gets into your bloodstream and attaches to the red cells so the oxygen cannot. Room deodorants, for example, are an unnecessary encumberment. All they do is produce fatigue of the olfactory system and add chemicals like formaldehyde to your environment. They overwhelm the smelling senses and fatigue them so that you cannot smell whatever it is you are trying to hide. Some people react to them with headache, nausea, irritability or mental sluggishness. The liver becomes overburdened and must detoxify them.

Likewise, inhaled molds react with cells on the nasal mucosa surface and cause symptoms. It is interesting that the U.S. hostage in Iran who was sent home with multiple sclerosis had been held captive in a moldy mushroom cellar before his disease began. Look at how many doctors at an annual Candida Albicans Conference raised their hands in response for a show of hands of physicians who had seen patients with MS who were markedly better after the Candida was appropriately treated with a mold-free diet, injections to mold and huge doses of nystating gradually started. It is known there is a decrease in T-5 cells in MS, so look further for the cause of the T-5 suppression

I am overwhelmed by the amount of arthritis I see that is caused by hidden food allergies and home chemicals. We know that a new carpet takes six to fifteen years to outgas and that particle board (used in kitchen cabinets and sub- flooring) takes about twenty years. Formaldehyde glue is very unstable and hydrolyzes with moisture and heat. In other words, when it is hot and humid, more of it gets into the air and enters the body through the lungs. Latex paint takes a couple of years to outgas and by then it is time to repaint again.

Medical journals are just now discovering the many serious symptoms from latex allergy, only because so many are suddenly using gloves to avoid AIDS. I wonder when it will dawn on them that this very latex is in wall paints? In the meantime, with this heightened exposure, people become more sensitized and are at greater risk of developing additional and more severe chemical hypersensitivities. The overload and compromised detoxification mechanisms develop deficiencies like zinc, B2, selenium, etc. As one deficiency leads to another, there is a domino or snowball effect - you've got it! The spreading phenomenon!

IgE may turn out to be the gatekeeper. The presence of such an antibody, that attaches to a cell and causes the release of histamine which then makes blood vessels leak, opens the gate for chemicals to enter and into contact with parts of cells which are normally protected. This may be the key action site for letting other types of immunologic reactions occur, such as immune complex reactions. That is why I feel compelled not to stop at helping you clear just your inhalant or pollen, dust or mold sensitivities.

In immune complex reactions (like arthritis, thyroiditis, colitis, glomerulonephritis) the body makes an antibody against a certain substance, for example an apple, and this antibody now attaches onto some surface. It could be the kidney causing glomerulonephritis, the skin causing severe eczema or the joints (synovial surfaces) causing arthritis, inflammation and joint destruction. When an antigen or a macrophage-digested piece of antigen, (such as an apple) gets into the blood stream and attaches to an antibody, there is then a chemical reaction leading to the joint destruction, or whatever bad thing that particular antigen-antibody does in that particular target organ in that particular person. That is one reason why even the smallest amount of cheating on the diet can keep a disease process going.

As you will read in the **LEAKY GUT SYNDROME,**

the leaky gut syndrome is the most common cause of all autoimmune diseases. And it is curable! Furthermore enzymes can digest and destroy the damaging auto antibodies that form immune complexes.

It is fascinating that we can turn on one symptom with one particular dose of a food or chemical and then turn it off with the next dose. Remember that these reactions are reproducible. The same has been known for years concerning natural body chemicals. A too low dose of thyroid produces exactly opposite symptoms of what a too high dose can produce. One dose of histamine causes inflammation; a different dose of the same chemical turns off the inflammation. The same occurs with serotonin. Currently, there is voluminous evidence for many body chemicals (histamine), nutrients (vitamin E) and parts of the immune system (complement) that have this same biphasic or dual action.

We already know that the body responds very differently to chemicals that undergo one minute change. Take an epinephrine or adrenaline molecule, for example. If we make one tiny little change at one particular position of the molecule and substitute one different chemical, we now have a molecule that the body now sees totally differently; the body reacts with a different duration of action and different side effects. So, it is easy to see how the body can pick out differences between inhaled chemicals and manifest a variety of symptoms. Indeed, it is a dated physician who denies that chemicals have potent effects on the immune system. It is no longer conjecture.

1) The **Journal of Allergy and Clinical Immunology** and the **Annals of Allergy** have had a plethora of articles in the last couple of years showing that the plastic industry's chemical TDI (toluene diisocyante) causes not only asthma but many other diverse body chemistry disturbances.

2) What doctor hasn't seen or read about the

symptoms of persons whose homes were insulated with urea-formaldehyde foam?

3) The January 1983 **British Medical Journal** cited forty-three patients with rheumatoid arthritis who were treated with penicillamine. The body reacted to the penicillamine and manufactured an antibody to the acetylcholine receptors of muscle, thereby mimicking the disease myasthenia gravis. The disease vanished when penicillamine was taken away.

4) Dr. Rea has much evidence of the role of chemicals and foods in causing vasculitis (see Resources) in the form of angina, phlebitis and more.

5) The February 10, 1993 **New England Journal of Medicine** (308, #6, p 331) explains that already two types of antibodies have been demonstrated in diabetes. They reflect that autoimmunity, such as diabetes, may be spontaneous or the consequence of some external factor such as a chemical agent in the environment. Just as we know some chemically- induced cancers can take twenty to forty years to develop, there is evidence that the antibodies involved in diabetes have been present up to eight years prior to the clinical onset of the disease. Again, a multitude of factors are involved - heredity, nutrition and environment. We know many cancers really start ten to thirty years prior to onset of symptoms. Point in fact: a few years later the same journal showed some children had made milk antibodies that attacked the pancreas, creating diabetes.

Jacoby's, **The Enzymatic Basis of Detoxification**, and Reeve's, **Toxicology**, explain how we can get all the bizarre symptoms of E.I. Each chemical is capable of forming over a dozen other chemicals once it gets in the body. The effects are staggering.

We have a system of macrophages or scavenger cells which clean up all the garbage and things that shouldn't be floating around in the bloodstream. They destroy excess rheumatoid factor, for example, and other harmful antibodies that we make. Maybe the chemicals knock out their scavengering ability as well. Maybe they are defective or overloaded by stress, food and chemical antigens. As a result, they can't clean up as well as they should and so these harmful antibodies settle into areas where they cause disease.

Why do people get worse when they begin fasting? When there is antigen excess of the food that gives you your symptom (you have overdosed on a food) much of the antigen- antibody complexes are in equilibrium and floating around in the bloodstream. So, you feel fine, you have no symptoms; you have had your "fix." When there is an antibody excess (not enough food antigen to bind it), the antibody tends to bind to the target organ and cause a temporary exacerbation of your symptoms (withdrawal phase when you crave your food). The immunologic evidence for this is in Penner, E., et al, Association of Immune complexes, etc., **Int. Arch. Allergy & Appl. Imm.**, 67: 245-253, 1982. Also, fasting depletes the monooxygenase detoxification enzymes in the gut and liver, so you can suddenly be more reactive to foods and chemicals.

Many of the opponents of the titrated method say that low doses do not work, but in his text on allergy by Dr. Elliott Middleton, **Allergy Principles and Practice**, (1978, Mosby and Co.) we see that low doses of antigen produce high affinity antibodies. Low dose therapy causes the production of antibodies that stick to the cell and work better than high dose therapy. In other words, when you use small doses (safer, titrated), you tend to make a more powerful antibody.

Dr. Rea presents a diagram in his article in Gerrard's **Food Allergy** which shows the various things that can happen when vessels leak due to allergic reaction. You can see that a small amount of leaking is called a hive. A larger amount is called a local swelling or edema. A still larger amount might be termed idiopathic fluid retention (we commonly see people who can gain ten to twenty pounds in one day from certain food antigens). Much larger amounts can cause purpura and hemorrhage. Vessel damage is the precursor to all arteriosclerotic disease whether it ends with senility, cerebral vascular accident (stroke) or myocardial infarction (heart attacks from clot or hemorrhage in cardiac vessels). Many chemicals also damage the sodium pump (swelling) and calcium pump (cardiac arrhythmia, high blood pressure). We are so loaded with evidence for the mechanism of E.I. we haven't had time yet to organize it. See the subsequent books for more.

One of the major problems still remaining for people with environmental illness is that if they do not lower their total antigenic load enough, they will experience no improvement whatsoever and then assume that they do not have ecologic illness. Even though they have taken care of the foods and are on an organic rotated diet, they may still never clear if they continue to use a gas heater, drink chlorinated water, wear polyester (formaldehyde) clothes, surround themselves with plastics or if they neglect to use foil and cotton materials on their beds.

We tell you all of this so that you can see how pitiful it is when some physician uses his authority to intimidate you then proceeds to denigrate environmental medicine. I merely want you to have enough knowledge to be able to see through this so that you can choose only those physicians and insurance companies that are truly interested in growing in knowledge, interested in truth, not politics in medicine, and interested in helping you attain maximum health.

E.I. SURVIVORS

In 1951, Dr. Barbara McClintock, working alone in a New York laboratory, made a discovery that was revolutionary. However, it took the scientific world thirty years to acknowledge it and in 1983 she received the Nobel Prize for her "jumping genes." Long before Watson and Crick introduced the DNA helix, and long before the correct number of chromosomes was known, this solo scientist discovered that genetic changes did not have to occur vertically (that is, down through generations) but could occur horizontally (that is, within an organism) and spontaneously. One of the many triggers that could initiate the jump of a gene from one locus on a chromosome to another was shown to be an environmental chemical that was presumed to be harmless. This was one more way nature had for allowing an organism to adapt to its ever-changing environment.

In the same year, 1951, another discovery was made that was also too difficult for scientists to accept. Dr. Theron Randolph in Chicago realized that many people reacted to simple, every day chemicals, such as formaldehyde and phenols found in furniture, carpeting, mattresses, plastics, construction materials and natural gas. The symptoms could be anything imaginable - they mimicked well-known diseases like rheumatoid arthritis, asthma, multiple sclerosis, ulcerative colitis, depression, migraines, angina and thrombophlebitis. Included also are such elusive symptoms as dizziness, panic attacks, nausea, inability to concentrate, chest pain, cardiac arrhythmia, poor memory, extreme unwarranted fatigue, muscle aches, cramps or weakness. Most of these victims had had exhaustive medical exams by numerous specialists who, at the peak of their frustrations, suggested psychiatric referral.

How then, did Dr. Randolph know these people's symptoms were due to chemical exposure? How did he prove they were reacting to levels that other people were comfortably unaware of? He designed a special unit in a hospital with strict environmental controls. No plastics, synthetics, polyesters or cleaning solutions were allowed. Only ceramic tile, metal and wood were allowed. Cotton mattresses (without insecticides or fire retardants), cotton sheets and cotton pillows were used; nurses wore cotton and were not allowed to wear scented cosmetics or toiletries; even patients showered upon arrival and wore only a cotton gown. The air supply was not connected with the rest of the hospital but came through a series of special filters that removed industrial and auto exhaust.

The patients fasted for a week in this chemically clean environment and then the miracles happened. Symptoms that had plagued them for years melted away. When they were totally clear (it varied from days to weeks, depending upon the individual) the testing began.

First, a safe water was found. This may sound incredible, but many had a recurrence of symptoms when they drank chlorinated water (chlorine which is by law added to all municipal water supplies). Nor could spring water be put in plastic containers, for the pthalates leeched into the water and precipitated symptoms in others. Next, foods were introduced, one at each meal to determine which ones were contributing to symptoms. Usually, only unusual or infrequently eaten foods were tested first so that the patient could be guaranteed of having something to eat. So, lion, gazelle or papaya might be on the menu. For it was quickly found and still is today, thirty-five years later, that the foods that also contributed to these people's symptoms were usually the things they loved and ate most often.

For example, many arthritics develop pain and swelling that can last for days and weeks after eating beef, potato, tomato or chocolate. Wheat and sugar have been found to be common causes of depression and hopelessness. Patterns as simple as these are difficult to come by since each person, even though he might have the same disease, has a totally different set of environmental triggers.

Next, when patients were tested to a variety of chemicals that are nearly impossible to escape in twentieth century life, such as phenols, formaldehyde, auto exhaust, toluene and xylene, their original symptoms again recurred.

In some way these twentieth century chemicals damage the immune system or the genetics and create a new sensitivity to environmental pollutants that formerly were tolerated. As this happens, a spreading phenomenon is triggered; now the person begins reacting not only to chemicals but also foods, dusts and molds. In other words, they become sensitive to nearly everything. Thanks to the dedication of Dr. Randolph and his followers, this multitude of sensitivities has been worked out for many and has given them a new lease on life.

How do they live once they return home from such a pure, environmentally controlled hospital unit? A restructuring of lifestyle is necessary. The house, for example, should be electric with heat pump and special air filters. No carpeting or furnishings with formaldehyde-containing foam and polyester. Only materials of wood and metal and hard wood or ceramic tile floors. Cotton mattresses can be special ordered without pesticides and fire retardants. Cotton bedding and clothes are used. No perfumes, scented toiletries or cleansers, only safe non-odorous ones of which there are increasingly more used. Special air filters are installed in an older car which has had foam-filled vinyl seats replaced with cotton.

The diet should be structured. Frequently, allergy injections are given to counter the concomitant dust, mold, pollen, food or chemical sensitivities, but it is a multi-pronged approach that restores the body to health. As you have probably already guessed, not everyone is able to accomplish so much change. Some are lucky and, because they have milder sensitivities, improve with little effort. Others are so sick that they must do all of the above and more in order just to survive. They may never reach a state of healing where they can leave their homes to visit less chemically clean environments, such as other people's homes, offices, schools, churches or stores.

One man I saw had the classic symptoms of chest pain, dizziness, nausea, depression, weakness and inability to concentrate. His symptoms completely stumped his physician and four specialists which included a family practitioner, pulmonologist, allergist, gastroenterologist and industrial hygienist.

Since he was highly intelligent and motivated to help himself, he figured out a temporary makeshift way to feel normal and continue working. He uses oxygen delivered through a ceramic mask with stainless steel tubing (plastic and tygon would cause symptoms) while operating on his patients at the hospital. At home, he sleeps in the garage with the door open despite our freezing New York winters. Is this a sacrifice not worth the price? Not when he is ecstatic to feel normal again and has abrupt recurrence of all symptoms when he stays in the house or office too long. He will soon obtain a house designed to meet his specifications. For those of us who have the disease, when we are sick enough there isn't anything we won't do to feel better.

Despite television coverage, lectures, several books and hundreds of papers over the years, Dr. Randolph's ideas are still vehemently opposed, much as Dr. McClintock's were for thirty years. Now that scientists are finally appreciative of her discovery that plants have clever ways to combat the environment, by having DNA segments or genes jump from one locus on a chromosome to another, they need to take a fresh look at all the contributory evidence now supporting Dr. Randolph's findings. For example, extensive studies have been published in the

Journal of Allergy and Clinical Immunology which demonstrate that simple chemicals found in the plastics industry can cause a plethora of immunologic responses. In one individual there will be asthma and demonstrable IgG; in another there will be totally new antigens created; in another there will be a change in the membrane chemistry so that sensitivity is heightened to specific mediators; and in another there will be no demonstrable antibodies but the symptoms will be just as devastating, if not more so.

We know that the mechanism of chemical hypersensitivity is not the simple IgE mediated type as it is in ragweed hay fever. First, IgE is rarely demonstrable. Second, we can't modulate symptoms with antihistamines or steroids; they are totally ineffective. However, Dr. Marvin Boris of New York has shown prostaglandin inhibitors do have a modulating effect.

If a physician chose to continue to ignore Dr. Randolph's work, he would have been hard pressed to do so after the 1970's. It was then that the urea foam formaldehyde insulation (U.F.F.I.) epidemic hit the U.S. and people flocked to our offices with symptoms that had begun after the installation of the U.F.F.I. There was no doubt in their minds as to cause and effect. They had headaches, dizziness, the inability to concentrate, unwarranted depression, muscle aches, nausea, rashes, irritated nasal passages and eyes, earaches, sinusitis, arthritis, panic attacks, sore throats, coughs and much more.

A physician didn't have to know anything about chemical hypersensitivity; the patient taught him. However, if they had been keen observers and historians, the physicians would have recognized the same cause and effect relationship in other people who had had the onset of these nebulous symptoms one or two years after the U.F.F.I. had been installed. These unfortunate victims and their doctors rarely made this association and diagnosis since the onset of symptoms was so far removed from the triggering event. Some people apparently require a longer exposure to damage their immune systems. If the stumped physician failed to ask about insulation, he usually made a psychiatric referral after all the tests proved negative.

The keener observers continued to advance. They saw people who sounded like classic U.F.F.I. victims, but when they questioned them, there was no confirmatory history. However, after testing them to formaldehyde, they knew they were sensitive to it. In addition, these patients related the classic experiences of such victims - an exacerbation of symptoms when in certain places of high formaldehyde, such as shopping malls, traffic, offices, new construction, buildings heated by gas forced air and usually their own homes.

The EPA collaborated with the National Center for Toxicologic Research (published in 1984 in **Environmental Health Perspectives**) to show us that many homes and offices have just as high, sometimes higher, levels of formaldehyde as a foam-insulated home. This is due to the outgassing of various twentieth century products - carpets, furnishings, construction materials, cleansers, etc. Especially high levels can be found in a new or newly renovated house. Rarely, however, does the patient correlate the environmental additions with his symptoms and oftentimes it takes months or years for the symptoms to become full-fledged. As a result, the event is completely forgotten, much less suspected as the incitant.

A peculiar fact of chemical hypersensitivity is this - as a person becomes sensitized and continues to be exposed, he becomes progressively more sensitive. It is as though his thermostat has been reset, because now it takes less of the chemical and a shorter exposure to turn on symptoms worse than ever before.

It is unfortunate that these victims of this twentieth century illness are caught in the middle of an egocentric battle among physicians. At present, there are less than four hundred trained physicians in the country who are qualified to diagnose and treat Environmental Illness (E.I.). It is not yet taught as a cohesive comprehensive discipline in medical schools. However, all of its component parts are taught - toxicology, pharmacology, nutrition (limited), physiology, biochemistry, etc. They just haven't yet stepped back to see the whole picture. Each academician is usually involved in some sub-microscopic aspect of a super-specialty. Therefore, the majority of physicians have never heard of it. As a result, its victims go from specialist to specialist without a diagnosis.

The most unfortunate are those for whom the nervous system is affected, for they are quickly shuttled off to the psychiatrist. Dr. Robert Feldman of Boston University School of Medicine has just begun to document a smattering of the neuro-psychological effects of these toxins, such as the more common headaches, inability to concentrate, confusion, exhaustion, unwarranted extreme depression, muscle weakness, dizziness and nausea (see **American Journal of Industrial Medicine** - 1980).

Now, biochemists have elucidated the pathways in the body that cause this "toxic brain fog." It seems that every chemical that enters the body through eating, contact or breathing can be broken down into over a dozen other chemicals. Some of these chemicals are more dangerous than the parent compound and even cause cancer, birth defects, genetic change or mutation (to E.I. or other illnesses).

The pathway a chemical takes is dependent on many factors, such as the availability of trace minerals and vitamins and the overload already present from other chemicals. Some of the pathways lead to the production of acetaldehyde and chloral hydrate, (Yes! The old Mickey Finn or "knock-out" drops.), both of which can cause the toxic brain symptoms seen with E.I.

Consequently, we now have a new generation of

people that are the first to be exposed to our twentieth century world. In an effort to conserve energy, they tighten up their homes and eliminate badly needed air exchange. They continue to amass modern possessions that continually offgas formaldehydes, toluenes, xylenes, benzenes and more. All bets are off as the rules of medicine and science are changing rapidly. The gene (at one time considered stable) can now jump around in an effort to adapt to its environment.

We have made a dreadful mistake and have ignored a major rule of biology. In our haste to modernize with renovation and the addition of thousands of chemicals, we have forgotten to stop and ask ourselves whether this biological organism has the ability to adapt to this changed environment. For every person who is experiencing acute symptoms, there are many more who are developing insidious, "degenerative diseases" for which we have been taught there is no treatment, only palliative chronic medication to mask symptoms.

Simple chemicals can trigger a plethora of antibody responses and even new antigens and they can change membrane reception sensitivity. If that is not enough, Dr. N.K. Jerne has shown us that these antibodies proceed to develop antibodies to themselves, called anti-idiotypic antibodies. As Dr. David Sacks of N.I.H. has shown, these anti-idiotypic antibodies can enhance or suppress a reaction, depending upon other concomitant factors. Still, the conventional allergist continues to ignore Dr. Randolph's work.

What should the poor victim of E.I. do while all this battling is going on? He should begin to read and learn some simple methods to pinpoint the cause and treatment of his symptoms.

Years ago, peculiar bouts of unwarranted depression and negativity would come over me suddenly and last for days. We had no idea what triggered them. Later, they would leave as suddenly as they had come. We finally identified all the triggers and my body healed. Do I feel angry or bitter to be the victim of E.I.? No. In fact I feel extremely lucky to know what I have and how to heal it. I enjoy teaching other people how to possess the tools to transform themselves from E.I. victims to E.I. survivors.

And every part of nutritional, dietary and environmental controls was necessary. Some people experience a step-wise improvement with every single thing they do. Others won't experience improvement until the last part of the total load has been dealt with. And others lie somewhere in between, improving sporadically when certain landmarks in the total load have been achieved.

SECTION X

Future

So, why did I bother to write this? I certainly have more than a complete life and can think of a thousand and one things I would have preferred doing in the many years I spent writing this. Plus, it was downright grueling since I obviously lack any training in journalism. (Fortunately, the subsequent books got progressively better and we apologize for this. But we had such an urgent need to fill before more people needlessly suffered and died, never to know what they had or how to get rid of it).

The reasons we wrote this are simple. I felt an overwhelming gratitude at first for having been cleared of my multitude of problems, which I thought were incurable. I couldn't bear the physical back pain, the mental anguish of brain fog and the nightmare of depression. I frankly thought my life was over in my 30's. I had visions of myself reaching fifty with a scarred and constantly eczematous face and I wondered how I could mentally cope with this. When I got more into the field of environmental medicine, I realized there were people much more desperate than I - they were dying. They had exhausted all that medicine had to offer. They were now labelled merely neurotic!

It became imperative I make this body of knowledge known because very few physicians are aware of it and most think an allergy is not life-threatening. It is one thing if the field of medicine is unaware of this knowledge and tells us nothing can be done (It is not even taught in one solitary medical school in the entire world yet); it is another thing if it refuses to acknowledge the now overwhelming evidence. When a person finally figures out what he had and how to help himself, it is unfortunate that his doctors and insurance company still refuse to believe him or become obsessed with proving to him that he is wrong. When he becomes sicker, they use rationalization to explain it and become more defensive and hostile. This is dangerous.

I think that the following incident is important because it teaches us chemically sensitive people several lessons and warns us about things that we had better be prepared to handle in the future.

You may recall I told you about one of my patients who was 27-years-old and had fourteen bloody bowel movements a day with his regional ileitis. This had begun when he was fifteen years of age. Each time he got bad he would be hospitalized and a small bowel resection was done. He had had three of these. Medicine tends to cut out and throw away parts that are not doing well rather than finding the cause. Following that logic, if you have a headache I guess the prescription would be a guillotine and if the diagnosis is V.D., well, you are tough out of luck!

Anyway, we tested him years ago and within two weeks he was totally clear and has since stayed clear. He could turn himself on and off like a faucet by just not rotating his foods or not giving himself his injections. When he and I told his gastroenterologists, they totally ignored us. How could food have anything to do with bowel disease!?! They were aghast that we could conceive of anything so unheard of.

Years later, however, he injured his knee and went into the hospital for an operation. When he awakened from the anesthesia, he had severe abdominal pain, cramping and profuse bleeding. His colitis had instantly returned, presumably as the result of the chemical assault to his body from the anesthesia, the I.V.'s in plastic bags, the plastic I.V. tubing and the many pre-operative drugs (not to mention hospital food).

The gastroenterologists were called in and they decided to do a barium enema. When he had the barium enema, he had worse cramping and bleeding. Then they decided to do an upper GI. He protested vehemently and said that he had never had any trouble with his stomach and didn't need to have that part x-rayed. He told them that he was reacting to the barium and that if he could just go home and return to his rotated diet (of organic foods) and his food and inhalant shots, he would be better. Not able to handle the possible fact that he could know his body better than they, he was ignored. They ordered an UGI anyway as part of their total canned standard workup (it is one of the only tools they have).

It was, of course, negative. The problem is that it created such horrendous cramps and bleeding that they took him to surgery the next day. When he awakened from surgery (after having a second anesthesia just days after the previous one) he had a day of convulsions and a day-and-a-half of blindness due to retinal artery spasm (and probable undiagnosed magnesium deficiency—actually we'll never know because they never checked magnesium). Needless to say, he was wise enough to get out of there as fast as possible and he cleared once he was back home on his rotation diet and injections. His asthma had returned while he was hospitalized and off his inhalant injections. However, this too he was able to bring under control. Later, he was lucky enough to have his job switched to a building that was much more chemically clean; his total load came under even better control.

This points out that we all have to be extremely cautious, depending upon our levels of sensitivity. Not only are there very few physicians who understand environmentally caused ecologic illness, but many of them are determined to prove that we are neurotic hypochondriacs and in the process of their proof, they could very well kill us, never knowing what they had done. This young man has very little bowel left (he has had four bowel resections - three before he started injections) and if he has to undergo another operation, he may end up with a colostomy bag for life, and he isn't even 30!

We hope that he will not require anymore anesthesia and can live out the rest of his life without the intervention of conventional medical treatment. Obviously, by now you see that "convention" means "practicing medicine without knowledge of environmental illness, and using drugs and surgery as the major tools."

By the way, none of his doctors believe him as of this writing. They think his diet and injections are bunk and that nothing that happened to him in the hospital has anything to do with a hypersensitivity. They think that his fast recovery after he left the hospital was due to their fine care.

Another reason for this book is that only a book can give the proper coverage. The environment causes illness in many people that is far too complicated a subject to cover on a talk show. It must be spelled out so that people can study it in the privacy and quiet of their homes. The tremendous individual variation of this disease must sound like science fiction to the uninitiated. If I did not suffer from E.I. myself and had not seen hundreds of people turn their diseases off, I am sure I would not believe it! Especially the back pain which left me bed-ridden for weeks, the incapacitating brain fog and the life-robbing depression!

The individual uniqueness does make the disease hard to swallow. Back in the seventies, while at an allergy meeting, I asked a prominent New York City immunologist, "What do you think about this stuff that is going on in the environmental unit in Dallas, where they have people sniff formaldehyde or phenol and they duplicate such symptoms as phlebitis, urticaria, cardiac arrhythmias and convulsions?" He just said, "Hah, it is a big hoax. If you give anybody enough of that stuff to smell, they'll have symptoms of some sort or another." It is this type of blind ignorance that has led me - has fueled me - to carry on the message. It is ironic that his specialty is urticaria, or hives, and he concludes every national lecture by telling us there is no cure. I would like him to meet Bill, who had been told this for thirty-one years! Within one month of being on inhalant and food injections, he was totally clear. He said, "Doc, you have no idea how great it is to get a full night's sleep without being awakened by itching!"

Many physicians also naively believe that no one dies from environmentally induced illness and they are blind to the person who disintegrates in the hospital for unexplainable reasons. They never draw blood to check the levels of xenobiotics and nutrients.

Another reason I have done this is to show that there are inexpensive ways for people to test themselves and identify the triggers that affect them. Certainly, I wasn't in a life-threatening situation, although I often wondered about the value of my life with the disfiguring eczema on my face and incapacitating back pain, not to mention the chronic toxic brain symptoms of unwarranted spaciness, depression, arthritis and exhaustion. Fortunately, the blinding headaches, burning eyes, chronic sinusitis, asthma and spastic colon were under control. Chronic misery does not exactly make someone a joy to be with. Luckily, the majority can manage with environmental manipulations and need no testing or injections. Only the very sensitive need testing and/or injections.

An additional reason is to help some people prevent further disease. I think any person with chemical allergies should want to read **The Politics of Cancer** by Samuel Epstein and **Consumer Beware** by Beatrice Trum Hunter. Not everyone is interested in prevention because, after all, prevention is one of the last things that we all want to look at. If we were good at prevention, there would be no diabetes, hypertension, obesity, etc., We are only interested in things after they affect us. Then, we want constant care.

Those who recognize that they have bodies that cannot handle this incredible chemical overload of the twentieth century should read as much as possible and become as knowledgeable as possible. This will help them to unload their systems and to enjoy freedom from symptoms. Everyone's sensitivities and total load are uniquely different, and to further complicate matters, these things change with time within the same individual.

Our efforts seem to be constantly tested as new problems arise. Currently, the government has initiated a program to irradiate foods. This lowers a great many vitamin levels. They think they will compensate. Will they omit the more expensive magnesium, vitamins E and B6 like they did from packaged cereals? What about the other small trace amounts of nutrients and minerals that they distort or change that they can't put back or are unaware of? Where are the ten to twenty year studies on the effects of eating irradiated foods? There are obvious molecular changes induced in the foods. Are pro-carcinogenic compounds produced? In what form are they going to replace these vitamins? Are they going to use vitamin C extracted from citrus to supplement a non-citrus, irradiated food so that now someone like myself who is sensitive to citrus can no longer eat that particular food? Are the same government organizations overseeing this that allowed carcinogenic pesticides to remain on the market for years and are still allowing others that have not been sufficiently tested?

These are unanswered questions about short and long-range effects. These are going to be solved by the very people that have decided it is better to let the food industry rake in huge profits and adulterate with additives, antioxidants, bleaches, tenderizers, dyes and a variety of chemicals that have been shown to cause a barrage of disease, least among which is cancer. Once you have read **Consumer Beware: Your Food and What's Been Done To It**, I doubt you will ever be as complacent again about how you feed yourself. You see, we take nutritional food for granted and allow others to think for us. The evidence is all there and our exorbitantly high level of degenerative disease is too. Obviously, we have "advanced" to a stage where the world needs many of these additives. But do you?

Conventional allergists are working on allergy injections made from gluteraldehyde which is a formaldehyde derivative. Urologists prescribe antibiotics that become formaldehyde in the bladder. Surgeons are putting plastic parts in hearts. Many patients would reject these plastic parts or be intolerably ill with them. Why not go to the source of why we are prematurely degenerating our parts to begin with? We see so many each week with resistant cardiac arrhythmias, for example, and they are often well within weeks; only because we realize the heart is merely another target organ, vulnerable to environmental triggers and biochemical defects.

The fourth reason for this book is to increase public awareness and urge doctors to get involved and understand what is happening so that if they get a patient who is traveling through their town who requests that he have no corn dextrose I.V., plastic IV tubing or plastic I.V. bottles, that they won't view him as crazy and worsen him.

We must respect individuality and not plunge obstinantly into our conventional habits. Hopefully hospitals will improve their design to augment healing and not retard it. The studies from Dr. Rea's Unit on thrombophlebitis are a clear example of people with chemically-induced susceptibility. Look at the life-threatening thrombophlebitis that occurs post-operatively in a highly chemical "regular" hospital environment.

The fifth reason is to educate people so that they can directly put pressure on insurance groups for recognition and coverage of environmental illness and on legislators for pollution control and decreased spraying of insecticides in public places and restaurants and improved ventilation in stores, businesses and schools so that more workers do not become ill from outgassing. Why not give a copy of this book to your doctor and start his wheels turning? In a few years he may be your area's leading specialist in environmental medicine, regardless of his initial specialty. Most people have consulted over twelve doctors before they reach us and never have so much as a diagnosis. However, they sure have large medical bills!

It is here that you might be interested in a little of the politics of medicine. Private practitioners like myself are busy seeing sick people. If we are not good, no one comes to us and we don't make any money. Academic allergists are paid by the medical schools to teach medical students and run the allergy clinic where poor people go. If they are not any good, it doesn't matter because the poor people have no place else to go. Also, they get to run their experiments on the clinic cases to see which treatments are best. These tests are usually regarding drugs, and funded by the pharmaceutical industry.

These doctors also sit on government medical and insurance boards and decide policy, such as what types of allergy treatments will be paid for by insurance companies. These doctors are thought to be in a good position to decide which treatments are best because they have residents and medical students do a lot of their work so they can read journals, plus they have large clinic populations they can do research on and learn from.

In order to do a research study you need money in the form of a grant to subsidize you. This can come from the government or the drug industry. The drug industry likes to support research that shows their products to be superior so they can sell more. The academic doctor likes to do any research he can that he gets a grant for, so that he is subsidized and gets notoriety from his findings. This is a marriage made in heaven, for the needs of the drug industry and academic physicians complement one another. On second thought, is this analogy an insult to the complementary richness and beauty of a marriage? Does this really more accurately resemble the relationship found in the worlds' oldest profession?

The academic allergists in medical schools determine what insurance companies pay for. The only drawback is they stunt the real progress in allergy. It took Dr. Miller years of trial and error in his office to work out the bugs of food testing. He had no grant for this. It was all his own time and money. In spite of the fact that we all benefit from it, no medical school is willing to go through the tremendous amount of work entailed in learning the technique. They could not humble themselves to go learn from the master in his office. They live by the unwritten rule that all great discoveries must have their beginnings in medical schools where the research is being carried out. After all, that is their justification for existence.

If they begin to be curious about our successes, they call our offices and demand that we give them references that have been published proving our methods work. The reasons we don't publish are many: 1) We are extremely busy taking care of sick people. 2) It costs several thousands of dollars to do a study. No one will fund us because they have nothing to gain. It doesn't sell more drugs; in fact, we get people off drugs. 3) When we do try to report our cases, the referee panel of the journal is made up of these same narrow-minded jealous academicians. They reject our papers saying, "When you prove this on one hundred people double-blinded, then we will consider looking at it." That means half the people get the real thing and half get water and they can't know which half they are. Now, who is going to pay me for a year of water injections? Even if I did it for free, why would they come back? How can you "double-blind" the tremendous effort that goes into the rotated diet?

Besides that, there is much dishonesty. **The New England Journal of Medicine** showed a study where giving 100 I.U. of vitamin E a day cuts cardiovascular disease in half. This was done on 85,000 people. But the FDA wants to take vitamins off the market in spite of no side effects. The same FDA allowed Claritin, a new antihistamine on the market. It was only tested on 12,800 people and has the side effect of cancer of the liver. And we already have 35 other antihistamines. I could go on.

Now you understand part of the bitter controversy that is hurting E.I. patients. The drug industry controls much of medical research and the purse strings of the academic allergist. He in turn sits on the governing bodies of insurance companies and determines what type of allergy treatment you will be able to be reimbursed for. The fact that ecologic treatment helps you after you have failed in the offices of three conventional allergists doesn't count. That is immaterial - until you get angry and become effective. Sadly enough, most people don't get motivated, even for matters of health and money.

What I guess we need is for many more people to become victims of environmental illness. The problem is, many are victims and don't know it. There are only a few hundred of us trained in the field and we can't treat all the people. Many are not fully trained yet and can only handle the simpler cases. Hence, the written word is one way of educating people to at least consider alternative medical therapy when all else has failed.

We have to be aware that medicine is putting doctors in increasingly narrower areas of specialization and that we have to go back to a wholism approach, because there are so many diverse factors which create illness in people with ecologic illness. One stress lowers the threshold to a second one, so that the total load gives the disease. Everything is part of an interacting spectrum. In ten years there may no longer be the specialties of neurology, endocrinology and metabolic disease separately. Instead, they will be part of an effort to reach down to the levels of molecular biology by studying nutrition, environmental xenobiotic (foreign chemical) metabolism, immunology above IgE reactions and basic biochemistry and psychoneuroimmunology. Even the psychiatrists will not be immune to having to learn about health and wellness.

It is like the old story of four men evaluating an elephant from a distance of six inches. Each one had a different view and a different idea of what it represented. It was only the man who could get off from afar and appreciate the entire animal who could make sense out of all the parts. Likewise, how can any of the narrow visions of any of the 38 ENT specialists, neurologists and gastroenterologists who examined the state trooper with dizziness, headaches and nausea ever diagnose his problem as formaldehyde hypersensitivity? If a plant is sick, we look at it's food, light and water. How about applying this approach to people instead of irradiating and drugging them. We need to scrutinize the current approach of x-rays, blood tests and drugs.

Physicians in environmental medicine realize also the many obstacles that they are going to have to face because our brand of medicine tries to help the patient become independent of the physician, independent of drugs and teaches him to shun the highly chemicalized universe which we are now in. There is a new chemical compound being discovered and brought into use every minute in the United States. There is mounting evidence that many of these chemicals cause adverse effects on genetically susceptible people. Many of these adverse effects have the fancy names of diseases which we are taught to advise people to "learn to live with."

Now it is time to let you in on some other secrets. If you are going to take far greater control of your health, you can no longer shelter yourself in naivete. You will find that there is tremendous resistance to environmental medicine. That is because many institutions and governments put your health second and money first.

Money from big industry is more important than the health of people who live in a polluted area. Look at all the examples of Love Canal, acid rain, food additives, carcinogenic pesticides, Times Beach and nuclear reactors where policing is lax. Look at the length of time it took to ban urea formaldehyde foam insulation, only to reverse the decision to unload the courts of lawsuits. Were there any tests for the effects of it on people before it's use? Yet, there were scientists who spoke up and warned and were ignored. A case of malignant neglect by intent.

There are literally volumes of books citing the lack of tests on additives which are allowed. Yet we do not have access even to the most meager of test data that were performed, by the food manufacturer himself, no less! Independent testing laboratories are not required, nor do all the additives even have to be stated on the label.

Environmental medicine attempts to have people drug- free. Do you think the powerful drug industry will not fight that in a surreptitious way? Just read how big industry and the FDA have managed the many indiscretions they have been granted in the name of the almighty dollar. The majority of medical school research is subsidized by the drug industry. There is no monetary motive to back research showing chemicals are not the way to stop disease and least of all to support vitamins.

When I say discredit, you might think that is being a little dramatic. After all, how could anyone discredit all this evidence? Very easily. First, by ignoring and refusing to believe it exists and second, by attacking the people who propose it. It is being done now.

I have never ceased to be amazed at how medicine can turn on anyone at anytime, regardless of staggering accomplishments. The Nobel prize winning Dr. Linus Pauling was denigrated as soon as he researched vitamin C. Dr. Rea was the cardiovascular surgeon selected to operate on Connely in Dallas. Now he is badgered for his leadership in ecology. Many doctors in ecology have a long list of impressive credentials which suddenly become invisible to their colleagues once they associate with frontiers of medicine.

I have seen some of the most intelligent, level-headed, truly well-adjusted people you would ever hope to meet labeled neurotic. I have witnessed it happening to doctors of excellent caliber once they stumble into environmental medicine. I have witnessed it in patients from all walks of life when they do the same. It doesn't matter if the patients are physicians themselves or lawyers, engineers, college department heads, millionaires, clergy or corporate heads. When they first present with their symptoms, they are treated seriously with all the respect they deserve. Then, as soon as the doctor realizes he doesn't know what they have, he panics, turns on them and labels them neurotic. As one V.P. of a major Fortune 500 corporation told me, "When I asked if my symptoms could be related to allergy, my doctor looked as though I had just bitten him on the leg."

Poor Dr. Feingold was only reporting an observation that some kids were indeed hyperactive with certain food additives. Yet, they attacked him more viciously than a communist. This is in spite of the fact that many of the parents of kids who improved on his diet were themselves pediatricians. Likewise, most ecologists are themselves victims of environmentally induced illness. I guess by necessity you have to be or have a relative who is suffering to be willing to commit yourself to the tremendous amount of resistance and work it entails. It was so much easier having been a conventional allergist for nine years. There is no comparison. You can make money much faster and with far less patient involvement and effort via the conventional route.

Yes, indeed, powerful drug industry having joined forces with the other industries continues to attempt to discredit us. When I say powerful, that is an understatement. In the last few years, two drugs that we were not exactly starving for, one a diuretic and the other an arthritis medicine, were withdrawn from the market because of hepatic or liver enzyme abnormalities within six months of their release. There have been several others since. You may not know it, but one of the very simplest parameters of all to monitor in a new drug are hepatic. All you do is draw a simple tube of blood every few weeks and see if the liver enzymes remain normal. Within six months of being on the market, after supposedly seven years of laboratory testing, these two drugs were withdrawn because they caused abnormalities of liver enzymes. How could it happen so quickly if they were tested seven years? It frightens me when I know this. It means there was the grossest neglect or self-interest where testing of the drugs was concerned. It makes me wonder just what they did test and how much money they were paid by whomever to get the drugs on the open market and making money? How many others are there with longer term effects that we ever dreamed of?

No, my friend, the building, manufacturing, chemical, drug, food and many other industries are going to find clever ways of discrediting this new branch of medicine, because it is unhealthy to their pocketbooks. They don't want people complaining of their smokestacks, toxic wastes, working conditions, contaminated food and water and their products. They like the uninformed, complacent Mr. John Q's ignorance.

Medicine itself doesn't want to find out you don't have to have certain diseases like arteriosclerosis. What are they going to do with all those plastic hearts? all those surgeons? all those cardiologists?

For example, Dr. Rea presented the following case at the 16th Advanced Seminar for Clinical Ecology in Banff in 1982. A young woman had had a 95% pancreatectomy at a leading Texas medical school for uncontrolled hypoglycemia and diabetes. She was on 80mg of prednisone and 80 units of insulin when he saw her. In the unit, if they gave her four figs, her glucose went over 600 milligrams percent. After three weeks in the unit on a controlled diet and in an environment clear of chemicals, they were able to feed her 16 figs with no problem and she required no medication and was off her steroids and insulin. Her sugar rose to 120 milligrams percent.

In other words, her chemical and food sensitivities triggered her immune system to be weak enough to be unable to handle the directives of her insulin molecules. She had wild swings of hyper and hypoglycemia. These could be duplicated in a chemical test booth in the environmental unit. They could cause wild swings in her sugar by exposing her to petrochemicals, insecticides, particular foods and molds and it is all so incredibly logical. Instead of her target organ being the mast cell in the lung causing asthma, or being the nasal mucosa causing rhinitis or the synovial lining causing arthritis, hers was the insulin receptor site of cells.

Dr. Rea presented another study in the 1981 Annals of Allergy of patients with phlebitis or blood clots in the legs. This disease gets so bad that usually people are not able to work and oftentimes they end up having amputations. They also spend thousands of dollars being hospitalized each year when the flare-ups get bad enough that they require intravenous heparin to control the clotting so that the clots do not flow to the lung or heart and cause death.

Half of the study wanted no part of ecology. The other half wanted to try it. At the end of five years, those who had investigated ecologic illness found that various foods and chemicals could trigger their phlebitis. In fact, eight out of ten could turn on their phlebitis when exposed to the test chemicals - phenol, formaldehyde, petrochemical ethanols, or pesticide - in the unit. They were all at work and they had had no hospitalizations. The other group had spent thousands of dollars being in and out of the hospital, just as they had previously, and they were not employed.

They had 60 episodes of thrombophlebitis treated at home and 41 episodes requiring hospitalization. The ecologically treated group had two episodes lasting less than 48 hours and both were treated at home. They occurred when they were inadvertently exposed to chemicals.

I might mention that I have never appreciated the meaning of the word dedication until I worked with such people as Dr. Joseph Miller, Dr. Doris Rapp and Dr. William Rea. These people are the most dedicated physicians I have ever had the privilege of meeting in my life. I think that they have a more thorough and deeper appreciation of what a tremendous discovery all of this is than I. They are obsessed with helping as many people as possible. They have been professionally slammed in as many ways as possible by their jealous and unquestioning colleagues. Yet they are all very calm, quiet, and extremely humble people. I don't know how they suppress the urge to run out and scream and shout their discoveries.

I don't know how, for example, someone like Dr. Rapp is able to maintain her quiet humility when she sees a child who has a diagnosis from the Buffalo Medical Center of attention deficit disorder. This is a high-falutin' word for hyperactive and lousy student, a "pain in the class." The only deficit in this type of disorder lies in the person who is making the diagnosis, because he has not studied the findings in the scientific literature, and has not taken the time to view the videotapes that she has made that show hyperactivity being turned on and off with injections of an offending food. Instead, they prescribe dangerous amphetamines to a child! These suppress growth, both mental and physical.

Many of us might feel secure in the knowledge that DDT was legally restricted in the States, but what people don't appreciate is that most of our food now, especially the luscious fruits and vegetables that we receive in the wintertime come from foreign countries where not only do they lack legislation to protect against the use of this, but oftentimes when they receive their huge drums of carcinogenic chemicals, they cannot even read the English label. Men applying it in the fields do not have education and do not understand the ramifications. They not only expose themselves but us as well.

There are instances where they have used the leftover barrels containing insecticides as rain barrels for a local school, from which the children can dip their cups and get a drink (see the book, **Circle of Poison**).

We are in a society that expects instant cure and many drugs, but now we know that chronic medications are not good because they are chemicals. These chemicals must be broken down and metabolized or detoxified just like any other. They further overload the already overburdened twentieth century xenobiotic (foreign chemical) detox mechanisms of the body, further straining the system and leading to easier vulnerability to E.I.

The symptoms masquerade as diseases with fancy names which we have been taught have no cause or treatment. We have been warned that anyone not associated with a big name medical school who alleges being able to help these people must be a quack. Yet, there is not one full-blown environmentally controlled hospital unit in the country in a medical school. If I got severely ill tomorrow, I would not go to our local medical school hospital, but directly to Dallas.

The body can be likened to an automobile; the doctor to a mechanic. As Dr. Ron Finn says, there are only three categories of malfunction. First, the car could be the result of a manufacturing error - a lemon. This in the body is analogous to a genetic defect. Second, the car could be abused and mistreated. In the body we call this degenerative disease, but fail to consider the diet, nutrition state and chronic ambient chemical exposure. Third, an accident can damage the car. In the body, damage occurs through chemical overload. We need to re-evaluate the way we view disease and be less involved with naming (it seems the name of the game in medicine is the name) and more concerned with cause. We doctors are great memorizers, but our problem-solving skills need honing.

Right now, the brain is the most commonly affected allergic target organ and the least appreciated. There are few blood tests or x-rays to even prove if a patient is malingering. Single blind provocation-neutralizations can prove a chemical hypersensitivity and xenobiotic levels are our best current tools.

Once a person becomes allergic, the immune system responds to anything, even its own hormones. We develop what is called an emerging or spreading allergic diathesis and people become universal reactors, or develop a total body allergy. Again, chemicals damage the membranes and other regulatory parts of the immune system and overburden the detoxification mechanisms, allowing the body to respond with a heightened hypersensitivity.

We have seen people with severe psoriasis totally cleared with ecologic management which consisted of $4.50 worth of an oil found in a health food store. As well, there are numerous cases of diabetes, phlebitis, arthritis, colitis, migraines and asthma that improved with serotonin injections, aluminum foil on the bed, screwy diets, treating a "harmless" yeast like Candida or taking vitamins. It sounds like a panacea but it is not. It is just that we have been looking at the wrong things. We are calling symptoms diseases and we are not looking at the basic individuality and hyper-responsiveness of people to a variety of environmental triggers. We have failed to sit back and look at the body as a whole then implement regeneration and total body healing. We do this by unloading the body so that it can heal on it's own. After all, if doctors can clear their own metastatic cancers with macrobiotics, (**Recalled by Life**, A. Sattillaro, M.D.), the E.I. should be a piece of cake. It is not instantaneous like a pill and it requires a major diet change, time and commitment. Many just don't feel their health is worth it.

Again, it is the difference between people, not the difference between disease, that is important. That is why people have cleared multiple sclerosis with Nystatin. In others it has done nothing. We don't all have the same cause for our problems. Others with eczema don't have the exact same foods and chemicals that cause mine.

We have reached the era of the powerless person. In an effort to control the masses and simultaneously control the purse strings and ultimate power, various authorities have been fabricated. No endeavor is exempt - politics, economics, manufacturing, banking, religion, pharmaceuticals, medicine, etc.

Why, right now the average person is so powerless that he allows his insurance company (not even his physician, but a business) ultimate authority over his health. He allows his insurance company to tell him what diseases he can and cannot have, how long he can have these diseases, who can be his doctor and what treatment he can use. And, he allows his
employer to bargain hunt for the cheapest one he can find.

For example, E.I. is not in the medical computer, so he can't have that. He can't have an hour of educational time in the office regarding his condition (because he is considered uneducable), but he can have hundreds and thousands of dollars of fifteen minute tests that don't help diagnose or treat him. He can't be hospitalized for three weeks in his local hospital to diagnose if he has E.I. and he can't go to the environmental hospital unit in Dallas. If he has cancer, he must have radiation, chemotherapy or surgery. That is recommended even though the cure rate is horrid, but he cannot have macrobiotics or the Gerson therapy, all of which have produced remarkable results. That, my friends, is your department. I have my own battles to wage. When enough of you get tired of being powerless over the destiny of your lives, you will band together to regain the power to make your own medical decisions.

This reminds me of Jeff, a fine young man in his 20's. He had an auto accident and required much medication for months to manage his pain and muscle spasms. Within a year he had deteriorated to such a state that he was unable to work. His parents took him to every consultant they could think of, but no one could make him better.

Some friends recommended he see me and I looked for only those things that I know all the other doctors were unaware of, since he had had everything else imaginable done. He had a rather simple case. He was abysmally low in over half a dozen vitamins and he was also quite mold sensitive. Within one month he felt better than he had before his accident and was back to work.

Three years later Jeff was periodically still sending me sweet little notes thanking the office for his care and recovery. All of the specialists that he had consulted had been paid by the insurance company. Mind you, none of them diagnosed his problem and none of them helped him and he was not able to work. However, he had not been fully reimbursed for my treatment because the insurance company couldn't understand (in spite of many letters and documented grossly abnormal blood tests for vitamin levels) how vitamins could help him when he could buy them without a prescription. What did mold injections have to do with weakness, headaches and inability to concentrate?

If you find that hard to swallow, a (surgeon) urologist and his R.N. wife brought their teenager in for undiagnosable, untreatable fatigue. For 4 years she saw 9 specialists in their university medical center area and no one could help. In less than 2 months on our program she was well for the first time in four years. But a year later, even though still well, the insurance company was still hassling the father, a doctor, about paying him back for our treatment that healed her. But they quickly paid for the 9 doctors who couldn't help her. You see, our values are askew. If you follow the protocol, you get paid even if the patient dies. If you save him and make him better, and even get him back to work making money so he can pay his insurance premiums, that doesn't count. That is why I treat people, not insurance companies. I do not select the company that each person has chosen to represent him and I don't have the time to deal with the bureaucratic mentality which conveniently sees only what it chooses. Educating them is your department. You have the knowledge and the vested interest and I have seen many who have been highly successful at it.

Many physicians are intimidated by nutrition because of sheer lack of knowledge. After all, we must know much more biochemistry to attempt to balance the whole body than to just prescribe a few pills from the PDR.

Some are afraid of losing control over you because you can get them without a prescription. Many people will never get better until deficiencies are discovered. We just finished a study showing over 55 percent of the people who walk through our doors are zinc deficient. This nutrient alone controls enzymes in every major system of the body - gene repair, detoxification, healing and growth, nutrient absorption, vision and taste, hormone and enzymes production, etc. In fact, its deficiency alone serves as a perfect model for the spreading phenomenon.

So, where do we go from here? It seems the sky is the limit. I am constantly researching for a better way to maximize to full potential the essence of healing power that each person carries inside him. We also know that although this is not a psychiatric disease, the mind is very powerful in healing. We know there is a subset of people with occult anger, hostility, guilt or fear who, regardless of how well they follow all the principles of ecologic or conventional medicine, will never get better. As soon as they learn to shed those destructive feelings and to give and receive for themselves God's unconditional love, they make remarkable improvements. How does this work? We have no idea. So, we call them miracles, but we are getting closer to understanding the mechanism day by day. It is utterly mind boggling the untapped power that each individual possesses.

People often ask me when they get stuck on a decision in medicine, what would you do if you were me? What would I do? Well, knowing what I know now, if I ever got a severe illness that I could not clear quickly, I would hot foot it to Dallas so fast you wouldn't know what hit you. Assuming I didn't know about E.I., I would never have thought about an environmental illness as the cause of my symptoms and if I were told about it, I wouldn't believe it and I didn't for many years. So I can't blame the many denigrators.

People can ask but it doesn't mean they are going to listen or learn from our mistakes. Many a person has been told what was needed to get to that 100% better mark, but they blocked it out. Years later many returned and enthusiastically reported they finally got sick of being sick and went the extra mile and feel great.

I guess we all have a special time when we are ready to heal. Just remember when Dr. Rea told me that my back pain could be due to chemical sensitivity; I resisted vehemently and even ridiculed the idea. I belligerently went along with the trial and, much to my surprise, there was method to his madness. For the first time in years I was suddenly free of pain medication. I could turn the pain on and off with environmental incitants. Even for several years after this discovery, I was still constantly testing it out, denying its reality. We humans are a stubborn and ignorant bunch sometimes!

Yearly patients from all over the country check back to learn of the advances that have occurred, for the whole field is moving tremendously fast. For the last few years there has been something new at least every 2-3 months. People we couldn't help three months ago can now have a second chance. The speed of constant new discoveries is breathtaking.

For instance, as you will read in **Tired or Toxic?**, we know a tremendous amount about the nutrients and where they fit into the detoxification pathways to make us more "normal." And in **You Are What You Ate** we showed how many, myself included, are no longer even 1/100th as chemically sensitive and no longer even need any injections. **The Cure Is In the Kitchen** takes over where that leaves off to show you how to reach maximum health. In fact, many people, doctors included, have used these programs to totally reverse and heal cancers when they were given just days to live and told that nothing more could be done.

Then **Macro Mellow** was designed for the rest of the family and also people who were just not that ill, but wanted to gradually get healthier.

In 1994 **Wellness Against All Odds** explored many problems from the leaky gut syndrome, celiac disease, how to clear arthritis and heart disease to, cancers, chronic back problems, chemical sensitivity, and much more. It went into spirituality, the carnivore diet (to save marriages split by diets and for those who cannot or refuse to do macro), as well as many resurrected powerful healing techniques that do not cost money and are non-prescription. Plus it is referenced for doctors. They all form a continuum, a growth, a medical education that shows people how to literally heal the impossible. And more are on the way as we speak.

So, if this work helps just one person, it is worth it. I know it will help many more because already these ideas have helped thousands of people. They certainly have saved my life.

We have an epidemic in disguise and only a handful of visionaries are aware of it. These survivors possess the lucky combination of great intellect and tremendous motivation. I am very lucky - I only see the most intelligent and motivated people. The rest get lost by the wayside. The people I have had the privilege of guiding have comprehended how the principles described in here could help them and they had the fortitude to carry out the program to prove it. In short, they were committed to wellness and optimistically embraced illness as a challenge to be conquered.

It is exciting to be a pioneer in the forefront. It is exhilarating to be in a position of hope, knowledge and power over our bodies as opposed to hopelessness. Most of us have experienced the despair of hopelessness and now can rejoice in our new found freedom from disease. We invite you to benefit from this major revolution in medicine and to lift your life to new levels of hope, health and happiness.

JUST THE BEGINNING!

SECTION XI
RESOURCES

Information For Environmental Hypersensitivities

BOOKS

The following books are of great help for people with environmental allergies. If your local bookstore cannot order them, they can all be purchased (most of them are in paperback) from Dickey Enterprises, 635 Gregory Road, Fort Collins, Colorado 80524.

Is This Your Child? by Doris J. Rapp, M.D. Practical Allergy Research Foundation, P.O. Box 60, Buffalo, NY 14223-0060.

Dr. Mandell's Five Day Allergy Relief System by Marshall Mandell, M.D. Paperback, for food sensitive.

An Alternative Approach to Allergies, by Dr. Theron Randolph. Paperback, required for chemically and food sensitive.

If This is Tuesday, It Must be Chicken, by Natalie Golas. If you are having trouble rotating, this is a must.

Chemical Victims, by R. MacKarness, M.D. Paperback version of the hardcover, "Living Safely in a Polluted World".

Coping With Your Allergies, by Natalie Golas. Deals with how to manage all the environmental controls.

Books on how to build your house:

Your Home and Your Health and Well-Being, by Rousseaux and Rea. Don Quixote Pub. Co., Inc., P.O. Box 9442, Amarillo, TX 79105

Sunny Hill, by Bruce Small. The story of an engineer and his family's long struggle to find out they had ecologic illness and how they were able to deal with it.

Why Your House May Endanger Your Health, by Alfred V. Zamm, M.D. with Robert Gannon.

The Household Environment and Chronic Illness, by Pfeiffer, Guy, Nickel, C..

How to Live With the New 20th Century, a resource guide for living chemically-free. L. Weiss & M. Culiss, D.D.S., P.O. Box 64, Franklin, MI 48025

Allergies and the Hyperactive Child and **The Impossible Child**,(Excellent) by Doris J. Rapp, M.D. Practical Allergy Research Foundation, P.O. Box 60, Buffalo, NY 14223-0060.

Consumer Beware: Your Food and What's Been Done to it, by Beatrice Trum Hunter (excellent).

Food, Mind and Mood, by Sheinkin, M.D., Schachter, M.D., and Hutton.

Not All in the Mind, by Richard MacKarness.

The Body Wrecker, by Nick Travis. Case histories of undiagnosable symptoms of chemically sensitive people. Don Quixote Pub. Co., Inc., P.O. Box 9442, Amarillo, TX 79105.

Supernutrition, by Richard Passwater, Pocket Books, 230

Avenue of America, New York, New York 10020.

Brain Allergies and **Victory Over Diabetes**, by William Philpott and Dwight Kalita, Keats Publishing, Inc., 27 Pine Street, New Canaan, Connecticut 06840.

A Diet To Stop Arthritis by Norman Childers, (1977), Horticultural Publications, Somerset Press Inc. , P.O. Box 699, Sommerville, NJ 08876 or 3906 N.W. 31st Place, Gainesville, FL 32601.

Seventy-three percent of over 700 patients who evaluated this diet derived great improvement over three to six months in all types of arthritis. It is certainly worth a try for anyone who hurts, and the odds are in your favor!

Maximum Immunity, by Michael Weiner, Ph.D., Houghton Mifflin Co., Boston, 1986.

Human Ecology and Susceptibility to the Chemical Environment, by Theron Randolph, M.D. Order from Human Ecology Research Foundation, 505 N. Lake Shore Drive, Suite 6506, Chicago, IL 60611.

The Susceptibility Report: Chemical Susceptibility and Urea Formaldehyde Foam Insulation, by Bruce Small. Order from Deco-Plans, Inc., P.O. Box 870, Plattsburgh, NY 12901.

The Household Pollutants Guide, by Center for Science in the Public Interest. Order from Environmental Action Foundation, 724 Dupont Circle Bldg., Washington, D.C., 20036.

Recommendation for Action of Pollution and Education in Toronto, A Report by Bruce Small, Ph.D., RR #1, Goodwood, Ontario LOC 1AO. Current data to help schools understand and respond to E.I. needs.

Indoor Air Pollution and Housing Technology, research Report by Bruce Small and Associates, Ltd. This report was originally available for free from the Canadian Housing Information Centre, Canada Mortage and Housing Corporation, National Office, Montreal Road, Ottawa, Ontario, Canada K1A OP7. Phone (613) 748-2367.

It's All In Your Head, by Hal Huggins, D.D.S. About mercury amalgam toxicity.

The Allergy Cookbook - Tasty Nutritious Cooking Without Wheat, Corn, Milk or Eggs, by Ruth A. Shattuck, New American Library, 1633 Broadway, New York, NY 10019, 1984. For mothers who need ideas for children's parties, school lunches, etc.

Solved: The Riddle of Illness, by Langer, S.E., Keats Publ., New Canaan, CT, 1984. Hidden hypothyroidism can mask ecologic illness.

Detox, by Saifer, Phyllis, Zellerback, M. How to get unhooked from chemicals and foods.
Silent Spring, by Carson, Rachel.

Tracking Down Hidden Food Allergy, by Crook, William G., Professional Books, P.O. Box 3494, Jackson, TN 38301. Excellent for figuring out what your child can eat.
Non-Toxic and Natural - How To Avoid Dangerous Everyday Products and Buy or Make Safe Ones, by Dadd, Debra Lynn. Non-Toxic Lifestyles Inc., P.O. Box 210019, San Francisco, CA 94121-0019. Excellent for making nontoxic substitutes for many home products, toiletries, cleansers, pesticides, etc.

The Yeast Syndrome, by John Trowbridge and Morton Walker, Bantam Books, 1986.

The Yeast Connection, by Crook, William G. Available through Future Health Inc., Box 846, Jackson, TN 38302 or dial 1-800- 835-1157. As you will see, Candidiasis can mimic or cause ecologic illness.

The PMS Solution, by Nazzaro, A., Lombard, D. Winston Press Inc., 430 Oak Grove, Minneapolis, MN 55403.

How to Improve Your Child's Behavior Through Diet, by Stevens, L.J. and Stoner, R.B. The New American Library, P.O. Box 999, Bergenfield, NJ 07621. Great ideas for kids meals and recipes.

The Chemical Feast, by Ralph Nader Study Group, Turner, J.S., 1970, Penguin Books, 625 Madison Ave., New York.

Against The Unsuspected Enemy, by Hill, Amelia N., New Horizon, 5 Victoria Drive, Bognor Regis, West Sussex, England.

How to Live With the New 20th Century Illness, by Weiss, D.D.S., L & M, Box 64, Franklin, MI 48024.
Aids for Recovery From Environmental Illness, Farnsworth, et al., Woods-Edge Press, P.O. Box 174, Polter Valley, CA 95469.

The Politics of Cancer, Samuel Epstein, M.D., Anchor Press, Doubleday, Garden-City, NY.

The Toxic Substances Dilemma, Edward Segal, M.D., Kamlet, K.S., Clark, B., Veraska, W., National Wildlife Federation, 1412 16th Street NW, Washington, D.C. 20036.

The Greatest Battle, Glasser, M.D., Ronald, Bantom Books, a division of Random House, 201 E. 50th Street, New York, NY 10022.

Cancer and Chemicals, Corbett, M.D., Thomas, Nelson-Hall, Chicago, IL.

Laying Waste - The Poisoning of America by Toxic Chemicals, by Brown, Michael.

Sugar Blues, by Dufty, William, Chilton Press, Chilton-Radner, PA.

Eater's Digest, by Jacobson, M.D., Michael, Anchor Press, New York, NY.

Eating Clean - Food Safety & The Chemical Harvest, Selected Reading Center for Study of Responsive Law, 1982, Center for Science in Public Interest, 1755 South Street NW, Washington, D.C. 20009.

The Great Nutrition Robbery, by Trum Hunter, Beatrice, Charles Scribner's Sons, New York, NY.

Nutrition and Physical Degeneration, by Price, D.D.S., Weston A., Lee Foundation for Nutritional Research, 2023 W. Wisconsin Ave., Milwaukee, WS.

There is a Cure for Arthritis, by Airola, M.D., Pavo O., Parker Publ. Co., Inc., West Nyack, NY.

Cancer: Causes, Prevention & Treatment, Pavo Airola, Ph.D., Health Plus Publ., P.O. Box 22001, Phoenix, AZ 85028.

Recalled by Life: The Story of My Recovery from Cancer,

by Santillaro, M.D., Anthony, Houghton Mufflin, Boston, MA.

Fasting As a Way of Life, by Cott, M.D., A., Bantam Books, New York, NY.

Fighting the Food Giants, by Stipt, Paul A., A Division of Natural Enterprises, P.O. Box 2107, Manitowoc, WS 54220.

Stocking Up, Edited by Stoner, Carol H., Rodale Press, Emmaus, PA.

Malignant Neglect, by The Environmental Defense Fund & Doyle, Robert H., Vintage Books, A Division of Random House, New York, NY.

Other Books of Interest

Clean Your Room! A compendium on Indoor Pollution, California Department of Consumer Affairs, 1982.

Work is Dangerous to Your Health, by Stellman, J.M., Daum, S.M.

Work and Health, by Polakoff, P.L.

The Effect of Air Ionization, Electric Fields, Atmosphere & Other Electrical Phenomenon on Men & Animals, by Sulman, F.G.

Light, Radiation and You, by Ott, J.N.

The Body Electric, by Becker, R.O.

My Triumph Over Cancer, by Bishop, Beata, Keats Publishing, New Canaan, Connecticut.

References on food and chemicals that have caused vascular disease:

Cardiovascular disease Triggered by Foods and Chemicals, Rea, W.J., Suite, C.W., p 99-143 in: **Food Allergy:** New Perspectives, Gerrard, J.W., Ed., 1980, Charles C. Thomas, Springfield, IL.

Rea, W.J., Environmentally triggered small vessel vasculitis, **Ann Allerg,** 38:245, 1977.

Taylor, G.J., Harris, W.J., Cardiac Toxicity of Aerosal Propellants, **JAMA,** 214:81, 1970.

Davies, D.R., Rees, B.W.G., Johnson, A.P., Elwood, P.C., Abernathy, M. (1974), Food antibodies and myocardial infarction. **Lancet,** I., 1012-1014.

Rea, W.J., (1976), Environmentally triggered thrombophlebitis. **Annals of Allergy,** 37, 101-109.

Rea, W.J., (1978), Environmentally triggered cardiac disease. **Annals of Allergy,** 40, 241-251.

Rea, W.J., et al., Recurrent environmentally triggered thrombophlebitis: A five-year follow-up. **Annals of Allergy,** 47, (5 Part I): 338-344, 1981.

COTTON - clothes, bedding, furnishings, cellophane bags, etc. Send for catalogues:

Environmental Health Shoppes
1-800-447-1100

KB Cotton Pillows, Inc.
P.O. Box 57
DeSoto, TX 75115
(214) 223-7193

The Cotton Place
P.O. Box 59721
Dallas, TX 75229
(214) 243-4149

Dona Shrier
825 Northlake Drive
Richardson, TX 75080

The Janice Corporation
12 Eaton Drive
North Caldwell, NJ 07006
(1-800-JANICE'S)

Also solid wood/cotton furnishing for the whole house:

Heart of Vermont
P.O. Box 183
Sharon, VT 05065
1-800-639-4123

CHARCOAL MASKS

Hand held cotton bag of activated charcoal to get those chemically sensitive through airports, traffic jams, etc.
Also, ceramic masks and stainless steel tubing for oxygen cylinders.

Environmental Health Center, Dallas
8345 Walnut Hill Lane
Suite 205
Dallas, TX 75231
1-800-428-2343

VITAMINS

Mostly all products we recommend can be ordered from N.E.E.D.S., 527 Charles Ave, 12-A Syracuse NY 13209 1-800-634-1380 or Emerson Ecologics, 14 Newtown Road, Acton, MA 01720, (613) 263-7238.

Specialty supplements - send for catalogues:

Vital Life, Klaire Labs,
PO Box 618
Carlsbad CA 92008-0110

Cardiovascular Research Ltd.
Box 6629
Concord, CA 94524.

Ecological Formulas
1064-13 Shary Circle
Oakland, CA, 94618

Nutricology/Allergy Research Group
400 Preda Street
San Leandro, CA 94577-0489

Organic Foods - send for brochures, not everything each one has is organic.

Discount Natural Foods, 2120 Burnet Ave, Syracuse NY, 13206 (off 690 Midler exit)

Goldmine Natural Foods
1947 30th St.
San Diego, CA 92102
1-800-475-FOOD (3663)

Walnut Acres
Penns Creek, PA 17862
Send for catalog: (717) 837-0601
("Everything from soup to nuts," dried fruits and nuts handy for travel and office).

Clear-eye Food Co-op
RD #1
Savannah, NY 13146-9790
(315) 365-2895
(some organic)

Dear Valley Farms
RD #1
Guilford, New York 13780
(meats, poultry, grains, vegetables, fruits)

Jaffee Brothers
P.O. Box 636
Valley Center, CA 92082-0636
Jaffee - nuts, dried fruits - excellent. Freight is expensive, best to get a group order.

Backbone Hill Farm
1496 Rt. 34B
King Ferry, NY 13081
(315) 364-5177
Delicious chicken, eggs, pork and lamb, free-range organic.

Schoenfield's Certified Organic Farm

5680 Old Oneida Road
Rome, NY 13440
(315) 337-0247
(many vegetables, fruits, herbs)

Organically Grown
Freedom Mall
Rome, NY 13440
(315) 337-9332

Espirit de Cure
7110 Greenville Ave.
Dallas, TX 75231

Mother Earth Health Foods
733 South Bay Road
North Syracuse, NY 13212
(315) 458-2717

Shiloh Farms
White Oak Road
Martindale, PA 17549
(717) 354-4936

Erewhon Catalogue
236 Washington Street
Brookline, MA 02146
(617) 783-4561 or 1-800-222-8028

On the Rise
109 Walton Street
Syracuse, NY
(315) 475-7190
(organic breads, muffins, cookies, yeast-free rice bread)

Briggs Way Co.
Ugashik, Alaska 99683
(Natural Alaskan salmon packed in glass.)

Ugashik Wild Salmon Co.
3423 West 100th
Anchorage, Alaska 99515

"Nuts to You"
24 South 20th Street
Philadelphia, PA 19103
(dried fruits, nuts, raw honey)

C. & M. Brichard
RD #5, Box 113
Montrose, PA 18801
(organic beef, fish, vegetables)

Snow Farms
2181 Warners Road
Warners, NY 13164
(fresh fruit and vegetables in season, pick your own)

Organic Farmers - ask any of the above or Rodale Press for address of National organic Farmers Association. Write and get names closest to you. Always approach with caution. We have not checked all sources and people's definition of organic varies. The list changes. Also, some have booths at the Syracuse Regional Farmer's Market on Park Street.

Other regional organic farmers:

Grindstone Farms, Tinker Tavern Rd, Pulaski NY 13142
(315)296-4139 great carrots, greens and other veggies

Gary Horton, Marcellus, NY

Janice and Michael Capulo, Aquarian Goods, 948 Old Seneca Tnpk, Skaneateles NY 13152 (315)685-1553

Bill Casey, Apulia (dairy, cauliflower, strawberries, broccoli)

Beth Rose, Trumansburg (sheep and chickens)

Doug Jones, Canton (vegetables)

Ann Miller, Baldwinsville, NY (carrots, grains, beans)

F & F Farm, Fulton, NY 592-9090

Mrs W. Marshall (Betty) Naylor
Ransom Road
Jamesville, NY
(315) 492-3056
(excellent organic beef, veal, chicken, eggs, mild and vegetables)

Sundance Farms
P.O. Box 375
Skaneateles, NY 13152
(rental ground for growing your own organic foods, organic pea pods, etc)

Clark's - Baldwinsville - apples, veggies, other fruits.

Remember to think of ordering in bulk with other H.E.A.L. members to save money. Organization and planning are a must. Fresh fish locally, and sometimes organic produce, will surprise you at the grocery. Keep your wants known to friends, relatives and grocer and they will be on the lookout for you too.

The macrobiotic catalogue from Mountain Ark Trading Post, 120 Southeast Ave., Fayetteville, Arkansas, 72701, 1-800-643-8909, has low priced organic grains and beans.

DeWitt Mall, Ithaca, NY has an organic food store, Somadhara.

Natural Lifestyle Products: 1-800-752-2775.

Other items of interest

Dr. John Laseter, Ph.D.
Enviro-Health Systems
940 N. Bowser Road
Richardson, TX 75081
1-800-558-0069
Your physician can write here and get information to draw your pesticide and general volatile chemical levels and have them determined with the most precision available at this time. Also:

Pacific Toxicology Labs
1545 Pontius Avenue
Los Angeles, CA 90025

AIR CLEANERS

Large care and home air filters, good for bedroom. Very reliable company. Shower water filter. Send for brochure:

E.L. Foust Company
P.O. Box 105
191 South Sunnyside Avenue

(312) 834-4952

"Hands-Free" unit to filter chemicals. Worn in malls, traffic, etc.:

H. Read Miner, P.E.
P.O. Box 616
Decatur, IL 62525

Ionizers for airplane, car office, home. Also have large variety air cleaners that remove chemicals from air in home, office or car. Reliable, responsible can rent to evaluate and apply cost toward purchase:

N.E.E.D.S.
527 Charles Ave., 12-A
Syracuse, NY 13209
1-800-634-1380

Electrostatic air filters and other E.I. needs from:

Environmental Health Shoppes
P.O. Box 239
Fate, TX 75137
(214) 635-9843

Mountain Valley Water, distributor, home delivery (free in Syracuse):
George Luttmann
106 Traister Drive
Liverpool, NY 13088
(315) 457-5055

TESTIMONY

Expert testimony and air testing throughout the United States:

Dr. Thad Godish, Ph.D.
Indoor Air Quality Services, Inc.
5008 Isabella Lane
Muncie, Indiana 47302
(317) 285-1302

Dr. William J. Rea and Associates
8345 Walnut Hill Lane, Ste. 205
Dallas, TX 75231

OTHER

Dupont Lucite paint, low off-gassing odor, discount stores. Formaldehyde Room Monitors - expose 24-hours in room for total formaldehyde level or, wear as lapel badge for 8-hour formaldehyde exposure determination at work. Order 3M Formaldehyde Monitor #3750 ($35.00):
3M Company
Department FH
Box 43157
St. Paul, MN 55764

Formaldehyde Spot Test

One vial does 100 tests. Apply a drop of solution to anything - clothes, paper, furniture, wallboard, ceiling tiles, building materials, etc. If formaldehyde is present in the amount of 10 ppm or greater, the spot turns purple. $30 for 100 test vial and 3 test solutions of formaldehyde so various colors representing various concentrations can be seen. 10 ppm turns very faint purple; 100 ppm turns medium purple. Available at our office.

For our periodic newsletter to which we all contribute news, recipes, articles, new sources of cottons, organic foods, questions and anything of interest to the multiply-sensitive person, write:

H.E.A.L. of CNY
Mrs. Eleanor Hathaway
337 Dorothy Drive
Syracuse, NY 13215
(315) 492-0091

They also have a resource book of where to find hypoallergenic items. Also, if you move away or live out of the area, it is useful to join because you can receive not only the newsletter, but audio tapes of our monthly meetings and guest speakers.

As well, Bruce Small, engineer and author of **Sunnyhill** has a retreat for patients and counsels prospective home builders.

Any resources you cannot locate can be found in our large folder in the office. It cannot be removed, but you can browse through for addresses for catalogues that will contain items you need, especially cottons. As you come across items you find useful, please write down all the particulars and send it to me. We will eventually have a printed, computerized resource list available.

APPENDIX
DIAGNOSING THE TIGHT BUILDING SYNDROME:
AN INTRADERMAL METHOD TO PROVOKE
CHEMICALLY-INDUCED SYMPTOMS

Published in and reproduced with kind permission:
Environmental Health Perspectives, the U.S. government's
National Institutes of Health medical journal,
Volume 76, pages 195-198, December 1987.

Sherry A. Rogers, M.D., F.A.C.A., F.A.B.F.P., F.A.B.E.M.
Northeast Center for Environmental Medicine
2800 West Genesee Street
Syracuse, New York 13219
Correspondence:
Box 2716
Syracuse, NY 13220-2716

ABSTRACT

Formaldehyde is but one of many chemicals capable of causing the tight building syndrome or environmentally induced illness (E.I.). The spectrum of symptoms it may induce includes attacks of headache, flushing, laryngitis, dizziness, nausea, extreme weakness, arthralgia, unwarranted depression, dysphonia, exhaustion, inability to think clearly, arrhythmia or muscle spasms. The nonspecificity of such symptoms can baffle physicians from many specialties. Presented herein is a simple office method for demonstrating that formaldehyde is among the etiologic agents triggering these symptoms. The very symptoms that patients complain of can be provoked within minutes, and subsequently abolished, with an intradermal injection of the appropriate strength of formaldehyde. This aids in convincing the patient so he can initiate measures to bring his disease under control.

INTRODUCTION

A survey of the literature indicates homes with indoor chemical problems have higher concentrations of volatile organic compounds than houses without problems. (1) The tight building syndrome is defined as a building in which worker complaints of ill health are more common than might be reasonably expected. (2) Furthermore, it is assumed that non- occupational explanations of symptoms have been ruled out. Some have called this illness in victims of the tight building the sick building syndrome. (3) Medical specialists relate better to the treatment of people.

Over 25 years ago Randolph (4) recognized that chemicals in the indoor air environment could provoke symptoms, but acceptance was delayed by lack of measurements and testing techniques which today abound. Since many of these indoor chemicals exist in outdoor air as well, a more accurate designation might be environmental Illness, or E.I.

Volatile organic hydrocarbons are but a part of the triggers of the tight building syndrome (TBS) or environmentally-induced illness (EI). With the installation of urea foam formaldehyde insulation (UFFI), a concordant dramatic increase in symptomatology provided a vast number of victims for study. This provided us with a prototype from which we could observe the evolution and diversity of symptoms associated with an acute increase in one quantifiable indoor chemical, formaldehyde.

Over the last six years increasing numbers of patients have presented with symptoms reminiscent of these UFFI victims (5), but with no history of UFFI exposure (6,7). Measurements of ambient levels of formaldehyde have shown that new mobile homes, newly constructed homes with particleboard sub-flooring, offices recently renovated with paneling or pre-fab walls, new clothing or even new carpeting and new furnishings, and homes with new beds and cabinetry can accumulate as much formaldehyde, as a result of off- gassing, as a UFFI home (8-11). A variety of other commonly encountered volatile substances are capable of inducing the same symptoms (12-15). For example, the mean reported levels for formaldehyde in indoor air in residences was reported as 0.03 ppm for houses without UFFI and 0.12 ppm for houses with UFFI (with and without complaints) (11). Some mobile homes were 0.4 ppm, and the mean level for several hospitals was 0.55 ppm.

Guidelines are needed to facilitate diagnosis and indemnification of the triggering agents. Attacks of headache, nausea, inability to concentrate, mental obtundation, dizziness, lethargy, arrhthymia, flushing, laryngitis, dopiness, irritability, dysphonia, unwarranted depression, arthralgia, and extreme weakness, although nonspecific, are some of the most common symptoms of E.I. and frequently lead to a sequence of diagnostic evaluations which are ineffective; psychiatric evaluation is often suggested.

With proper questioning, the victim will often be able to associated the onset of disease with the purchase of new carpeting, furniture, beds, cabinets, renovation of the home or office, moving into a new dwelling, or insulating with UFFI. We now need a test that would substantiate that formaldehyde (or other chemicals) was among the triggers.

Methods and Materials

In this study, U.S.P. 37% reagent grade formaldehyde was diluted 50% with Hollister-Stier diluent and was used as a "concentrate". One ml of this concentrate was added to 4 ml of sterile water; this made dilution #1 a 3.7% formaldehyde solution. One ml of dilution #1 and 4 ml of diluent made dilution #2, which was thus a 0.7% solution. Five-fold serial dilutions as described by Miller and Morris

(16,17) were thus prepared out to #9, a solution containing just under one-one hundred thousandth of 1% formaldehyde (0.0000094%).

Testing of patients, who in all cases had failed to obtain relief with medical treatments elsewhere, was initiated with an intradermal injection of 0.01cc of the #3 dilution (0.15% formaldehyde); this created a 4mm x 4mm wheal. After 10 minutes the symptoms and wheal size were determined. If no symptoms and no growth in wheal size were observed, 0.05cc of #3 dilution was injected creating a 7mm x 7mm wheal. If after another 10 minutes both parameters were again negative, then the test was considered negative. If either parameter was positive, then 0.05cc of #4 (0.03% formaldehyde) was tested. If positive, then 0.05cc of #5 (0.006% formaldehyde) was used. Negative wheal growth and negative symptoms determined the point at which testing was terminated. If symptoms were produced with positive wheal growth, and were subsequently eliminated by the dose that had no wheal growth, the test was considered positive.

All tests were done in a single-blind fashion, and were preceded by at least one placebo control. Patients were never aware of what they were being tested with until all tests had been completed.

In some cases the blood serum level of formic acid, a metabolite of inhaled formaldehyde, was measured (Smith-Kline Laboratories, King of Prussia, PA). In others, a 24 hour level of formaldehyde in the ambient air of a suspect room was measured with a passive (badge) monitor.

Selected Case Examples

For brevity, only 2 of 24 cases are presented: C.P. was a 39-year-old consulting engineer who traveled extensively. Two years ago he moved into a brand new home in this area. There were new carpeting and particleboard sub-flooring throughout the house. Six months later he experienced an insidious onset of joint pain. He consulted an internist, and a rheumatologist, and in spite of their treatments, he reported a year and a half later that he had the same symptoms. He also indicated that he ached more after he had been home for the weekend, but felt well whenever he was out of town for a few days.

His blood serum level of formic acid (a metabolite of formaldehyde) was 10 mcg/ml after a weekend at home and 6 mcg/ml after a day at work. A passive (badge) monitor showed an ambient 24 hour formaldehyde level of 0.06 ppm in his home. Note that the current recommendations for maximum ambient air formaldehyde exposure levels range from 0.25 ppm (National Academy of Sciences) to 0.12 ppm (ASHRAE, the American Society of Heating, Refrigeration, and Air-conditioning Engineers), while concentrations below 0.06 ppm are considered of limited or no concern (18).

Single-blind testing with normal saline produced no symptoms. An injection of 0.01cc of #3 dilution (0.15% formaldehyde) produced wheal growth and a "warm feeling"; 0.05cc of #4 (0.03%) produced ringing in the ears and achy joints. With 0.05cc of #5 (0.0006%) after 10 minutes all of his symptoms were clear and there was no wheal growth. Another normal saline produced no wheal growth or symptoms.

M.B. was a 41-year-old teacher who had worked in the same school for eight years. Over summer vacation renovations were done in the school. When she re-entered the building in the fall, she started having symptoms that with each subsequent entry came on more quickly and more severely. She would eventually lose her voice as it gradually became more hoarse over the first few hours. She also experienced a sore throat and tender submandibular lymphadenopathy. She would have a feeling of achiness as though a flu were starting, and become exhausted.

These symptoms persisted for a day or two after leaving the building and were proportional in duration and severity to the amount of time she spent there. At home she was without symptoms. Her serum level of formic acid was 10 mcg/ml after a day at school and 6 mcg/ml after a weekend at home. This measurement was repeated with the same results on subsequent days. The 24 hour level of formaldehyde in the school air, measured with a passive (badge) monitor, was 0.06ppm. Single-blind testing to formaldehyde duplicated her symptoms in the office, with administration of 0.05cc of #5 (0.0006% formaldehyde), producing visible facial flushing and the patient's voice became weaker. The next dose, 0.05cc of #6, cleared the symptoms.

All patients described were universally and unquestionably freer of symptoms after they had been through an intensive educational program to teach them how to lower their ambient levels of formaldehyde exposures.

Discussion

The last half decade has provided us with over a thousand patients with "undiagnosed" chronic symptoms, refractory to a wide variety of treatments. Single-blind testing to various chemicals generally identified a suspect chemical and provided convincing enough duplication of symptoms in patients to enable them to make inconvenient and costly environmental changes which appear to be a necessary part of a comprehensive program to bring about symptom relief for the first time. Obviously we have extended these techniques to include other difficult to avoid chemicals such as toluene, benzene, xylene, ethanol, trichloroethylene, natural gas and more, and in many instances have paired the intradermal skin tests with serum measurements before and after exposure to the suspected environmental xenobiotics (Enviro-Health Laboratories,

Richardson, TX).

In patients requiring legal proof of chemical exposure, serum levels of these chemicals are obtained after a day at work and another set after a day at home. When the levels at home are comparatively lower, we have been able to provoke and duplicate symptoms with the particular chemical, single blind or double blind, and then neutralize or terminate symptoms with the non-reacting intradermal dose in our office, which is exceptionally free of potential chemical pollutants.

To accomplish a pollutant-free environment in our office, carpets have been removed and replaced with hard wood or quarry tile floors. Wooden cabinets and synthetic chairs have been replaced with metal. As many extraneous materials as possible are kept out of the testing room. Metal lockers are provided in another area for purse, coats, and packages. No people are allowed into the office who do not pass the sniff test by chemically sensitive nurses. Nurses and all patients must be free of fragrances, from fabric softeners, polyester clothes, dry-cleaning fluid, cosmetics, toiletries, tobacco smoke, home cooking odors, work odors, and in fact any detectable odors. Air depollution devices with charcoal and potassium permanganate filters to absorb chemicals are used extensively and outdoor air is continually filtered and pumped inside.

It is evident that a super-sensitive individual cannot be tested, for example, by a nurse wearing perfume. He can react to this trigger shortly after coming into contact with her, confusing the test results. The major problem is that the treatment dose for the chemical being tested will not stop his symptoms, because it is not the chemical that initiated them. This has been repeatedly demonstrated and has helped us attain a progressively less contaminated office and in particular, testing area. Many people happily note the relative paucity of symptoms that they experience after they have been in our office for a period of time.

It seem that multiple changes in the immune system are triggered in part by the increasing environment overload (19,20). The mechanism of this technique may involve in part the prostaglandin system (21). Many have pondered over why only one specific dose of the same agent that causes the symptom can also abolish it, while all other doses trigger the actual symptom or are without effect. Many biological systems have dose-dependent diverse actions. Certainly we know various biological responses have a dose that enhances and a dose of the same substance that suppresses (22). Likewise many biological systems have a bell-shaped response curve where there is an optimum dose for response and those too high or too low will be ineffective. As well, non-immunologic mediator release can even be triggered by a change in substrate concentration (23).

Two characteristics of environmentally induced illness are perhaps most worrisome; the phenomena of spreading and of heightened sensitivity. Illness in these patients was usually triggered by an overexposure to one chemical, such as formaldehyde; prolonged exposure to the initial stimulus will frequently result in the development of hypersensitivities to other chemicals, "spreading" to foods, or inhalants such as dusts and molds. Furthermore, once sensitized, the patient gradually reacts with heightened sensitivity to increasingly lower levels of the insulting agent.

The practitioner dealing with this select patient population is thus presented with a set of diagnostically baffling symptoms, which, despite accepted medical treatments, may become worse as weaker and less intense exposures to the initial chemical triggers symptoms. All the while other chemicals and antigens may become triggers as well.

Formaldehyde exposure can be related to the level of formic acid measured in the blood. Formic acid is also a metabolite of endogenously produced formaldehyde. Form-aldehyde of endogenously produced formaldehyde. Form-aldehyde oxidase normally rapidly converts aldehydes into acids, since aldehydes are harmful to the body in promoting cross-linking. But formaldehyde oxidase is limited in it's production and with ambient overload, production is unable to keep up with the increased demand. Once this is exceeded, the biochemistry switches from an oxidation reaction to a reduction reaction with alcohol dehydrogenase. This may explain the preponderance of cerebral or toxic brain symptoms as the aldehydes are reduced to alcohols (24-26).

Since these reactions require folic acid (27), often a folic acid deficiency was observed, as well. Certainly as deficiencies progressed with continual exposures, other biochemical systems would be adversely affected by a domino effect. This may explain the spreading phenomenon whereby other sensitivities develop and other target organs became involved. It is an interesting observation that rats cannot get formaldehyde toxicity since formate does not accumulate in this species. Hence, it would appear to be an invalid animal in which to do formaldehyde toxicity studies (27).

The diversity of symptoms of E.I. victims is more easily appreciated with the understanding of the extent of the damage that is rendered by inhaled xenobiotics or toxic chemicals. They interfere with cellular energy metabolism by inhibiting glycolysis, and mitochondrial respiration. They inhibit ATP synthesis and other enzymes, decrease the efficiency of the sodium pump, disrupt cell membranes, produce free radicals, overload the cytochrome - P450 detoxication system, and damage DNA (28). Each person's biochemical uniqueness serves to amplify the possibilities.

This paper presents a simple method for determining if a patient is sensitive to formaldehyde. We do not know the percentage of sensitivity or accuracy, nor do we understand the mechanisms, but in testing over a thousand patients with these baffling symptoms, those reacting positively have all improved after being shown how to reduce their environmental chemical overload. Treatments were based on avoidance of chemicals that were shown to duplicate symptoms.

One important caution: The testing method will not work if the physician's office has an ambient level of formaldehyde or any other triggering agent that provokes the patient's symptoms. This may explain the major cause of failure of clinical investigators who have tried these techniques and been unable to reproduce these results. The need to lower the total load or total burden of chemicals presented to the patient (in his system and in the test area) is fundamental to the success of this technique and cannot be over-stressed. The same subjects, tested double blind to the same chemicals in a normal office or hospital, do not respond in a predictable manner. Whereas in an office such as ours, where special measures have been taken to omit many commonly occurring chemicals, the technique appears able to turn symptoms on and off like a switch.

Basic principles used to create a safe testing environment are; decreasing the amount of synthetic materials used, markedly increasing the ventilation, and filtering the air. It is important to reiterate the variability in sensitivity and target organ of man and the need to focus attention on the importance of indoor air quality on health.

BIBLIOGRAPHY

1.   Molhave L, Bach B, Pedersen O F Dose-Response relation of volatile organic compounds in the sick building syndrome, **Clinical Ecology** IV, 2, 52-56, fall (1985)

2.   Finnegan M J. Pickering C A C, Burge P S, The sick

611

building syndrome: Prevalence studies. **Brit. Med. J.** 289: 1573-1575 (1984)

3.   Lindvall M D, The Sick Building Syndrome, **Clinical Ecology**, III, #, 140-164, fall (1985)

4.   Randolph T G, Domiciliary Chemical Air Pollution in the Etiology of Ecologic Mental Illness, **Intern J Soc Psych**16: 223-65 (1970)

5.   Bardana E J, and Montanaro A, Tight Building Syndrome, **Immunol. Allergy Pract.** 3: 17-31 (1986)

6.   Rea W J, Environmentally triggered cardiac disease, **Ann Allergy** 40: 243-251 (1978)

7. Godish t, Formaldehyde and building-related illness **J Env Health** 44: 116-121 (1981)

8. Dally K A, Hanrahan M A, Wordbury M A, and Kanarek M A, Formaldehyde exposure in nonoccupational environments, **Arch Env Health** 36, 277-284 (1981)

9.   Gupta K C, Ulsamer A G, and Preuss P W, Formaldehyde in indoor air: Sources and toxicity, International Symposium on Indoor Air pollution, **Health and Energy Conservation**. Harvard University Press, Boston (1981)

10. Hollowel C D, and Miksch R R, Sources and Concentrations of Organic Compounds in Indoor Environments. **Bull New York Acad Med.** 57 962-977 (1981)

11. Hart R W, Terturro A, and Neimet L, ed. Report on the Consensus Workshop on Formaldehyde, **Environ Health Persp** 58: 323-381 (1985)

12. Andelman J, Human exposures to volatile halogenated

organic chemicals in indoor and outdoor air, **Environ Health Persp** 62: 313-318 (1985)

13. Feldman R G, Ricks N C, and Baker E L, Neuropsychological effects of Industrial toxins: A review, **Am J Indust Med** 1:211-227 (1980)

14. Randolph T G, **Human Ecology and Susceptibility to the Chemical Environment** Springfield, IL, Charles C. Thomas (1962)

15. Rea W J, and Mitchel M J, Chemical sensitivity and the environment. **Immunol Allergy Pract 4**, 21-31 (1982)

16. Miller J B, **Food Allergy. Provocation Testing and Injection Therapy**, Charles C. Thomas, Springfield, IL (1972)

17. Morris D L, Recognition and treatment of formaldehyde sensitivity, **Arch Soc Clin Ecol 1**, 27-30 (1982)

18. **World Health Organization Report** 78. WHO, p.24 (1983)

19. McGrath K G, Zeiss C R, and Patterson R, Allergic reactions to industrial chemicals, **Clin Immunol Rev** 2: 1-58 (1983)

20. Street J C, and Sharma R P, Alteration of induced cellular and humoral ummune responses by pesticides and chemicals of environmental concern, **Toxicol and Appl Pharmacol** 32: 587-602 (1975)

21. Boris M, Shiff M, Weindorf S, and Inselman L, Bronchoprovocation blocked by neutralization therapy (abst), **J. Allergy Clin. Imunnol.** 71:92 (1983)

22. Vogt C, Schmidt G, Lynen R, and Dieminger L, Cleavage of the third complement component (C3) and generation of the spasmogenic peptide C3a in human serum via the properdin pathway: Demonstration of inhibitory as well as enhancing effects of epsilon amino-caproic acid, **J Immunol** 114:671-677, Part I (1975)

23. Findley S R, Dvorak A M, Kagey-Sobotka A, and Lichtenstein L M, Hyperosmolar triggering of histamine release from basophils, **J Clin Invest** 67: 1604-1613 (1981)

24. Rea W J, **Chemical Sensitivity**, Lewis Publ, of CRC Press, Boca Raton, FL (1992), vol II, 1994

25. Reeves R A, **Toxicology, Principles & Practice**, Wiley and Sons, NY 29-47. 93-143 (1981)

26. Jacoby W B, **Enzymatic Basis of Detoxication**, Vol I 26-366 Academic Press, NY (1980)

27. Billings R E, Tephly T R, Studies on methanol toxicity and formate metabolism in isolated hepatocytes, **Biochem Pharmacol**. 28:2985-2991 (1979)

28. Parke D V, Mechanisms of chemical toxicity A Unifying hypothesis, **Regulat. Toxicol. & Pharm** 2: 267-286 (1982)

Key Words

Tight Building Syndrome
Formaldehyde
Environmentally-Induced Illness
Provocation-Neutralization
Xenobiotic
Spreading Phenomenon

Office-Based Testing
Sick Building Syndrome
Toxic Brain Symptoms

RESOURCES

For an excellent video tape of Dr. Rogers with many patients as well describing their recovery from environmental illness, with diagnosis and treatment, contact

> Robin Kormos Productions
> 149 Avenue A
> NY, NY 10009-8921

This tape is suitable for television, schools, doctors' offices, private individuals, businesses, etc.

Week-long residential seminars are also available at the Kushi Foundation in the Berkshires. These are excellent for patients with end-stage cancers who need a crash course in macrobiotics. For information, write:

> Kushi Foundation Berkshire Center
> Box 7
> Becket, MA 01223
> (413) 623-5741

They also have week-long seminars for physicians which I highly recommend.

For courses for physicians in nutritional biochemistry and for names of physicians (in various stages of learning) near you who may practice some of this form of medicine, write to:

> The American Academy of Environmental Medicine
> 4510 W. 89th St
> Prairie Village KS, 66207

Support and informational group for people with E.I., regardless of whether or not they use macrobiotics:

Human Ecology Action League of Central New York
377 Dorthy Drive
Syracuse, NY 13215

For physicians wanting courses on chelation, as well as patients who want to know the location of the nearest chelation physician:

American College for Advancement in Medicine
23121 Verdugo Dr., Ste 204
Laguna Hills CA 92653
ph. 714-583-7666

For books, tapes, and seminars on alternative ways to heal,

Cancer Control Society
2043 N Berendo St.
Los Angeles CA 90027
phone 213-663-7801

The address to our office is:

Northeast Center for Environmental Medicine
Sherry A. Rogers, M.D., Medical Director
2800 W. Genesee St.
Syracuse, NY 13219
(315) 488-2856

but address correspondances to:
Box 2719
Syracuse NY 13220-2716

We also have a bimonthly newsletter, called **HEALTH LETTER**, in which we publish up-to-date findings regarding macrobiotics, nutritional biochemistry (vitamins, minerals, amino acids, essential fatty acids and accessory nutrients) and environmental medicine. There are original and new articles and all is referenced so it is of use for physicians as well. All diseases and aspects of health and medicine as well as politics and insurance items of interest are covered. There is nothing else like it!

Articles from Environmental Medicine column, edited and written by Sherry A Rogers, M.D. Available from **INTERNAL MEDICINE WORLD REPORT**, 322-D Englishtown Rd.,Old Bridge NJ 08857

1. Rogers SA, Chemical sensitivity: Breaking the paralyzing paradigm. Part I, INT MED WORLD REP, 7:4, pp 1, 15-17, Feb 1- 15, 1992

2. Rogers SA, Chemical sensitivity: Breaking the paralyzing paradigm. Diagnosis and treatment. Part II, INT MED WORLD REP, 7:6, pp 2, 21-31, Mar 1-15, 1992

3. Rogers SA, Chemical sensitivity: Breaking the paralyzing paradigm. How knowledge of chemical sensitivity enhances the treatment of chronic diseases. Part III, 7:8, pp 13-16, 32- 33, 40-41, Apr 15-30. 1992

4. letters to the editor May 1-15, 1992

5. Rogers SA, When stumped, think environmental medicine, INT MED WORLD REP, 7:10, pp 24-25, May 15-31, 1992

6. Rogers SA, Is it senility or chemical sensitivity?, INT MED WORLD REP, 7:13, p 3, July 1992

7. Rogers SA, How cost effective is improving the work environment?, INT MED WORLD REP, 7:14, p 48, Aug 1992

8. Rogers SA, Is it recalcitrant arrhythmia or environmental illness?, INT MED WORLD REP, 7:19, p 28, Nov 1- 14, 1992

9. Rogers SA, (ed.) Chester AC, Sick building Syndrome and the Nose, INT MED WORLD REP, 8:4, p 25-27, Feb 1993.

****

SCIENTIFIC PUBLICATIONS
OF SHERRY A. ROGERS M.D.
IN PEER REVIEWED MEDICAL JOURNALS

1. Indoor Fungi as Part of the Cause of Recalcitrant Symptoms of the Tight Building Syndrome, **Environment International** 17,4,271-276, 1991.

2. Unrecognized magnesium deficiency masquerades as diverse symptoms, evaluation of an oral magnesium challenge test, **International Clinical Nutrition Reviews**, 11:3, 117-125, July 1991.

3. A practical approach to the person with suspected indoor air quality problems, **International Clinical Nutrition Reviews** 11:3, 126-130, July 1991.

4. Zinc deficiency as a model for developing chemical sensitivity, **International Clinical Nutrition Reviews**, 10:1, 253-259, January, 1990.

5. Diagnosing the Tight Building Syndrome or Diagnosing Chemical Hypersensitivity, **Environment International**,

15, 75- 79, 1989.

6. Diagnosing Chemical Hypersensitivity: Case examples, **Clinical Ecology** 6,4, 129-134, 1989.

7. Provocation-Neutralization of Cough and Wheezing in a Horse, **Clinical Ecology,** 5,4, 185-187, 1987/1988.

8. Resistant Cases, Response to Mold Immunotherapy and Environmental and Dietary Controls, **Clinical Ecology, Archives for Human Ecology in Health and Disease,** 5,3, 115- 120, 1987/1988.

9. Diagnosing the Tight Building Syndrome, **Environmental Health Perspectives,** 76, 195-198, 1987.

10. A Thirteen Month Work, Leisure, Sleep Environmental Fungal Survey, **Annals of Allergy,** 52, 338-341, May 1984.

11. A Comparison of Commercially Available Mold Survey Services, **Annals of Allergy,** 50, 37-40, January, 1983.

12. In-home Fungal Studies, Methods to Increase the Yield, **Annals of Allergy,** 49,35-37, July, 1982.

13. A Case of Atopy With Inability to Form IgG, **Annals of Allergy,** 43,3, 165-166, September, 1979.

14. Is Your Cardiologist Killing You?, **Journal of Orthomolecular Medicine,** 8:2, 89-97, 1993

15. Is It Chronic Back Pain or Environmental Illness, **Journal of Applied Nutirtion** 48: 4; 106-109, 1994

SCIENTIFIC ARTICLES BY SHERRY A. ROGERS IN PROCEEDINGS OF INTERNATIONAL SYMPOSIA

1. A Practical Approach to the Person With Suspected Indoor Air Quality Problems, The 5th International Conference on Indoor Air Quality and Climate, Toronto, Canada, Canada Mortgage and Housing Corporation, Ottawa, Ontario, volume 5, 345-349.

2. Diagnosing the Tight Building Syndrome, an intradermal method to provoke chemically induced symptoms, Man and His Ecosystem, Proceedings of the 8th World Clean Air Congress 1989, Brasser, LJ, Mulder, WC, editors. The Hague, Netherlands, Society for Clean Air in the Netherlands, P.O. Box 186, 2600 AD Delft, The Netherlands. 199-204, volume 1.

3. Case Studies of Indoor Air Fungi Used to Clear Recalcitrant Conditions, Healthy Buildings, '88, CIB conference in Stockholm, Sweden, September, 1988, Swedish Council for Building Research, Stockholm Sweden, Berglund, B, Lindvall, T, Mansson, L-G, editors, 127, 1988.

4. Diagnosing the Tight Building Syndrome, an intradermal method to provoke chemically induced symptoms, IBID, 371.

5. Diagnosing the Tight Building Syndrome, Indoor Air '87, Proceedings of the 4th international conference on indoor air quality and climate, West Berlin, Seifert, B, Esdorn, H, Fischer, M, Ruden, H, Wegner, J, editors, Institute for Water, Soil and Air Hygiene, D 1000 Berlin 33, volume 2, 772- 776.

6. Indoor Air Quality and Environmentally Induced Ill-

ness, A technique to revoke chemically induced symptoms in patients. Proceedings of the ASHREA conference, IAQ 86, Managing Indoor Air for Health and Energy conservation, 71-77, ASHRAE, 1791 Tullie Circle, NE, Atlanta, GA 30329.

Also listed in Indoor Air Referenced Bibliography, United States Environmental Protection Agency, Office of Health and Environmental Assessment, Washington, D.C., July, 1990, pg. C81 and C162.

BOOKS BY S.A. ROGERS, M.D.

1. **The E.I. SYNDROME** is a 650 page book that is necessary for people with environmental illness. It explains chemical, food, mold and Candida sensitivities, nutritional deficiencies, testing methods and how to do the various environmental controls and diet in order to get well. Many docs buy these by the hundreds and make them mandatory reading for new patients, as it contains many pearls about getting well that are not found anywhere else. In this way it increases the fun of practicing medicine because patients are on a higher educational level and time is more productive for more sophisticated levels of wellness. It covers hundreds of facts that make a difference between E.I. victims versus E.I. conquerors. It helps patients become active partners in their care while avoiding doctor burnout. It covers the gamut of the diagnosis and treatment of environmentally induced symptoms.

2. **TIRED OR TOXIC?** is a 400 page book, and the first book that describes the mechanism, diagnosis and treatment of chemical sensitivity, complete with scientific references. It is written for the layman and physician alike and explains the many vitamin, mineral, essential fatty acid and amino acid analyses that may help people detoxify everyday

chemicals more efficiently and hence get rid of baffling symptoms. The program shows how to diagnose and treat the majority of everyday symptoms and use molecular medicine techniques. It also gives the biochemical mechanisms of how Candida creates such a diversity of symptoms and how the macrobiotic diet heals "incurable" end stage metastatic cancers. It is the best book of the 4 for the physician.

3. **YOU ARE WHAT YOU ATE** is a book to show patients how to begin the macrobiotic diet, with which so many universal reactors have lost their food, mold, Candida and chemical sensitivities, as well many other people have healed the impossible with this diet.

4. **THE CURE IS IN THE KITCHEN** is the first book to ever spell out in detail what all those people ate day to day who cleared their incurable diseases, undiagnosable symptoms, relentless chemical, food, Candida, and electromagnetic sensitivities, as well as terminal cancers. Dr. Rogers flew to Boston each month to work side by side with Mr. Michio Kushi, as he counseled people at the end of their medical ropes, as their remarkable case histories will show you. If you cannot afford a $500 consultation, and you chose not to accept your death sentence, why not learn first hand what these people did and how you, too, may improve your health.

5. **MACRO MELLOW** is a book designed for 4 types of people: (1) For the person who doesn't know a thing about macrobiotics, but just plain wants to feel better, in spite of the 21st century.
(2) It solves the high cholesterol/triglycerides problem without drugs and is the perfect diet for heart disease patients.
(3) It is the perfect transition diet for those not ready for

macro, but needing to get out of the chronic illness rut.

(4) It spells out how to feed the rest of the family who hates macro, while another family member must eat it to clear their "incurable" symptoms.

The delicious low-fat whole food meals designed by Shirley Gallinger, a veteran nurse who has worked with Dr. Rogers for over a decade, use macro ingredients without the rest of the family even knowing. It is the first book to dove-tail creative meal planning, menus, recipes and even gardening so the cook isn't driven crazy.

WELLNESS AGAINST ALL ODDS

Here is the 6th and most revolutionary book by Sherry A. Rogers, M.D. It contains the ultimate healing plan that people have successfully used to beat cancer when they were given 2 weeks, some even 2 days to live by some of the top medical centers. These people had exhausted all that medicine has to offer, including surgery, chemotherapy, radiation and bone marrow transplants. And one of the most unbelievable things is that the plan costs practically nothing to implement and most of it can be done at home with non-prescription items.

Of course, in keeping with the other works and going far beyond, this contains the mechanisms of how these principles heal and is complete with all the scientific references for physicians. Did you know, for example, that there are vitamins that actually cure cancer, and over 50 papers in the best medical journals to prove it? Likewise, did you know that there are non-presciption enzymes that dissolve cancer, arteriosclerotic plaque, and autoantibodies like lupus and rheumatoid? Did you know that there is a simple inexpensive but highly effective way to detoxify the body at home to stop the toxic side effects of chemotherapy within minutes? Did you know that this procedure can also reduce chemical sensitivity reactions (from accidental chemical exposures) from 4 days to 20 minutes? Did you know that there are many hidden causes for "undiagnosable" symptoms that are never looked for, because it is easier and quicker to prescribe a pill than find (and fix) the causes?

The fact is that when you get the body healthy enough, it can heal anything. You do not have to die from labelitis. It no longer matters what your label is, from chronic Candida or fatigue, or MS to chemical sensitivity, an undiagnosable condition, or the worst cancer with only days to survive. If you have been told there is nothing more that can be done for you, you have the option of kicking death in the teeth and healing the impossible. Are you game?

THE SCIENTIFIC BASIS FOR SELECTED ENVIRONMENTAL MEDICINE TECHNIQUES

This book contains scientific evidence and references for the techniques of environmental medicine. It is designed with the patient in mind who is being denied medical payments by insurance companies that refuse to acknowledge environmental medicine. With this guide a patient may choose to represent himself in small claims court and quote from the book showing, for example, that the Journal of The American Medical Association states that "titration provides a useful and effective measure of patient sensitivity", and that a U.S. Government agency states that "an exposure history be taken for every patient". Failure to do so can lead to an inappropriate diagnosis and treatment.

This book is designed for patients who choose to find the causes of their illnesses rather than treat their symptoms with drugs for the rest of their lives. It is also for those who have been unfairly denied their insurance coverage.

625

CHEMICAL SENSITIVITIES, Keats Publishing, 1995, Available from Sand Key Publishing, PO Box 40101, Sarasota, FL 34242

PRESTIGE PUBLISHING   P.O. BOX 3161   Syracuse, NY 13220
(800) 846-ONUS (315) 455-7862

Please send the following books: Quantity Sub-total

The E.I. Syndrome Revised....... $17.95   _____   _____

You Are What You Ate.............. $ 9.95   _____   _____

Tired or Toxic?.......................... $17.95   _____   _____

Macro Mellow............................ $13.95   _____   _____

The Cure Is In The Kitchen....... $14.95   _____   _____

Wellness Against All Odds...... $17.95   _____   _____

Scientific Basis for Selected Environmental

Medicine Techniques $17.95   _____   _____

HealthLetter(bi-monthly)newsletter

U.S.   1 year $30.00   _____   _____

                       2 years $50.00   _____   _____

International   1 year $38.00   _____   _____

                       2 years $58.00   _____   _____

Mold Plates (one room).............. $25.00   _____   _____

Formaldehyde Spot Test (50 tests +).. $45.00   _____   _____

Physicians Slide Presentation with

Script "Chemical Sensitivity"....... $305.00   _____   _____

Non-Patient Telephone Consultation$100.00   _____   _____

                                    Sub-total   _____

                          *Quantity discount   _____

              NY State residents add 7% sales tax   _____

**Shipping/handling $4 for one book   _____

$1 each additional..   _____

Total enclosed...   _____

**Ship/hand $4.00 each item in the continental
U.S., then $1 for each additional up to 5.
After 5 books call for pricing on quantity orders.
*Discounts available on ten or more books.

INITIAL SUBSCRIPTION OR RENEWAL
NORTHEAST CENTER
FOR ENVIRONMENTAL MEDICINE HEALTH LETTER
P.O. Box 3161, Syracuse, NY 13220-3161
(315) 455-7863
1-800-846-ONUS (6687)

_____Please start my subscription for _____years.

_____Please renew my subscription for _____years.

Bimonthly Subscription rates:
(United States)One year, $30.00
Two years, $50.00

(International) One year, $38.00 (U.S.)
Two years, $58.00 (U.S.)

_____Charge to: _____VISA_____MasterCard

#_____Exp._____

Signature:_____

Name_____

Address_____

City_____State_____Zip_____

Telephone _____
Northeast Center For Environmental Medicine Health Letter
is published bimonthly by Prestige Publishing,
P.O. Box 3161, Syracuse, NY 13220.

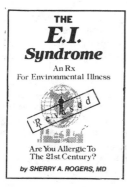

THE
E.I.
Syndrome
An Rx
For Environmental Illness

Are You Allergic To
The 21st Century?
by SHERRY A. ROGERS, MD

This book is 650 pages crammed full of pearls and spells out the entire workup for the most mildly allergic person to the universal reactor, which Dr. Rogers, herself was. It goes through everything the patient needs to know about mold and other inhalant allergies, food allergies, chemical allergies, Candida syndrome, nutritional deficiencies, toxicities of xenobiotics, and the psychoneuroimmune connection. It shows you how to diagnose your own food and mold allergies and chemical sensitivities. Then it tells you how to treat them, with environmental controls and diet changes you can do at home. This is required reading for all people with environmental illness, regardless of the stage.

$17.95

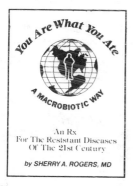

You Are What You Ate

A MACROBIOTIC WAY

An Rx
For The Resistant Diseases
Of The 21st Century
by SHERRY A. ROGERS, MD

This book is macrobiotics modified for the chemically sensitive person and people with mysterious undiagnosable illnesses as well as those who have been told they just have to learn to live with it. It is for people who have severe cravings, resistent Candidiasis, or who have had food injections, rotation diets, vitamins and everything they can think of, but are still not functioning at 100%. With this modified macrobiotic program, many suddenly no longer needed their masks or Nystatin and could tolerate progressively more foods and chemicals within a few weeks. This is required reading before tackling the more advanced stage in " The Cure Is In The Kitchen."

$9.95

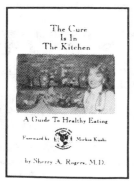

The Cure
Is In
The Kitchen

A Guide To Healthy Eating

Foreward by Michio Kushi

by Sherry A. Rogers, M.D.

Did you ever read the books about people who cleared their cancers with macrobiotics and find yourself asking " Well, what did they eat and do exactly day to day?" Dr. Rogers did and went straight to the highest source to find the answer. This is the first book to ever spell out in detail what all those people ate day to day who cleared their incurable diseases, undiagnosable symptoms, relentless chemical, food, Candida and electomagnetic sensitivities, as well as terminal cancers. Dr. Rogers flew to Boston each month to work side by side with Michio Kushi as he counseled people at the end of their medical ropes, as their remarkable case histories will show you. If you cannot afford a $500 consultation, and you are a medical mystery, have been told there is nothing more medicine has to offer, or you'll have to live with your condition and its medication for the rest of your life, or have been told your days are numbered, why not learn first hand what these people did and how you, too, may improve your health. It also contains the latest information on cholesterol and heart disease treatments.

$14.95

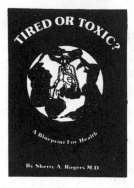

Here is the first book, complete with references that provides in terms that everyone can understand, the biochemical explanation and verification of chemical hypersensitivity, Candida sensitivity, and how to heal all of these, including some cancers.

It explains the most common biochemical blunders of medicine, and how they actually promote aging, Alzheimer's and arteriosclerosis. These blunders include the prescription of foods and drugs to lower cholesterol, the prescription of blood pressure medication, the recommendation of calcium for osteoporosis, and drugs for arthritis.

Medicine is on the threshold of another stage in its evolution. NO LONGER IS A HEADACHE A DARVON DEFICIENCY. We now have the tools to identify and correct the environmental triggers and nutritional and biochemical deficiencies that cause disease, rather than just drugging or covering up symptoms. If you want to bring your doctor into the 21st century, this is the book to give him.

This book will most likely have the most significant and long-lasting impact on your life of all the books you read this year. Come bring your mind, your body and your health into the 21st Century.

$17.95

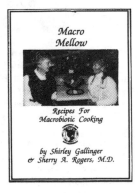

This book is designed for 4 types of people:

(1) For the person who doesn't know a thing about macrobiotics, but just plain wants to feel better, in spite of the 21st century.

(2) It solves the high cholesterol/triglycerides problem without drugs and is the perfect diet for heart disease patients.

(3) It is the perfect transition diet for those not ready for macro, but needing to get out of the chronic illness rut.

(4) It spells out how to feed the rest of the family who hates macro while another family member must eat it to clear their "incurable" symptoms.

The delicious low-fat whole food meals use macro ingredients without the rest of the family even knowing. It is the first book to dove-tail creative meal planning, menus, recipes and even gardening so that it doesn't drive the cook (who used to have to run 2 kitchens, "normal" & strict macro) crazy!

$12.95

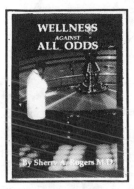

Here is the 6th and most revolutionary book by Sherry A. Rogers, M.D. It contains the ultimate healing plan that people have successfully used to beat cancer when they were given 2 weeks, some even 2 days to live by some of the top medical centers. These people had exhausted all that medicine has to offer, including surgery, chemotherapy, radiation and bone marrow transplants. And one of the most unbelievable things is that the plan costs practically nothing to implement and most of it can be done at home with non-prescription items.

Of course, in keeping with the other works and going far beyond, this contains the mechanisms of how these principles heal and is complete with all the scientific references for physicians. Did you know, for example, that there are vitamins that actually cure cancer, and over 50 papers in the best medical journals to prove it? Likewise, did you know that there are non-presciption enzymes that dissolve cancer, arteriosclerotic plaque, and autoantibodies like lupus and rheumatoid? Did you know that there is a simple inexpensive but highly effective way to detoxify the body at home to stop the toxic side effects of chemotherapy within minutes? Did you know that this procedure can also reduce chemical sensitivity reactions (from accidental chemical exposures) from 4 days to 20 minutes? Did you know that there are many hidden causes for "undiagnosable" symptoms that are never looked for, because it is easier and quicker to prescribe a pill than find (and fix) the causes?

The fact is that when you get the body healthy enough, it can heal anything. You do not have to die from labelitis. It no longer matters what your label is, from chronic Candida or fatigue, or MS to chemical sensitivity, an undiagnosable condition, or the worst cancer with only days to survive. If you have been told there is nothing more that can be done for you, you have the option of kicking death in the teeth and healing the impossible. Are you game?

$17.95

The
Scientific Basis
for
Selected
Environmental
Medicine
Techniques

by

Sherry A. Rogers, M.D.

This book contains scientific evidence and references for the techniques of environmental medicine. It is designed with the patient in mind who is being denied medical payments by insurance companies that refuse to acknowledge environmental medicine. With this guide a patient may choose to represent himself in small claims court and quote from the book showing, for example, that the Journal of The American Medical Association states that "titration provides a useful and effective measure of patient sensitivity", and that a U.S. Government agency states that "an exposure history be taken for every patient". Failure to do so can lead to an inappropriate diagnosis and treatment.

This book is designed for patients who choose to find the causes of their illnesses rather than treat their symptoms with drugs for the rest of their lives. It is also for those who have been unfairly denied their insurance coverage.

$17.95

EVIDENCE FOR FIGHTING INSURANCE COMPANIES

Sherry A. Rogers, MD

There is a new book now full of the evidence for the environmental medicine approach to medical problems. It has been designed with the patient in mind, so he could conceivably go to small claims court and represent himself. Even though an insurance company might send an attorney in an $800.00 suit to fight this fellow, he should be able to merely show the judge, page by page, the various evidence of the techniques.

For example, he can show him pages of references demonstrating the benefits of titration and that there are no published studies of deaths of patients receiving titrated extracts. And furthermore, he can show him pages of evidence that do show him deaths using conventional, "one dose for all" treatments. Then he can quote from the **Journal of the American Medical Association** where it says titration has scientific merit.

Then he can show him where U.S. government agencies conclude it borders on malpractice for a physician to fail to take an environmental history regardless of his specialty. And on and on it goes.

This is available through Sand Key Publishers, Box 40101, Sarasota, Fl 34242. The title is **The Scientific Basis For Selected Environmental Medicine Techniques** (1994). Cost $17.95 plus $4.00 shipping and handling. It will be updated periodically with new evidence as it comes in.

Prestige Publishing

THE SCIENTIFIC BASIS FOR SELECTED ENVIRONMENTAL MEDICINE TECHNIQUES

by Sherry A. Rogers M.D.

This book contains scientific evidence and references for the techniques of environmental medicine. It is designed with the patient in mind who is being denied medical payments by insurance companies that refuse to acknowledge environmental medicine. With this guide a patient may choose to represent himself in small claims court and quote from the book showing, for example, that the Journal of The American Medical Association states that "titration provides a useful and effective measure of patient sensitivity", and that a U.S. Government agency states that "an exposure history be taken for every patient". Failure to do so can lead to an inappropriate diagnosis and treatment.

This book is designed for patients who choose to find the causes of their illnesses rather than treat their symptoms with drugs for the rest of their lives. It is also for those who have been unfairly denied their insurance coverage.

_____ copies of THE SCIENTIFIC BASIS FOR SELECTED
        ENVIRONMENTAL MEDICINE TECHNIQUES
                                @ $17.95 _____

    add $4 each postage and handling
    ($1 each for additional book.)   _____
    * Orders of 5 books or more are shipped U.P.S.
    (call for pricing)
    add 7% N.Y.S. tax (NYS Residents)   _____

                         total enclosed _____

INDEX

By now you realize there are two types of medicine.

(1) The old or standard type that you are accustomed to where "a headache is a darvon or aspirin deficiency". Everything is treated with drugs.

The emphasis is on blood tests and x-rays so you can get a fancy name or **label** for your problem. Once you have that label, it is merely a **cookbook** exercise to find the corresponding drugs or surgery.

(2) Or you can do environmental medicine which incorporates the era of molecular medicine and all we know about the biochemistry of the body. In an environmental medicine approach to symptoms, every symptom is important. And you are not expected to see a different doctor for every different body part that is affected.

But most fundamental of all is the approach to the patient. First we want to **find the cause for all symptoms, not cover them up with drugs.** Second, we want to **educate** the patient as much as he is willing, so that he can learn how he got sick, how to get well, and how to stay well.

Hence **the name of the disease is really inconsequential.** It is the **cause** which concerns us the most. With this basic difference in mind, an index diminishes in usefulness. For example, if we had a "normal" index, under a listing for "chemical sensitivity" I would have to put "pgs 1-633". The same would go for multiple sclerosis, cancer, fatigue or any other problem.

As you see, there is no point in putting names of specific symptoms or diseases in it, because every page has to do with every illness. **Medicine has evolved from a**

catalogue to a process. Therefore we leave several blank pages for you to jot the page numbers of things you would like to find later and thereby create your own index. With that and the table of contents, you should be able to retrieve whatever you need expeditiously.